SIGN OF PATHOLOGY

RSA·STR

THE RSA SERIES IN TRANSDISCIPLINARY RHETORIC

The RSA Series in Transdisciplinary Rhetoric is a collaboration with the Rhetoric Society of America to publish innovative and rigorously argued scholarship on the tremendous disciplinary breadth of rhetoric. Books in the series take a variety of approaches, including theoretical, historical, interpretive, critical, or ethnographic, and will examine rhetorical action in a way that appeals, first, to scholars in communication studies and English or writing, and, second, to at least one other discipline or subject area.

Nathan Stormer

SIGN OF PATHOLOGY

U.S. Medical Rhetoric on Abortion, 1800s–1960s

THE PENNSYLVANIA STATE UNIVERSITY PRESS
UNIVERSITY PARK, PENNSYLVANIA

Library of Congress Cataloging-in-Publication Data

Stormer, Nathan, 1966– , author.
  Sign of pathology : U.S. medical rhetoric on abortion,
  1800s–1960s / Nathan Stormer.
    pages cm — (The RSA series in transdisciplinary rhetoric)
Summary: "Examines the medical discourse on abortion in
the United States from the 1800s to the 1960s. Demonstrates
that abortion was seen as a sign of social pathology indicating
undoing of civilization"—Provided by publisher.
Includes bibliographical references and index.
ISBN 978-0-271-06555-7 (cloth : alk. paper)
1. Abortion—United States—History.
2. Rhetoric.
I. Title.

HQ767.5.U5S769 2015
362.1988'80973—dc23
2014034004

TO BUELLER and MCLOVIN, my cats,
one or the other of which has watched me
write almost every word of this manuscript
(with closed but attentive eyes).
Here is another book to sleep on, made
especially for you.

Contents

Acknowledgments

I have been working on this book for so long that it feels like its unfinishedness is what I am, a book in waiting. I thought I would knock it out in five years after my first book, tops. It took thirteen. Working as the sole author, particularly on a long, complicated research project, can be very isolating. I began to lose hope of ever finishing it and I reconsidered what I was doing, but finally I found my footing again. I never stopped working on it, yet looking at it now it seems to have taken rather a long time for an ordinary-sized book. You'd expect more of a doorstop from that much effort.

I don't mean to be maudlin about a completed book that I am proud of; there was no wailing or gnashing of teeth (well, a bit), and my slowness is of little meaning to anyone but my partner, Naomi, and me. What I want to say is that if it were not for many people who were kind to me, I might have given up and I am so happy to have this space to acknowledge that help and support. Whatever is good in this work is a reflection of the friends and colleagues whom I am so fortunate to have.

I am grateful to the many librarians and archivists who have helped me over the years at the Allegheny Special Collection on Women and Medicine, the American Medical Association Medical Fraud Archive, the Biddle Law Library, the Francis A. Countway Library of Medicine, the Frederick J. Taussig Papers at Washington University, the National Library of Medicine, the Schlesinger Library, the Sophia Smith Collection, the Wangensteen Historical Library, and the Western Historical Manuscript Collection. I am also grateful to Taylor and Francis for allowing me to reprint some portions of several of my essays within chapters of this manuscript ("A Likely Past: Abortion, Social Data, and a Collective Memory of Secrets in 1950s America," *Communication and Critical/Cultural Studies* 7 [2010]: 337–59; "Mediating Biopower and the Case of Prenatal Space," *Critical Studies in Media Communication* 27 [2010]: 8–23; "Recursivity: A Working Paper on Rhetoric and *Mnesis*," *Quarterly Journal of Speech* 99 [2013]: 27–50). I am very thankful for my colleagues Michael Socolow, Liam Riordan, and Constanza Ocampo-Reader, who read several chapters from this manuscript and helped me focus on audience so much better than I could have otherwise.

The friends and colleagues who bolstered my confidence over the years humble me and deserve mention as well. I am acutely aware that it is a privilege to have anyone pay heed to your work at all, let alone to tell you that they value it. So I want to express my gratitude for simple civilities and friendship, not the usual stuff of acknowledgements. These were the counterweights to necessary critiques and for that reason they are very precious to me.

Kirt Wilson, such a brilliant and thoughtful person, let me know right after I tenured that I was not working in a vacuum. Jeremy Engels paid a great compliment by including me in his circle of colleagues; it meant a great deal to have remarkably talented, meticulous scholars like Kirt and Jeremy believe in me. To round out the Penn State crew, Michelle Kennerly told me in passing that she looked forward to my next project—a small gesture, but you would be surprised what a remark like that can mean. Carole Blair and Majia Nadesan, scholars for whom I have great admiration, have recommended my work and shown me nothing but kindness. Carole in particular reviewed my first publication positively and I still carry that vote of confidence with me. Phaedra Pezzullo has said such flattering things about my research that I blush. Chuck Morris never fails to give a good word; Josh Gunn includes me in his high jinks; Ron Greene quietly lets me know that I am doing all right and, since I met him when I was nineteen in a debate elimination round, that matters. Dylan Dryer, a colleague at Maine, passed on praise from Carolyn Miller (which can lift anyone who studies rhetoric to the clouds). Kent Ono has vouched for me when it counts most and included me in the 2007 National Communication Association Critical/Cultural Studies conference planning. John Sloop has shown respect and friendship from the first moment we met; at that stage of my career it was significant to have such a terrific, accomplished scholar accept me. Barbara Biesecker and John Lucaites invited me out of the blue to contribute to an anthology on materiality and rhetoric. Ray McKerrow, Bonnie Dow, Mari Boor Tonn, and Tom Nakayma have been unflagging in their support and each has done me such kindness. Bonnie actually wrote me a fake recommendation letter with all the key words missing (like a MadLib) that is possibly the funniest gift I have ever received. Mari taught me how to accept compliments. Tom has shown me what it means to be professional, including writing a letter on my behalf to my dean and provost after the 2007 conference. And Ray is just nice to me. Always. Among my circle of friends and colleagues who have given me that needed pat on the back, I also count Greg Goodale, Erin Rand, Brad Vivian, Susan Schulz-Huxman, Brian Ott, Greg Dickinson, Lisa Flores, Angela Ray, and David Cisneros. None of these moments or relationships connects directly to this book, and some are just passing words, but I hold on to them.

I also have the benefit of close friends and mentors who do more than share a kind word or a generous opportunity. They look out for me. Zornitsa Keremidchieva, well, she is a bundle of love and support and though we don't see each other much, a little dose of Z is good for anyone who can get it (doctors recommend). Karlyn Campbell, my advisor, is with me always, although we don't talk frequently these days; her fierce support and love are never forgotten. Megan Foley has been inspirational; her stunning intelligence, spot-on comments, and good humor are so necessary. Bridie McGreavy is a little giant in my life and a gift in every way; I think differently because of her. Aric Putnam reminds me that being ridiculous is my true calling and that being so serious about scholarship is not really all it's cracked up to be. Diane Keeling is the colleague I always hoped for and her validation and friendship are like a river running full with the spring runoff. Laura Lindenfeld makes a dangerous cocktail and shares her home weekly, always ready to give a kind word or listen. Rob Brookey, my constant, mentorly, hysterically funny friend from grad school, has been more concerned for my career at times than I have been, and such love and concern is to be cherished.

Without Naomi Jacobs, though, I would be cooked. My love, my friend, my partner, she has read and edited virtually everything I have written, endured endless conversations about this book, and pushed me gently to be better. Really, thirteen years of me whining? That is some love right there, some sweet, generous, tolerant, sarcastic, queen-sized love in a tiny package. In one particularly trying moment she kindly urged that I take a semester leave to really dig in on the project. She made it possible for me to regain my focus on the professional commitment to research that gets me up in the morning. She also let me know I would be OK whether I finished the project or not. Naomi is the all and the every. I am so lucky.

So to everyone who has helped me with the work proper, you are remembered and appreciated. To everyone who has taken the time to show kindness, you don't know how important you are. And to people who love me, I don't deserve it but I will take it and try to make it up later. Probably with some pie.

Introduction | Struggling Through Life

> Official discussions about reproductive politics have rarely been women-centered. More often than not, debate and discussion about reproductive politics—*where the power to manage women's reproductive capacity should reside*—have been part of discussions about *how to solve certain large social problems facing the country.* These social or economic or political problems have changed over time. And the fertility of different groups of women has been associated with solutions to different problems. But across time, the social-problem approach for female fertility has prevailed.
> —RICKIE SOLINGER, *Pregnancy and Power*

Abortion became a public problem in the United States during the antebellum era, and it has been a site of struggle ever since.[1] It has been an enduring pathway for conflict and a critical vector for exerting pressure on ways of living. Rhetoric about abortion is, therefore, not only about *fighting over* the practice, but also about *fighting through* it, making it a thing by which and for which there is struggle.[2] This subtle difference in language expresses a significant difference in outlook. The *fighting over* perspective focuses on near-term goals and assumes that the issues contested via abortion, such as the limits of women's self-determination, can be addressed to some degree by the right policy or the right normative structures. This perspective is primarily concerned with the immediate act of ending a pregnancy, as well as the knowledge and decision-making authority involved with this act. Within this solution-oriented mentality, conflict tends to be defined by success in achieving specific goals. The current antiabortion strategy of raising barriers to access is a good example. Winning the contest to restrict access is seen as a partial solution to the perceived evils of abortion.

By contrast, the *fighting through* perspective explored in this book shifts attention away from battles won and lost and instead emphasizes the conditions upon which struggle continues. I am concerned with what makes it possible for abortion to function as a medium of power: the fact that practices for ending pregnancies (and all the legal, moral, and ideological entanglements thereof) rest firmly at the center of debate over many fundamental institutions and concepts, namely, the individual, the family, the state, human rights, and indeed, the human. Certainly the health and well-being of women is at stake in abortion's regulation and the fate of unborn embryos as well, but more broadly so are relations between genders, classes, races, immigrants, citizens, and religions. The family's purpose in regard to the state is also central to the regulation of abortion. Population growth is clearly linked to abortion practices and with it all the problems of too many people. Poverty, pollution, economic power, and climate change can all be implicated in interrupting pregnancy through its impact on population. For a disturbing portion of the public, too few of certain kinds of people make abortion a different kind of population problem relative to cultural/ethnic superiority. Conflict flows continually through women's bodies when modes of power adopt "life" (expansively construed) as the mechanism for shaping the conduct of whole peoples. If, when, and how pregnancies can be ended become critical skirmish points for efforts to remake how people live.[3]

We need to examine how we fight through, not just over, abortion, and the significance of interrupting pregnancy in medical rhetoric is a crucial dimension of how we struggle. Discussion of post-*Roe* pro-life and pro-choice advocacy usually alights on emotional, rational, ideological, and aesthetic tools and strategies but takes the medicalization of abortion's harm for granted. A potent assumption that persuasive words and images about abortion could solve something lingers in the background of such discussions, that we are trying to move toward or *should* be moving toward some kind of resolution of the conflict. With the right words, the right appeals, the right reasons presumably some sort of working consensus could be had, even if temporarily. The unspoken understanding is that rhetoric about abortion seeks and is capable of closure, or at least of putting key issues to bed. This assumes that determining what abortion is and does to people and to communities is essentially a factual disagreement that can be refereed by experts. Recognizing this some years ago, I began investigating the history of medical rhetoric on abortion. How had experts come to understand abortion's danger in the first place? When did disagreement over the consequences of abortion begin? Had there been consensus before? What had happened?

These were my initial questions and they lead to the nineteenth century because it was physicians of that era who first treated abortion as a disease that enervates society. A standard, thumbnail narrative about abortion's appearance on the U.S. national scene matches the perspective of a *fight over* the advisability of intentionally terminating pregnancies and begins with physicians' efforts to criminalize the practice. In the antebellum United States, most people did not believe that ending a pregnancy before quickening was wrong. Quickening is the ancient doctrine enshrined in English common law that life begins at first fetal movement, usually between fifteen and twenty weeks.[4] Northeastern doctors, most notably Horatio Robinson Storer of Boston, took the lead in changing that view. In 1859, after nearly two decades of mounting evidence that women were ending pregnancies in greater numbers, the new, professionally weak American Medical Association staged a medical campaign against the practice, spearheaded by Storer and like-minded colleagues. Exhibiting a diverse range of fears and aspirations, physicians combined political advocacy and public condemnation, echoed by some religious leaders and newspapers, to make abortion a public scandal. Most states criminalized abortion by the 1870s and the federal Comstock Law of 1873 censored salacious materials and licensed seizure of literature and items related to fertility control sent by mail.[5] Whereas in 1809 the "Massachusetts State Supreme Court dismissed an indictment for abortion because the prosecution had not reliably proved that the woman was 'quick with child,'" by century's end all states had criminalized the practice from conception onward.[6] The U.S. abortion underground was born.

Rather quickly, however, it became pointless to follow this tidy version of the story to find the bases of factual dispute *because* such inquiry is premised on abortion's being something we fight over. The relative harm from terminated pregnancies was always contested, but contestation was a function of abortion's serving a rhetorical purpose as the symptom of something else, a means to leverage broader struggles, not a result of shifting knowledge over which disagreement percolated. I found a relentless connection of abortion to world historical place-in-time, which lead me to question why abortion presented physicians with a problem of emplacement, or rather displacement from a better future we should already be occupying, and how fundamental struggles about power and order were refracted *through* the practice.[7] This is not easy to explain but it does suggest that a resolution of differences about induced abortion's risks to individuals and communities is improbable because abortion is not an issue that can be concluded. History does not lead to some prior medical consensus (there was none) or even to the sense that consensus could be achieved (there never has been any).[8] Because abortion, from ancient times to the contemporary world, is an ever-present activity that is intimately connected to the values, organization, and structure of societies, to find some consensus on its legitimacy would mean finding consensus on an extraordinary range of other issues.[9] The same might be said for birth control except that abortion involves the termination of pregnancy, not its prevention, and if done improperly or by unskilled hands, can be quite dangerous. The morbidity and risk associated with abortion and the fact of ending a pregnancy are materially different from contraception.[10]

Since my initial finding that abortion existed in medicine not as a dispute awaiting resolution but rather as way of orienting struggle around new ways of living, my research has been about how the material aspects of induced abortion function within medical discourse about it, particularly how abortion has been constituted as a problem by virtue of its morbidity and how its consequences are put to use broadly to contest ways of life. I have put aside the understanding of rhetoric as argument because, as a paradigm, it is incapable of explaining the way abortion practices and consequences serve as a conduit of contestation (as opposed to a topic to be debated). To couch the rhetoric of abortion in terms of public argument shoehorns its material aspects into a confining model of discourse, *dissoi logoi*, which is the concept of disputation derived from ancient Greek philosophy as a match between two sides.[11] It is a system that imagines opposing forces linked together through limited, specific concepts of communicative action within the public sphere; the ligature that produces clash between these forces, the point of connection that simultaneously divides them, is the process of civic and cultural dispute. Abortion in the United States today is a quintessential example of rhetoric as wrangling, or twofold discourse, to the point of demonstrating the futility of such rhetoric, for not even the most carefully crafted entreaties of the opposing sides seem capable of resolving the controversy, or even of satisfactorily defining the problem. Further, abortion can seem like an isolated disagreement, but this misleading view is a function of contemporary American politics that treats it as a "wedge issue" or a "special interest" concern. As an explanation for abortion conflicts, *dissoi logoi* can do little more than describe it as "intractable."[12]

Against this paradigm, I have found abortion practices and consequences to be rhetorically "weaponized," that is, made into a mechanism of struggle, by their medicalization. Specifically, medical experts constituted the occurrence and possible harm of abortion as a *sign of pathology*, by which I mean a measure of an afflicted society, one that threatens itself by interfering with pregnancy because of cultural stresses, limitations, and negative influences. Physicians made the state of affairs regarding abortion into a diagnostic that could situate a community in time and evaluate its overall progress. More broadly, they made it possible to use abortion as a means of inhabiting time. We know "where" and "when" we are based on how common and dangerous the practice is. Are we civilized or not? Are we advancing or sliding backward? Since the nineteenth century, the state of abortion can tell us, because now it signals if a community is generally doing well, given that its practice implicates institutional and cultural foundations. However, abortion as a sign of pathology became useful for more than judging the wisdom of present ways of life, and that is the key to its becoming a medium for contestation; a diagnostic of the contemporary moment is a modality for exerting power. Conflicts over how to live can be mounted based on the pathological indications of abortion. We know we need to live differently because they occur, so based on why and how they occur, we can surmise what needs fixing. As a bellwether, abortion came to operate as something like infant mortality rates but differently tangled up in power relations.[13]

To account for the ways in which ending pregnancy became a charter of who we are as a people, whether we are improving or getting worse, and how we might live differently, I analyze how indefinite conflict is sustained through the trauma linked to the practice. Hence, this book is intended to reposition one's sense of rhetoric about abortion, not to flatter it, by directing attention to the conviction that abortion is evidence of something wrong with the world, perhaps the least considered aspect of the rhetoric. In the process, I demonstrate something more fundamental: *abortion, as a broad indicator of problems, has become a way to inhabit the present as a moment of risk.* The privileged mode for this is to treat abortion as a sign of pathology and so it is important to attend to the crucible in which this mode was fashioned, professional medicine. Recognizing that abortion has been conceived as a measure of collective disorder and locating its germinal site is one thing; explaining why that matters is another and requires an unorthodox perspective on rhetoric.

By *unorthodox*, I allude to a capacity to produce memories as a core feature of rhetoric. Not memory as understood by the scholarly "tradition of inwardness,"[14] namely, studies of personal or cognitive memory, and not memory as understood by collective, social, or public recognition of the past, but memory understood as orientation in time and place.[15] Once abortion as a practice tells us something definitive about the wisdom or rightness of our ways of life, we can use it to remind ourselves how far we have come or how far we have fallen. The extent and danger of abortion become *recursive*, by which I mean a recurrent phenomenon that acts as a touchstone for memory work. Analyzing the recursive value of terminated pregnancies makes it possible to understand abortion's intractability not as a bug in the rhetoric but as a medicalized feature. The fact that abortion is ever present, but that its numbers and risks change depending on the conditions of its practice, offers the possibility of reconstructing what those conditions are or have been at any point in time. Fighting through abortion depends on this recursive capacity for recollection because it is impossible to position and evaluate the present *by virtue of abortion* without it. Functionally, abortion's material aspects make it possible to plot the trajectory of the present moment as part of *opening* and *waging* conflicts that can alter that trajectory and that often range beyond the practice itself. Only by attending to the persistent *pathologization* of induced abortion does the capacity for memory work undergirding incessant struggle become visible—not by attending to the persistent wrangling over its specific harms that follow from its being pathological.

Physicians did not avail themselves of any precise theory of pathology when discussing induced abortion because it is not strictly a physiological problem. They used available pathological models to discuss patients' somatic troubles, but the practice of abortion was itself a social problem expressed through physiological consequences. Nonetheless, physicians used the concept of sickness in ways broadly consistent with Georges Canguilhem's findings in his history *The Normal and the Pathological*. Reviewing modern theories of pathology, Canguilhem argued that "diseases are new ways of life" that are sensed as discomforting or harmful.[16] By "way of life," he meant that disease is a relative concept embodied within humans' experience of "their relations with the whole of their environment," corporeal and cultural. "To be sick means that a man [*sic*] really lives another life, even in the biological sense of the word."[17] Pathology is thus not a measurable divergence from normal health but a qualitative evaluation that a different way of existing is negative or undesirable. Disease is not the absence of health so much as "another norm but one which is, comparatively speaking, pushed aside by life." Or, sickness is "the feeling of life gone wrong," which is the sense that physicians used when describing induced abortion as pathological.[18]

The relational quality of "life gone wrong" is the condition for illness to function as a kind of signal: "pathogenic stimuli or agents are never received by the organism as brute physical facts, but are lived by the consciousness as signs of tasks or tests" that result from immersion in a lived environment.[19] Canguilhem points out that paradoxically it is the signs of pathology that produce concepts of the normal and the healthy. In other words, visions of normal, healthy ways of life are memory projects that have "recourse to disease as the only touchstone."[20] A normative view of life involves remembering *the loss of health* relative to future well-being; hence, it is the "nature of the normative that its beginning lies in its infraction."[21] In the abstract, the logic is straightforward: the promise of a different, healthier future depends on a normative judgment that the present state of things is afflicted in some way. "Now" is located temporally and spatially through the memory of disease. This requirement to *place* the present in order to *judge* the present as disordered is obligatory in the "social-problem" approach to fertility that Rickie Solinger describes in the epigraph to this chapter. When induced abortion becomes a public problem it brings with it the corresponding rhetorical problem of needing memory-related practices sufficient to place the current state of affairs as getting worse, or at least not improving.

Matters become complicated when you focus not just on the hazards of extant means of ending unwanted pregnancy but also on the details of *how* these practices participated in memory work. There was no special recollective medical practice that materialized a sense of place, no moment when physicians said, "We must position the contemporary world as failing in order to ground our calls for change." There neither is nor was a genre of discourse consciously devoted to remembering public health threats; medical experts did not principally turn to memoirs, commemorations, or reminiscences to build a case for action. Rather, patients became cases, cases became data series, and series became vital statistics.

In this book, I follow the descent of abortion as *pathognomonic*—that is, as a sign of pathology—from its emergence in medical discourse of the mid-1800s up to the 1960s, tracking the unintended memory work inherent to physicians' professional discourse. This is a tightly limited study because I am concerned with a particular rhetorical functionality relative to abortion practice. I deal exclusively with abortion's career as a sign of pathology, not with abortion in medicine generally, modern discussion and disagreement about which extends back into the eighteenth century. I also limit my study to the United States for practical reasons; a cross-cultural analysis would be too sprawling given the fine-grained analysis I have in mind. Along the way, I will wend through the discourse of *anti-Malthusians*, who opposed small families, and who saw in abortion an indicator of collective moral amnesia, to the emergence of a counterdiscourse among *neo-Malthusians*, favoring small families, who relied on the same pathognomonic logic to find in abortion an unscientific, retrograde society. Although the same recursive dynamic is active today, it has changed since the mid-1960s. The decline in maternal mortality and the rise of fetology introduced critical differences too complex to address in this work, so I will leave off my investigation at the moment when protection for unborn bodies displaced protection of women's bodies as a primary touchstone of medical discourse on abortion.

Capacity Is Not Strategy: Progress and Disease

Although not about the present, this study traces the history of a recursive dynamic that has everything to do with the present, or rather, with how we learned to locate the present in the damage from abortion. Thus, the dynamic I discuss is not a genre, an episteme, or an ideology, although it lends power to these. To call this dynamic a *capacity* instead refers to layered aspects of rhetorical power: an ability to produce discourse, and that discourse's ability to address the course of events, which is not the same as the effectiveness of a particular discursive strategy to achieve its intended goal. It is a matter of both the potential for future discourse to be created and the potential futures that discourse will create. In the case of abortion as a sign of pathology, that capacity turns out to be a rather flexible, robust ability to generate assessments of sociohistorical trends through the fate of pregnancies. Although this ability is not wedded to strategic goals for any given discourse, it is a necessary condition for strategic action regarding the politics of life that surround abortion. It is not possible to produce alternate futures by way of the practice without first constituting the capacity to situate the current state of affairs (whatever those may be).

Accordingly, the capacity I describe has served contradictory strategic visions of reproductive control even though it emerged when physicians first built their opposition to abortion on moralistic grounds. For example, you can hear the dynamic at work quite early in an 1839 lecture to obstetrical students by Hugh Lenox Hodge, in which he characterizes ancient Greece, Rome, and all nations "deprived of the light of Christianity" by their tolerance of "the hideous, unnatural crime" of abortion. "Would, gentleman, that we could exonerate the moderns from guilt on this subject!"[22] You hear it when J. B. W. Nowlin, reflecting on the biblical exhortation to "'multiply and replenish the earth'" before the Tennessee State Medical Society in 1887, says that the "demands of society . . . upon our modern women are so imperative that this injunction is ignored."[23] You hear it when Kentucky practitioner Frank K. Green, in 1914, argues that civilization is marked by the increasing protection of human life but that "modern ultracivilization" displays an "inevitable tendency" toward "race extinction" by tolerating induced abortion.[24]

Yet the same dynamic can be deployed to fulminate against antiabortion laws, as when urologist William Robinson writes in 1933 that abortion is "the lesser of two or three evils" because it demonstrates civilized advancement over infanticide ("a thing of the past" common only to primitive societies).[25] Similarly, you hear it when Regina Downie declaims in her 1939 presidential address to alumni of the Woman's Medical College of Pennsylvania that the "doctrine that the mother is to be sacrificed or risked for the benefit of the unborn child is a resuscitated relic of the dark ages and is, biologically speaking, unsound."[26] And you can hear it in 1965 when Alan Guttmacher, addressing the International Conference on Family Planning Programs, describes abortion as "clandestine rebellion" against "antiquated abortion laws" that, "like the prohibition laws of the twenties, can never work."[27] Although the dynamic in question is not exclusive to medical writings, it remains inherently medicalized; it turns on the state of harm to women and to the unborn to indicate how the nation is doing.

This capacity depended on notions of progress being lashed to disease, which required both that a metric put societal betterment in ratio to abortion and that abortion indicated collective disorder. When these elements fell into place, medical discourse conformed to what Charles Rosenberg dubs the rhetoric of "civilization as risk." It is a rhetoric of "progress-as-pathology," which maintains ambivalence toward human progress, finding that natural materials and processes altered in the name of progress are "inimical" to biological life, human life in particular. A nature-culture opposition structures judgment within such rhetoric, assuming "a rightness inherent in the biologically given and an arbitrariness unavoidable in the culturally constructed," such that "disease incidence becomes an argument for social reform, an indictment of a pathogenic society."[28] Rosenberg's analysis is a more specific, less tropological estimation of what Susan Sontag recognized about the rhetoric of illness: "Illnesses have always been used as metaphors to enliven charges that a society was corrupt or unjust."[29] Although illness as metaphor is an incisive way to convert the analytical power of pathology to cultural critique, more than a flexible transference of connotation subtends the rhetoric of progress as pathology. Taking civilization as risk involves determining threat vectors and remedies for disease. It consolidates analysis of hazards within governance of public health and is more exacting than invoking cancer, for example, to damn the peculiar dangers of individual or social repression.[30]

Consistent with the rhetoric of civilization as risk, the secretive practice had pathological significance beyond the patient's body for U.S. physicians, although the health and well-being of the mother and the unborn were always of primary, if variable, importance. Abortion signaled that something had changed for the worse with notions of womanhood, with immigration rates, with poverty rates, with access to medical care, and so on. Thoughts on the exact cause of the illness and the best remedies varied, sometimes dramatically, as one would expect. Nevertheless, conservative and progressive physicians alike understood that abortion was an undesirable event that revealed deeper problems of a nation.

Further, physicians right from the beginning of public controversy developed an airtight alignment between abortion as pathognomonic and a scale of civilization derived from the political economic theory of Thomas Malthus. Malthus famously argued that reproduction always (eventually) outstrips resources, leading to misery and vice to manage the numbers of mouths to feed. His calculation assumed that means of population control indicate relative progress.[31] Appropriating his calculus, physicians made abortion a direct and primary indicator of the health of American civilization and equally a direct and primary indicator of when and where the United States lay in global history relative to other nations. Interrupting pregnancy became a component of what Wendy Brown calls "civilizational discourse."[32] The fact and frequency of the practice betrayed a backward movement, the undoing of civilization; yet remedies themselves could contribute to the pathology and exacerbate it and so were evaluated by the extent to which they restored civilization to its proper place, advanced it, or aggravated its fall.

One notable example was the 1871 "Report on Criminal Abortion" by D. A. O'Donnell and W. L. Atlee, published in the *Transactions of the American Medical Association* at the height of early antiabortion fervor among physicians. More stringent laws were being passed at the state level and antiabortion orthodoxy had become the unyielding, public face worn by the American Medical Association, as well as by many doctors practicing "irregular" medicine like homoeopathy or Eclecticism.[33] O'Donnell and Atlee wrote, "It is not a little surprising that at this late date in the nineteenth century; in these days of boasted civilization, of science, and literature; in these days of steam navigation, railroad travel, and telegraphic communication—that we must, notwithstanding these and many other advantages, look to days gone by for examples of that which, above all others, should interest us most—a proper appreciation of human life."[34] Induced abortion was not just out of step with notions of a modern or good society; it fixed that society's location in comparison with others on history's stage.

Decades later, in 1936, Robert Latou Dickinson, physician, sexologist, and mentor to Alfred Kinsey, wrote the foreword to Norman Himes's magisterial

Medical History of Contraception. At this time, support for liberalized abortion laws and for better birth control as a means to reduce abortion was rapidly evolving among doctors and medical experts. But Dickinson's rhetoric is remarkably similar to that of the earlier report:

> In virtually every culture which is of historical importance the author discovers the presence of a *desire* to control fertility by artificial means. . . . It is shown that disproportionate attention has been focussed on abortion and infanticide, and relatively little heed has been given to the more elusive evidence bearing on widespread and consistent *groping* toward artificial control of conception. Whereas advances made in the process of civilization are forever characterized by economy of effort, abortion and infanticide are conspicuous examples of extravagant waste. If progress means anything, it means prevention curtailing destruction.[35]

The total progress of a civilization is pegged to a decrease in abortion. The work of this book is to account for what makes possible statements like those of Dickinson as well as O'Donnell and Atlee. Each treats abortion as pathognomonic, yet the authors evoke different understandings of the pathological, incompatible memories of civilization and, consequently, divergent strategic assessments of the present.

Secrecy was a crucial factor in the civilization-as-risk rhetoric threaded through abortion's harm. The practice was well known but hidden, which radically heightened its danger and confounded attempts to develop effective protections against its spread. It was not enough that abortion could be dangerous. Its threat was protected by subterfuge, which complicated the pathogenesis of the practice. People tend not to hide the fact that they have the flu, for instance (its not being illegal probably helps). Implicitly, and often explicitly, physicians wondered what it says about a people that they would flaunt the law and take such risks in defiance of medical opinion. More important, they transformed a concealed practice into a palpable measure of the nation's relative progress. Hence, medical study and treatment of abortion was a form of memory work organized around extracting secrets from individuals, their bodies, and the population. From this memory work came an anonymous, medicalized assessment of the state of civilized life.

Without such an event ever being the explicit goal, practices devoted to lifting the mantle covering abortion—as a function of trying to do something about it—created a particular capacity to place the present temporally and spatially vis-à-vis abortion's morbidity. So when Mary Steichen Calderone, one of the great champions of sex education and a medical director of Planned Parenthood, wrote in 1960 that "in calling illegal abortion a disease of society, I point to the very existence of illegal abortion as a departure from a state of total health of that society," she was enunciating as principle a rhetorical capacity that had been mutating within the medical profession for over a century.[36] Abortion had become recursive, affording the past, present, and future a passageway through which to shuttle back and forth tirelessly, thus enabling different people, groups, customs, and civilizations to be judged as enlightened or barbaric (as one hears in Dickinson or in O'Donnell and Atlee). Although physicians gradually refined abortion as a sociohistorical metric, they never agreed on what the metric should be or what constituted forward or backward movement—only that abortion *was* a yardstick.

Rhetorically, this linkage between abortion as a collective disorder and a scale of civilization was a capacitating development for strategic struggle *through* abortion about other, large-scale social problems. The linkage has a specific history and is not the inevitable outcome of two sides' believing different things about the same phenomenon. In fact, each side is derived from the other. They have developed together, turning ways of discoursing inside out to serve opposite ends. In the nineteenth century, medical observers reacting to greater family limitation developed induced abortion as an index of moral decline that one hears yet in "culture of life" rhetoric. In the twentieth century, physicians, sociologists, demographers, and psychologists turned that index to different purposes by contending that abortion's persistence indicated that the moralistic criminality adopted in the previous century was itself backward, all the while reinforcing the understanding that to interrupt pregnancy was an indication of "social disease."

Sidelong Glances: A Genealogy of Emplacement

Because this is a study of rhetoric, I avoid replicating the exceptional histories of abortion that have documented the impact of medicine on women and society. I could not hope to do better than Janet Farrell Brodie, N. E. H. Hull and Peter Charles Hoffer, Carol Joffe, James Mohr, Leslie Reagan, and Rickie Solinger in that regard.[37] My goal is to provide some greater sense of what in medical practice has made the discourse of the abortion conflict possible in itself and, further, its ability to support other conflicts. The best way to do that is to step away from the worn habits of treating abortion as a two-sided public controversy and try a different analysis that attends to medicine as rhetorically capacitating rather than as disagreements come and gone, and that highlights unexpected commonalities and ruptures within the rhetoric.

Up to this point, I have characterized the recursive dynamic in question in a thematic sense to familiarize readers with the broad issues to be elaborated. To understand how this dynamic operates requires more than thematic awareness. It requires that remembering and forgetting be understood as basic to the capacity to produce any discourse and not as specialized forms of communication, as in commemorations or public acts of forgiveness. Remembering and forgetting are essential to rhetoric, posing a fascinating problem that one can describe as a need born of a dilemma. The dilemma is that the present is always emerging from a receding past, which generates an endless need for discourse to reconstitute where and when "now" is. The present simply is not stable; it is constantly moving, repositioning itself on the heels of the future. So memory as I will discuss it is not an image of the past, with forgetting being its faded loss. Remembering and forgetting are constantly at work as we make sense of where and when we are, which in turn makes communication possible, certainly communication addressing large-scale social problems. Therefore, remembering and forgetting are treated as integral factors to all discursive practices, including medical ones such as case reports or statistical series from hospitals. In that sense, physicians did not cultivate some novel capacity unseen before in the history of rhetoric. Instead, they responded to the needs of their own dilemma, trying to determine and evaluate perceived threats amid dramatic changes in reproductive control, by finding harm from a specific practice to be a distinctive trait of any time and place.[38]

Furthermore, to think of remembering and forgetting in terms of rhetorical capacity requires that one consider them as clasped together rather than as separate phenomena. Memory needs forgetfulness, appearing not in the absence of forgetting but because of it. In other words, forgetting exists in a mutualist relationship with memory; it is not memory's parasite, as is often imagined.[39] Greek mythology is useful here because the Greeks imagined this mutualism as endless flow. The Titan Mnemosyne, mother of the Muses, granted the capacity to discourse by endowing humans with reason, naming all things, and fashioning memory as a place to keep thought and its objects. Mnemosyne had a "counterpole," Lesmosyne, and together they constituted "the entire being of the Goddess." Where water from a spring belonging to Mnemosyne granted a ceaseless fount of memory, Lesmosyne's spring, Lethe, induced ceaseless forget-fulness. Remembering and forgetting were knotted together "as equals *requiring each other,*" an "indissociable pair" whose combined powers created a perpetual inflowing and outflowing of life.[40] Steadying oneself amid the constant flow of life so that one can direct one's own and others' endeavors and thoughts, perhaps to organize a nation to change its reproductive practices, is the kind of capacita-tion of remembering and forgetting that I am interested in: together remember-ing and forgetting work in highly changeable, complicated ways to create our sense of the present, which is incumbent on addressing where we have been, are, and are going.

Apposite for this study, for the state of abortion to signal the present "being-at-risk" depends on a strong bond between abortion's morbidity and a mutualist remembering/forgetting. When W. J. Fernald of Chicago wrote in 1903 that Nature judges those who violate its laws by harming them unto death, echoing Nathan Allen, from 1868, who noted that physiology was the tablet of God's law, he saw in broken bodies a living memory of life's divine order that women had forgotten. For him, social mores and structures induced amnesia regarding the laws of life written into the body, compounded by the strategic amnesia of abortions conducted in secret; only the body could remind women of truth through the physiological punishments visited on them for ignoring Nature. If the body's reactions to damage were punishments and judgments, modern America was diseased with moral ignorance and in decline. By contrast, the concluding statement of Planned Parenthood's 1955 conference on abortion also found abortion to indicate a diseased society, but one afflicted by a lack of birth control and adequate medical care. Abortion's morbidity again functioned as a cache of memory—revealing unseen truths about contemporary life—but those truths were social and economic, not physiological. Forgetfulness lay not in the desire to limit childbearing but in an anonymized, statistical view of abortion rates and dangers upon which one could devise policy; piercing the secrets of abortion within the social body ironically obscured the faces of those involved.

In that memory and forgetfulness are indissoluble, it is therefore critical to this analysis to observe how they operate in tandem. However, no term in cur-rent use names the interdependence of remembering and forgetting as such, so rather than repeatedly use the cumbersome mash-up of *remembering/for-getting* I will refer to their interdependent operations as *mnesis*. Although an obscure Greek word for "memory related," *mnesis* has a breadth of reference that is useful for designating the combined, interactive powers of remembering and forgetting. Mnesis is the root for many concepts pertaining to memory. *Amnesia* (memory loss) and *anamnesia* (recollection) are well-known terms, but there are many others, such as *paramnesia*, mistaking illusions for memory, or *cryptomnesia*, mistaking memory for a novel thought, or *hypermnesia*, abnormally enhanced memory. The symbolic range of mnesis makes it a good candidate for a term of terms.[41] The word names the simultaneity of memory *and* its loss with no preference for one state or another, of having remembered over having forgotten. It highlights arrangements of remembering and forgetting that enable rhetoric to function, not the conservation of memory as a genus of rhetoric, as with commemorative sites and ceremonies. Discourse needs a sense of place to be addressed, and that depends on memory *and* forgetfulness. The analytical framework of this book, described more fully later, looks at the *mnestic* aspects within medical practices because they are the key to the rhetorical functionality of abortion as a sign of pathology.

Finally, a fundamental ingredient of the analysis is a genealogical sensibility. In the parlance of Friedrich Nietzsche and Michel Foucault, genealogy is a way of historicizing events, particularly those surrounding the rise of "morals, ideals, and metaphysical concepts."[42] Rather than seeking the pure origin for these sorts of objects, genealogy looks to moments when they emerge, descending from "numberless beginnings" that are tangled and obscured in the "details and accidents that accompany every beginning."[43] Origination is never a singular achievement, and tracing the many beginnings within a beginning is the basic task of a genealogist. Two principles guide the task: first, one must attend to the manner in which "descent attaches itself to the body," which means that "the body and everything that touches it: diet, climate, and soil—is the domain" of descent.[44] *Genealogy is a history of touch,* such that ideas, morals, and concepts descend through the body's encounter with a living world. Second, one must recognize that "emergence is always produced through a particular stage of forces," which means that emergence always occurs in "the endlessly repeated play of dominations."[45] Concepts like liberty emerge from power struggles, often lowly rather than noble ones, from which their history cannot be divorced—so, too, with the rhetorical capacities that undergird discourses, like political struggles mediated through "life."

The genealogy presented here investigates how a power of emplacement emerged from the stage of forces that propelled abortion into the national spotlight, keeping a close eye on the minute "touches" between the human body and the larger world manifested in the practices of medical rhetoric (the relation between morbidity and civilization's progress, in other words). New rhetorical possibilities emerge continuously as we struggle over and through discourse; what powers rhetoric may have are always changing and surfacing from within the struggles that discourses are used to affect. Thus, this volume is a "material history, not [a] history of ideas."[46] The emphasis on the materiality of rhetoric is the chief, perspectival difference between critiquing what U.S. physicians did to *fight over* abortion at various points and examining how they constituted and maintained an ability to *fight through* abortion. Rather than render hermeneutic analyses of physicians' texts at critical junctures to determine their impact on professional and public decision making, I pursue a history of the placements made possible by basic medical knowledge production about abortion. The reason is simple: the recursive dynamic in question exceeds any particular moment of medical influence and, in fact, is not best revealed by such moments. Analyzing rhetoric according to "a logic of influence," Barbara Biesecker explains, "blinds us to the discourse's radically historical character."[47] Abortion developed a sign of pathology within the mundane internalities of medical practice and independent of specific persuasive obstacles. Again, recursivity is not a strategy to shape a particular outcome but a capacity for emplacement needed to say anything to anyone regardless of purpose. More important, the complicated mutation of abortion's pathognomonics over time were responses to changing conditions of morbidity, a thread that is easy to lose when concerned with who influenced whom, so I keep a weather eye on what physicians did with the harm to capacitate emplacement. Influence is sometimes noted but not the point.

The approach I have adopted is necessarily indirect *because* I am looking at how medical rhetoric made a place from which discourse addresses the present rather than how rhetors persuaded specific audiences. In that regard, I am more concerned with how "rhetoric allows for a governing apparatus to make judgments about what it should govern, how it should govern, as well as offering mechanisms for evaluating the success or failure of governing," as Ronald Walter Greene put it.[48] The indirect form of attention needed for such a study is what I mean by "sidelong glances." The conflicted, antagonistic discourses of physicians shared a desire for a future without abortions, but the point from which they charted a course, the ever-changing place physicians felt themselves presently occupying as they moved toward that future, was produced by the mnestic dynamics of their medical practices. As a result, I work by persistently looking away from the overt purposes of physicians as they steam along toward their goal so that I might observe the churning operation of remembering and forgetting that powers their passage. So if the end that physicians set themselves was to bring the harm of abortion to light so as to justify changes in policy and practice, then my field of vision extends laterally to that goal. I inspect the shallow angles of memories gained and lost as they trail away from physicians' discourse as it plunges onward. Most important, however, I assume that abortion does not *have* to tell us about who we are or where we are in time. Only then may I question how the rhetorical capacity to do so emerged.

Then and Now

It would be inappropriate to draw contemporary conclusions from material that is a half century to the better part of two centuries old; too many significant events have affected how rhetoric on abortion operates in the interim. Given the current intensity of conflict over abortion, it is highly tempting to gloss over those differences and apply this work's observations to today's world. Nonetheless, it is important to acknowledge that the capacity to place the present via abortion—as a condition of struggling with one another—is not an artifact of bygone times and it is not contained solely within medical texts. Tracing how and when abortion as a disease of society was adopted as a recursive dynamic into rhetorics beyond medicine and how those rhetorics have evolved would require several conjoined analyses, which is well beyond what I can offer. My hope is that in becoming familiar with the early, core history of its development in medicine, the reader may gain not only a greater appreciation of medicine's importance in the history of abortion rhetoric but also "an eye" for when the present is being staked by abortion as a sign of pathology, even when medical terms and data are not in sight. For instance, in *Decoding Abortion Rhetoric*, Celeste Condit noticed what I term abortion's pathognomonics in public discourse from the mid-1960s to the 1980s. She refers to abortion rhetoric that located the present historically as a "heritage tale," noting a Catholic version that placed the United States within an ancient narrative of the respect for life relative to the Church, and a Protestant version that placed *Roe v. Wade* "within a strand of 'evil' in history."[49] She also noted that pro-choice reformers contested these heritage tales as value-laden, historical misrepresentations.[50]

These narrative forms are premised on the pathological value attributed to abortion. Indeed, recent rhetoric on the "culture of life" absolutely depends upon abortion as a sign of pathology; such thinking underwrites the apocalyptic imagery common to pro-life discourse. For example, Ronald Reagan, whom Condit identifies as an exemplar of the Protestant heritage tale, wrote for the *Human Life Review* in 1983 that "we cannot diminish the value of one category of human life—the unborn—without diminishing the value of all human life." He compared *Roe v. Wade* to the *Dred Scott* decision, likening a post-*Roe* America to a nineteenth-century, slave-holding one, which threatened the future of the entire nation: "We cannot survive as a free nation when some men decide that others are not fit to live and should be abandoned to abortion or infanticide."[51] Notable for a president, yes, but he simply made use of an ability common to abortion discourse, whether employed by pro-life activists of the 1980s or later national figures, such as Newt Gingrich, Speaker of the House from 1994 to 1998. As we will see, it was physicians, not theologians, who developed this orientation to time and place.

Indeed, abortion as evidence of the nation's trajectory permeates even the most run-of-the-mill statements about abortion today, whether those statements come from pro-life *or* pro-choice advocates. Take just the period between 2010 and 2012. In the 2010 elections, large numbers of hard-right legislators and governors were elected in the United States, many identified as Tea Party conservatives. They began a concerted effort to deny access to abortion, proposing unprecedented numbers of state provisions to restrict the practice.[52] The number of policies designed to obstruct access had been rising steadily since the mid-1990s, after the 1992 *Casey* decision, in which the U.S. Supreme Court declared that the state has an interest in persuading women to carry a pregnancy to term, but the push after 2010 was unparalleled.[53] Paired against the Right's term "culture war," the Left popularized the "war on women" to capture the late avalanche of restrictions as a return to the past.[54]

In the back-and-forth of the renewed legislative fight, advocates necessarily have staked their ground on the fate of the nation as estimated by abortion's regulation. For those on the right, as expressed in a spring 2012 editorial for the National Right to Life Committee (NRLC), the possibility of President Barack Obama's reelection signaled a further decline of the nation, because he exemplified "an anti-life mentality on a mission" that inevitably leads to "'after-birth abortion'—infanticide" and discounted "RU486 abortions—with the price slashed even more if you kill the kid on Sunday."[55] Increased availability of abortion is seen as the measure of an encroaching, barbaric evil that blights the nation and as a mark of moral degeneracy, if not of full-blown descent into genocide. On the left, by contrast, the National Organization for Women (NOW) wrote in a policy brief that there are "46 million abortions worldwide each year, with 26 million taking place under unsafe conditions, resulting in the death of 78,000 women. Millions are injured or disabled because of medical complications." For NOW, high rates of abortion are evidence of inadequate family planning and therefore a measure of insufficient cultural and legal development as well as of the state of women's rights and health. NOW placed the United States between Western and Eastern Europe in its development, regarding a downward trend in abortion rates as a positive indicator for increased birth control.[56] The fact of abortion is a measure of necessity, not an anti-life mentality, but its relative frequency still places nations on a scale of civilization. The difference is that NOW's scale registers policies forwarded after the 2010 elections as moving the United States backward, returning to dangerous, clandestine times before *Roe v. Wade*.

In fact, it is almost impossible to think that the state of abortion in America is *not* a measure of America in one way or another, because of the common understanding that abortion is undesirable at best or downright evil at worst. This assumption has rarely been as apparent as in 2006, when poet and essayist Katha Pollitt rebuked journalist William Saletan for a column in which he promoted the idea that a world without abortions was an achievable, better world. "The trouble with thinking in terms of zero abortions is that you make abortion so hateful you do the antichoicers' work for them," Pollitt wrote.[57] Such thinking, she argued, contributes to attacks on doctors and women, ignores birth control's imperfections, and hangs its hat on an impossible goal of no unintended pregnancies. Saletan countered that "abortion can be morally opposed but legally protected, which is what most Americans believe"; to take any other stance makes "pro-choicers" seem irresponsible, even blithe. Pollitt had the last word, asking why abortion is so bad relative to other problems people face. "You don't explain why, exactly, you, a pro-choicer, find abortion so outrageous, so terribly morally offensive, so wrong."[58] Yet Pollitt proceeded to argue that "the pro-choice movement has been making the more-contraception-equals-less-abortion connection" for quite some time. "It's been decades since the visible, mainstream pro-choice groups defended abortion as anything but a sad necessity and/or something that had to be legal because women have a right to make their own mistakes. . . . That is a way of emphasizing women's moral agency but also a way of saying that abortion is a morally serious, very unfortunate event."[59] After calling Saletan out for assuming that abortion is bad, she demonstrated that the pro-choice movement *agrees* with him; they are just more realistic and balanced.

Ultimately, though, Pollitt proved Saletan correct on a point neither he nor she was even trying to make, and that point animates this book. Pro-life and pro-choice advocates alike situate cultures and societies in time by how common abortion is and by its consequences, as grounded in a broad assessment that abortion is to be avoided. Whether it is to be avoided (a) because it is deemed a corrupting evil or (b) because it is seen as unfortunate yet necessary is critical to the unending struggles waged through abortion. The former position supports struggle for increasing criminalization, decreased reproductive freedom, and punishments unevenly distributed to and among women for active sex lives; the latter supports struggle for more extensive family planning services and sex education, with greater bodily control for women and healthier, safer reproduction. All the same, these opposed projects turn on a shared, vague commonplace—that abortion is bad. As a sign of pathology, induced abortion is a reminder of life gone wrong.

No doubt it seems a point so obvious as to bear no remark. *Of course* abortion is undesirable and less of an undesirable thing is always a sign of better times. But the nature of abortion's undesirability is nearly impossible to pin down, varying so much over time from person to person, group to group, as to make a mockery of the shared agreement that it is undesirable. This is an agreement about which there has been precious little accord. No one wants an abortion just for the sake of having one, and nobody wants one for other people (claims from some right-to-life supporters to the contrary),[60] but the reasons *why* this is so defy easy categorization. Similarly, the manner in which abortion acts as a sign of the times is highly flexible, because the practice can be linked to so many issues. For reasons of scope and method, I cannot address every permutation of abortion as a sign of pathology. Instead, this book burrows down into medical rhetoric prior to *Roe* wherein the undesirability of abortion was developed as a way to pinpoint the world's decline and, so, weaponized for continual struggles over life.

Preview

In a previous book, *Articulating Life's Memory*, I examined the early period when abortion was initially taken up as an issue in modern medicine, roughly 1850 to 1880. That volume explored the perceptual practices by which early physicians constituted the female body as a wellspring of truths in the hope of stabilizing culture against change. The analysis of this book overlaps with the first book but focuses less on perceptual practices in relation to the pregnant body and more on the relation of memory, forgetfulness, and morbidity as ingredients of rhetorical capacity. This book is a historically grounded analytical argument, and so the chapters are ordered in terms of their argumentative purpose. My relationship to the material is not uniform across the chapters because I need to treat different literatures in diverse ways to produce the analysis, and not every chapter advances in chronological fashion.

In part 1, I establish the analytical framework to be applied in chapters 3 through 5. Both chapters in this part are not of the genealogy but preparatory to it, establishing the politics of civilization implicated in abortion as sign of pathology and the theoretical understanding of mnesis that structures the chapters in part 2. Chapter 1, "When Abortion Became a Political-Economic Problem," operates as a belated postscript to the previous book, drawing out in more detailed fashion the politics that I discuss in chapter 2 of *Articulating Life's Memory* and extend throughout that work. Here I situate the control of abortion generally within what Foucault called "biopower" and specifically in relation to the political economics of Thomas Malthus, marking key intersections with other discourses as I do; however, I do not elaborate on those discourses or their internal divisions. My purpose is to familiarize the reader with Malthusian politics among early antiabortionists because it profoundly shapes later iterations of the rhetoric; I do not pursue a genealogy of Malthus in nineteenth-century U.S. medicine. Physicians of the time concerned about abortion adopted from Malthus the theory that civilization's advancement was scaled to fertility control, but they inverted Malthus's theological premise, contending that God's Providence demanded fecundity, not restraint. To limit numbers of children, especially by abortion, was a measure of un-Christian barbarism. Further, key physicians argued that the proper role of government was to aid in the struggle to protect life from itself. Accordingly, many physicians saw themselves in this abortion-specific political economy as leading the fight in a war to defend society from the internal threat posed by intentional abortion.

Having isolated the political theory that underlies medical rhetoric on abortion, I turn to theories of memory in chapter 2, "Remembering, Forgetting, and the Secrets of Life." This chapter is conceptual, not historical, and elaborates the critical tools used in later chapters to explain medical knowledge production in terms of *mnesis*. Mnesis is defined more fully as the confluence of remembering and forgetting and placed within broad concepts of memory theory. I also situate the concept of mnesis relative to biopower and the secrecy surrounding the abortion underground, closing with a discussion of how the construct is operationalized within my engagement of the archive. Readers less interested in theory may want to skip this chapter; however, the following chapters are organized and executed based on the parameters and concepts set forth in it. The genealogy that I have produced is not descriptive; it is critical and analytical and this chapter is my effort to be transparent about my thinking. Further, my approach is unusual within the literature on remembering and forgetting and explaining it is not easily blended into later chapters so I have elected to treat it separately.

In part 2, I begin the genealogy, picking up the rhetoric in the decades following the crusade, roughly 1880, and tracking through the 1960s the manner by which medical practices supplied a suitable sense of place for political judgments within an evolving medical Malthusianism. Chapter 3, "'White Man's Plague': Anti-Malthusian Memory Work at the Fin de Siècle," looks at the moment after the successes of the early crusaders. In James Mohr's view, the wind went out of the antiabortionists' sails from a policy as well as a motivation standpoint.[61] The rhetoric seemed listless as well, with little movement in the operative rules governing what were intelligible statements about abortion. However, as criminal statutes failed and the abortion underground flourished, turn-of-the-century physicians began to sharpen their critique of abortion as a sign of pathology, specifically of a moral disease, given the great many scofflaws in their midst. Anti-Malthusian physicians stressed that a physiological memory of God's Providence had been forgotten and called on one another to live up to a pastoral ideal wherein doctors might as medical shepherds guide women to recall their purpose.

Chapter 4, "'More Wisdom in Living': Neo-Malthusian Memory Work at Midcentury," looks at the change in medical discourse on abortion following the emergence of the birth control movement. By the 1930s, many physicians saw abortion not as a moral disease that flouted natural law, but rather as a social disease caused by privation. Like their predecessors, they believed that fewer abortions would demonstrate that the United States was becoming more civilized, but their belief was based in support for limited fertility rather than opposition to it. These physicians turned to more refined statistical data to position the United States as now falling behind its modern peers, Scandinavia in particular, because of outmoded laws and moralism. In place of a medical pastorate shepherding women back to God, neo-Malthusians imagined that abortion control regimes would reduce abortions through counseling centers, liberalized laws, and diverse other policies and prescriptions.

However, abortion was not *always* viewed as bad; sometimes it was deemed necessary and tolerable. Chapter 5, "'The Lesser of Threatened Evils': Therapeutic Amnesias," addresses the conundrum of the "therapeutic," or medically sanctioned, abortion, which existed before criminalization. Even model laws, such as those forwarded at the very beginning of the physicians' crusade, made an exception for the life of the mother, as did state laws that followed. When the disease becomes a cure, confusion follows regarding the value of abortion as diagnostic of an internal threat and a front in conflicts over biological, social, and cultural life. Therapeutic abortions never indicated that society was advanced, and yet their allowance was so understood.

Although they may have a roughly linear feel, chapters 3 through 5 are organized first by distinctive recursive variations within the rhetoric, second by chronology. For example, there are a few (very few) neo-Malthusian voices on abortion at the turn of the twentieth century, but I discuss them in chapter 4 when I consider neo-Malthusian memory work. There is a general turn in the rhetoric from anti- to neo-Malthusianism after World War I, which contributes to the chronological feel, but it is a mutation, not a revolution. Moreover, my purpose is not to tell a linear story but to highlight the shared, recursive entanglements of competing discourses. That a submerged variation emerged to replace the dominant form is an important narrative detail but not the analytical point of those chapters. Chapter 5 is different still because it discusses the crosscutting problem of therapeutic abortion that affects both anti- and neo-Malthusian memory work. This chapter ranges across the late nineteenth century to the 1960s, focusing mostly on the 1930s forward when therapeutic abortion became a more acute issue to the profession. However, I make a visit to the eighteenth century because a critical threshold for therapeutic abortion is crossed at that time; it is off key and distracting to discuss this threshold earlier such as in chapter 1.

The concluding chapter, "Seeking Immunity," explores the implications for rhetoric on abortion when the practice becomes a collective wound that never heals. Ultimately, rhetoric about abortion is directed not at seeking closure but at seeking immunity from and for women as part of defending society from itself. To limit abortion was to seek immunity for women in that restrictions were to protect women from harm; limitations also sought immunity *from* women in that they were to protect society from the consequences of women's actions. Also, as harm to women from elective abortion subsided, immunity *for* the unborn gained new significance in organizing the rhetoric. Regardless, immunity never came. The persistent failure of strategies to stop abortion was what capacitated rhetoric for biopolitical struggles *through* abortion. The search for remedies to the incurable sickness of interrupting pregnancy provides stability amid endless variations of conflict over how to live.

The material supporting the analysis is drawn from an extensive survey of the medical literature and selected archives as well as the secondary literature on abortion. In addition to the medical journal literature on abortion from the 1800s through the early 1970s, I have reviewed relevant conference proceedings, medical textbooks, and polemics from physicians. In certain cases, I examined the personal papers of key figures such as Mary Steichen Calderone, Robert Latou Dickinson, Alan F. Guttmacher, Abraham Stone, Hannah Stone, Horatio Robinson Storer, Margaret Sanger, and Frederick J. Taussig. I also examined the Allegheny Special Collection on Women and Medicine, the American Law Institute archives, the American Medical Association's Medical Fraud archives, the National Committee on Maternal Health archives, and the Planned Parenthood Federation of America archives.

Part 1

1

When Abortion Became a Political-Economic Problem

The principles or laws of physiology, when rightly interpreted, are a part of the will and government of God in this world. The law of increase, as here based on physiology, explains the free agency of man and human accountability as in perfect harmony with the divine government.

—NATHAN ALLEN, "The Law of Human Increase"

Consonant with abortion's being something we fight through, not just over, one of the first things historians note about abortion is that it has been consistently leveraged as a way of addressing issues that exceed the "immediate medical act": fertility rates, civil rights, immigration, disabilities, alcoholism, free speech, medical expertise, federalism, global development.[1] Carroll Smith-Rosenberg argues that abortion is leveraged universally, not just in modernity or postmodernity. Whenever "forces in society catapult the issue of abortion to a position of political and moral centrality. . . decisions surrounding abortion become the central drama of a culture, a play dealing with basic fissures in the social structure, one that raises fundamental issues concerning the distribution of power and the nature of social order." Abortion may be a "socio-sexual constant"[2] practiced in all known societies and its dramatic potential may have existed in all of them. However, the specific qualities of rhetoric about abortion within current struggles in the West, spanning two centuries, are not historical constants. "On every level, to talk of abortion is to speak of power," as Smith-Rosenberg observes, yet forms of power are not eternal, which compels one to ask about the "particular stage of forces" that catapulted abortion from obscurity to its current status.[3] In the United States, abortion became a problem of political economics, not just morality or health, which affected its significance beyond the immediate act.

Physicians who initially mobilized against abortion conceived and problematized the personal and collective dangers of the practice within modern philosophies of socioeconomic power and population dynamics. To be sure, ideological

explanations of the possible significance and meaning of abortion were ubiquitous. Fears about changing gender norms, the racial/ethnic composition of the
nation, and physicians' professional power saturated the discourse,[4] but relative
to abortion those fears were organized by a specific understanding of the purpose of creating new life for the nation. The fact that ending pregnancy consistently provides purchase for addressing issues other than women's health care is
connected to a medicalized political economic theory specific to abortion that
emerged before the Civil War and was refined immediately afterward.

In this chapter, I discuss the rise of abortion as a sign of pathology in the
nineteenth century relative to political economy. The new recursive capacity associated with abortion heavily depended on theories of that era that stipulated
the proper relationship between reproductive life and civilization. I begin with
a "wide shot" of the politics of life in modernity, then narrow the focus to a
particular model of political economy that physicians used to explain abortion's
pathognomonic value, and then narrow again to a close-up of physicians' revised, abortion-specific political economy. I conclude by noting that physicians
presented abortion control as part of a war to defend society from itself, such
that the purpose of governance was to detect and remedy threats born of the
social body. Throughout I make note of genealogically relevant tributaries that
feed the emergence of elective abortion's political economics, but this chapter is
not itself a genealogy of medicine or political theory. The following prefaces the
analysis to come in terms of abortion's significance when it became a problem
for the state.

The Politics of Life

The changed medical status of abortion in the United States was part of its general emergence as a central drama among many northern nations, and by extension their colonies and satellite states, from the early 1900s continuing through
to today. This is because strategies of governance were changing to focus on
the biological condition of the citizenry, such that reproduction had become a
critical practice for nation-states to manage. In modernity, "natural life begins to
be included in the mechanisms and calculations of State power," such that humans became "animals whose life as living beings is at issue in their politics, but
also—inversely—citizens whose very politics is at issue in their natural body."[5]
Abortion was more than a controversial issue propelled into the limelight by

doctors; it became a problem at a specific point in time when managing populations through life processes turned into a political focal point. Induced abortion emerged as a nodal point of *biopower* and the politics of life.[6]

The most important thinker on biopower is Michel Foucault, although he was not the first or the last.[7] His work is too sweeping (and for some too familiar) to review here without fatally sidetracking the argument, so I will instead discuss pertinent concepts as they become relevant. However, to set the table: Foucault contended that early modernity saw an expansive, new *modality* of power emerge from the intersection of Christian pastoral traditions, public health concerns, and changed views of the state (from a territory to be defended to a population to be secured). Broadly speaking, biopower arose in the shift from the religious "government of souls" to the modern, secularized "government of men" (and women).[8] This secularized government is characterized by institutional and normative forces directed at the conduct of groups or individuals, so as to shape ways of life that are deemed better, healthier, more productive, and so on. Ways of life marked as nonproductive or productive for the wrong groups were seen as threats to the well-being or survival of the collective. Biopower intertwined with, but did not supplant, existing legal authorities and the watchful eye of disciplinary institutions—instead, it was characterized by the flexible integration of knowledge about life, death, and well-being into the purposes of government. Biopower governs people in and by way of their daily lives, not by issuing sovereign edicts alone but by mobilizing pressures, incentives, and prohibitions to cultivate (and contest) ways of living in the name of a better world, where "better" is grounded in knowledge of life itself. As Foucault writes, "The fact of living was no longer an inaccessible substrate that only emerged from time to time, amid the randomness of death; part of it passed into knowledge's field of control and power's sphere of intervention."[9] For Foucault, then, *government* refers generally to "administration" or "management," not exclusively to the state, and potentially involves all public or private institutions and normative practices.[10]

Giorgio Agamben qualifies this history, noting that the problem of government to which biopower is applied is inherited from eighteen centuries of Western theology and politics, namely, managing a general and a particular economy. *Economy*, or *oikonomia* in ancient political philosophy, refers expansively to dynamic, relational order and not narrowly to commerce. The word *oikonomia* has led a complex and freighted life in theology and politics, being a key term for explaining God's Providence, but the specific lexical history of *economy* itself is not relevant at this point. What is important is that Agamben puts his finger on the fundamental task of biopower: the reconciliation of two orders, a transcendent *oikonomia* that, "while remaining transcendent," founds the governance of a worldly *oikonomia*. Or, how does a higher order of life operate within and guide mundane life (where the mundane "coincides with the history of humanity")?[11] Determining higher principles of how to live, which are presumably embedded within the order of everyday things and beings, and then putting those principles to work managing the conduct of people is an ancient formulation of the task of governance. In modernity, as Foucault showed so well, knowledge of sex and reproduction became conspicuously central to aligning the mundane order of society with a general order, providing knowledge of a transcendent economy by which to organize quotidian life, whether the general order was deemed a divine, natural, or humanly drafted plan, or whether those were understood as one and the same thing. Knowing the facts of life became a chief conduit for managing political economy and, as a result, engaging in power struggles.

Consequently, the ubiquitous phrase *the abortion problem* only hints at how fighting through the practice has been a fulcrum for attempts to reconcile a higher with a mundane order of life. Reframing abortion's rise to infamy in terms of biopower helps make sense of abortion's establishment as a national metric and, concomitantly, of the relentless investment in abortion control as a way to solve sociocultural problems as well as medical ones. To imagine what the rhetoric of fighting through abortion relative to biopower looks and sounds like, one might think of the linguistic codes developed around abortion being used to sculpt the contours of other issues, such as poverty.[12] For example, Smith-Rosenberg argues that in the nineteenth century medical discourse on abortion created a "sexual language" by which to speak about fundamental changes within gender, race, and class at a sociocultural level.[13] Edwin M. Hale's 1867 pamphlet, *The Great Crime of the Nineteenth Century*, is an archetype of the use of abortion as a sexualized language to talk about basic changes in the way of things. He identified its causes as "Poverty, Ill Health, Moral and Physical cowardice, Loss of beauty, Love of fashionable life, etc., Adultery, Seduction, Prostitution, Rape, Disgrace of Maternity." Hale discussed each of these, noting a woeful turn for the worse regarding women's views of family and maternity. His section on maternity as disgraceful to moderns is indicative: "Among the most ancient nations, especially the Jews, also the best and noblest of all countries, maternity was a crown of honor. . . . Has not a great change taken place. [*sic*] I have seen and heard weak-minded and fashionable wives, [*sic*] sneer at a neighbor because of her large family."[14] As code, abortion is made into a paradigmatic sign through its perceived causes; it becomes an ideographic terminal that links and expresses different ideologies critical of modernity, the foremost being a patriarchal view of women's proper place in the scheme of the world.[15]

However, abortion as a "sexualized" lingua franca for ideology is not what I mean when I say that the practice became a *sign* of pathology. I use *sign* in a medicalized sense of index or measure, not in the semiotic sense of the *term* abortion being used as conjunctural device for ideological work.[16] Mine is not a semiotic or an ideological analysis. Physicians used diverse, divergent terminologies to discuss abortion and its consequences over time; further, ideological investments in elective abortion's governance differed widely as well.[17] The syntactics, semantics, and pragmatics of language about women aborting and the oppositions and identities traced by their actions were marked by significant drift and permutation, yet an enduring rhetorical function persisted that gave different lexica and ideologies a sense of place. To say abortion as a practice—its occurrence, its motives and methods, its consequences—became culturally pathognomonic is to say simply that it was seen to evidence afflicted ways of life, much as Mary Steichen Calderone described in 1960: "It is a morbid process in the social structure, having a characteristic train of symptoms."[18] The diagnostic here is more robust than a sort of "canary in the coal mine," though. One does not affect the toxicity of the air by regulating the use of canaries in mines. By contrast, the pathognomonic function of abortion was directly connected to developing remedies for whatever institutional and normative factors purportedly contributed to women's ending unwanted pregnancies.

The extent and character of the practice, particularly its harm, became a metric for applications of biopower (such applications are referred to as *biopolitical projects* in this volume). With regard to biopolitical projects, "fighting through" depends on a reciprocal, productive relationship between knowledge and power. Biological and cultural knowledge of life provides a terrain of risks and opportunities on which power can be organized and activated; conversely, power arrangements enable production of the very knowledge of life necessary to deploy power.[19] In the mid-nineteenth century, medical discourse was on its way to becoming a standard lexicon for talk about abortion, but that shift established more than common linguistic tools in a signifying network. It established a way to estimate the threats posed by medicinally or surgically terminated pregnancies, to assess their relative danger, and to configure distributions of power to ameliorate those threats.

Explained in light of Georges Canguilhem's analysis of pathology, diseased ways of life are crucial to the political economics of biopower "in the sense that only the normal man [sic] can become sick, as only the ignorant man can become wise." Disease reveals living error, something awry integral to a mode of being, such that wrong living is the prime orienting condition for ethico-political projects. Hence, "recourse to disease [is] the only touchstone" for the memory work that propels biopolitical contestation from a fractured present and toward a mended future.[20] However, "there is a difference between an organism and a society, in that the therapist of their ills, in the case of the organism, knows in advance and without hesitation, what normal state to establish, while in the case of society, he [sic] does not."[21] To discriminate normal from erroneous social life is the thing by which and for which there is struggle. The relative "good" driving this or that project is functionally a mobilization of harm to end harm.

Malthusian Political Economics

To make sense, the use of abortion as a collective diagnostic required a scale that linked civilizations to standards of biopolitical progress, a temporal-spatial continuum on which to place estimates of abortion's dangers and, so, place nations and cultures relative to one another by virtue of their sophistication in addressing those dangers. Such a scale was implicit both in Hale's comment about the superiority of ancient Jews and D. A. O'Donnell and W. L. Atlee's remarks on the degeneracy of modernity; it is explicit in Robert Dickinson's designation of progress as the decrease in abortion. When abortion came to signal that something had changed for the worse, the specifics of what was worse and why it mattered were situated within a "Malthusian world."[22]

Thomas R. Malthus, English parson and political economist, argued at the turn of the nineteenth century that "the power of the population is infinitely greater than the power of the earth to produce subsistence for man [sic]."[23] In *An Essay on the Principle of Population*, published in 1798 and revised five times by 1826, he recognized that food and sex are necessities but argued that passion was the greater force, which inevitably led to misery and vice as numbers of people eventually outstripped available resources.[24] For Malthus, *positive* (as in productive) and *preventive* (as in preemptory) checks limited population growth—more deaths and fewer births, respectively. *Misery* and *vice* named the two primary kinds of limits on growth. On the miserable side of things, starvation and disease were positive checks on population because they killed people, whereas delaying marriage and celibacy were preventive miseries that decreased the number of new mouths to feed. War also kills people, and many of them, but for Malthus it was a vice precipitated by a "population extended beyond the means of supporting it,"[25] whereas the other vices of concern, abortion and birth control, prevented new births. Malthus also considered prostitution a preventive vice. However, this one is redundant in that female prostitutes curtail reproduction only by abortion or birth control; sex acts outside marriage do not affect population. The outcomes of sex are what count.

You will not find the term *scale of civilization* in Malthus's *Essay*; however, such a scale based on the efforts of a people to manage population levels undergirds his political economy, and it is this implicit hierarchy that matters for my analysis (which is why I have given it a name). The challenge of too many mouths to feed, Malthus argued, was God's engine for inspiring human improvement, endlessly cycling as civilizations grow and die away in the face of the mortal necessities created by passion and hunger: "The facts seem to show that population increases exactly in proportion that the two great checks to it, misery and vice, are removed, and that there is no truer criterion of the happiness and innocence of a people than the rapidity of their increase."[26] Yet there could be no perfection on Earth, no condition under which a civilization might transcend the principle of population to achieve such "happiness and innocence," only constant exertion to control numbers in the face of inevitable overpopulation, else a people be "crushed by the recoil of this rock of Sisyphus."[27] Catherine Gallagher observes that his was "a strange new story about how healthy bodies eventually generate a feeble overall population," which may be why his contemporary Thomas Carlyle called the *Essay* "dismal."[28] For Malthus, the continuous current of new life, rising, rushing, checked by unceasing demise, falling, fading, was the tidal clock of human time.

Malthus believed that human *im*perfectability was God's Providence, expressly rejecting the positions of philosophers William Godwin and Antoine-Nicolas de Condorcet (and implicitly the ethos of the Enlightenment) that humans are perfectible and can transcend misery and vice.[29] A civilization that failed to address the unbalanced ratio of fecundity to food was savage, ruled by a divine law of population but unable to take from it the lessons God intended. A civilization that took up the boulder presented by the principle of population and strove for the "full cultivation of the earth" and for sexual restraint was realizing the "general purpose of Providence": the excitation of human genius, industry, and moral excellence.[30] Although a civilization could never become perfected, by dedicating itself to the laws set forth by God, it could better align itself with "Christian virtues," which made it morally and spiritually superior.[31] More than that, it was more rational, since sexual moderation is a sign of Reason, "that faculty which enables us to calculate consequences."[32] It was an intensely materialist theo-politics.[33]

Relative advancement in this system was determined by measuring key criteria of populations. Malthus described what Foucault might call a biopolitical history; these measurements allowed a civilization's position in the world to be evaluated:

> A satisfactory history of this kind, of one people, and of one period, would require the constant and minute attention of an observing mind during a long life. Some of the objects of enquiry would be: in what proportion to the number of adults was the number of marriages; to what extent vicious customs prevailed in consequence of the restraints of matrimony; what was the comparative mortality among the children of the most distressed part of the community, and those who live rather more at their ease; what were the variations in the real price of labour; and what were the observable differences in the state of the lower classes of society, with respect to ease and happiness, at different times during a certain period.

Having conducted such histories, one can "elucidate the manner in which the constant check upon population acts and would probably prove the existence of the retrograde and progressive movements that have been mentioned,"[34] such as limiting fertility to prevent poverty (progressive) but also turning to contraception and abortion to do so (retrogressive). Adopting a well-established colonial logic, Malthus categorized societies as barbarians (e.g., Hottentots and North American Indians), shepherds (e.g., Scythians), and civilized nations (e.g., Europeans) according to the manner in which they managed misery and vice relative to overall numbers of people.

Malthusianism had a profound impact on nineteenth-century political economy and fertility control.[35] It was immediately contentious in England and spawned a more radical version, neo-Malthusianism, which held "not only that population could be controlled but that its control could provide a key to the creation of a good society." Against Malthus, who felt that delayed marriage and celibacy were the proper forms of sexual restraint and opposed birth control and abortion, neo-Malthusians (led by activist Francis Place)[36] advocated contraception as a means of addressing poverty. Malthusian thinking found its way to the United States through neo-Malthusian radicals, a trail that Linda Gordon diagrams as "[from] Malthus to radical democratic neo-Malthusians; through [Scottish socialist Robert Dale] Owen to U.S. utopian socialists; through the cluster of reformers and radicals in the United States in the 1840s to the women's rights movement."[37] Janet Farrell Brodie meticulously traces neo-Malthusian influence following Owen's immigration to New York, where he started the *Free Enquirer* and began to promulgate his worldview with the publication of his influential book, *Moral Physiology*, in 1830. Early feminist Frances Wright was Owen's coeditor and a notable public intellectual around 1830. Charles Knowlton, a doctor in western Massachusetts, was inspired by Owen and wrote the *Fruits of Philosophy* in 1832, which unlike Owen's work stressed male agency in fertility control and promoted contraception. Other writers emulated Owen and Knowlton, and lecturers on the lyceum circuit such as Sarah Coates and Mary Gove Nichols would promote birth control even if they did not teach it.[38]

The theology of perfectionism is a central aspect of early neo-Malthusian thinking in the United States that is relevant to antiabortion biopolitics. As described by Gordon, "American 'perfectionism' referred to the belief of a group of upstate New York and western New England Christian revivalists in the 1830s that human beings could, through conversion, become perfect while still on Earth." John Humphrey Noyes, founder of the Oneida utopian community in 1848, was a primary thinker among American perfectionists. Unlike Malthus, perfectionist utopians typically rejected traditional class structures, "the seeming eternalness of human suffering," and the idea that progress was paid for by "the misery of many." Perfectionists generally held that changing sex practices through self-control could lead to mastery of reproduction and produce "a perfectly tuned society."[39] Reception of neo-Malthusianism was not uniform among U.S. radicals, who held conflicted opinions about contraception: perfectionists preferred methods such as coitus interruptus or male continence, unlike "their British counterparts," and others advocated vaginal douching, condoms, and occasionally abortion.[40] The point of accord in the United States and in England, though, was "an enthusiasm for reproduction control as a means of creating larger social change."[41] Regarding abortion and medicine in the United States, the critical factor was the appropriation by traditionalist physicians of the linkage between fertility control and social change.

Nineteenth-Century Malthusianism and Abortion

The incorporation of Malthusianism into U.S. medical rhetoric on abortion was neither immediate nor, by all indications, particularly careful or deliberate until the campaign was launched.[42] However, the construct of the population, a dynamic unity made up of reproductive motives and countervailing pressures on fertility, became a proxy for the nation in physicians' discourse. Physicians absorbed the broad Malthusian framework of judging a nation's progress by the manner in which it balanced life and death, especially by way of procreation. In most cases, physicians embraced a Malthusian world, using a discourse already circulating in the United States rather than by acknowledging their debt to Malthus or neo-Malthusians; they opposed Malthus's dismal prognosis for perfectability on Earth, regardless.

Turning Malthusianism against itself would come later, as the initial concern over abortion did not need a world characterized by too much sex and too little food to make sense. As early as 1821, Connecticut criminalized prescription of abortifacients such as the herb hellebore after quickening on grounds that they were potentially poisonous.[43] Connecticut revised its law to include manual induction of "miscarriage" after quickening and by 1841 thirteen other states would pass similar laws aimed at regulating "the activities of apothecaries and physicians," as historian James Mohr tells us, and "not [at] dissuading women from seeking abortions."[44] Initially, then, the problem was framed not as abortion itself but as risky medicine. The growing concern for public health was not yet a governing mentality, or *governmentality* in Foucault's vernacular,[45] that was overly concerned with cultivating different reproductive habits among the population.

Around 1840 and after, amid waves of immigration from northern Europe, substantial increases in westward emigration, and ruptures to traditional family structures resulting from industrialization and urbanization, abortion quickly took its seat as a problem in a world "after Malthus."[46] Mohr observed that "dozens of medical societies and scores of medical writers all agreed that abortion became an open and pervasive practice in the United States after 1840."[47] Physicians began to understand abortion within a political economy of vital and morbid practices distributed throughout the population, including but well exceeding the concern that drugs or procedures could harm women. Hugh Lenox Hodge, a Philadelphia specialist, titled his introductory lecture to his 1839 class on obstetrics and women's diseases "Foeticide, or Criminal Abortion."

The lecture, later published and republished, is something of a founding text for U.S. medical rhetoric on abortion. Hodge engages certain basic, enduring formulas. His first words, "The history of almost every nation is blackened by this hideous, unnatural crime of infanticide," are shortly followed by the statement that "criminal abortion is almost as prevalent." From there he indicts modernity: "In our cities and towns, in this city, where literature, science, morality, and Christianity are supposed to have so much influence, where all the domestic and social virtues are reported as being in full and delightful exercise; even here individuals, male and female, exist, who are continually imbruing their hands and consciences in the blood of unborn infants."[48] Hodge was not in dialogue with Malthus, yet he evaluated contemporary U.S. history by the manner in which, as Malthus put it, "vicious customs" prevailed in relation to marriage, and by the mortality of children (keep in mind Hodges saw abortion as equal to infanticide). For Hodge, abortion was a vice whose presence called into question the advancement of a nation.

Moreover, Hodge compared abortion across classes, another Malthusian analytic: abortion afflicted all levels, Hodge argued, from poor and uneducated women to "educated, refined, and fashionable" ones.[49] Although he did not base his observations in data, he was clearly discussing populations. Most physicians of his time "preferred extremely general adjectives in estimating just how high [the abortion] incidence rate actually was."[50] It was not long, though, before medical observers began to attend to census data and to comparative fertility and mortality rates. They also variegated the matrix of differences between people, segmenting the national population into complex combinations of gender, class, region, religion, ethnicity, and race. To physicians' alarm, it became evident that native-born, advantaged, white Protestants in New England were not multiplying as before.[51] For instance, the *Boston Medical and Surgical Journal*, forerunner of the *New England Journal of Medicine*, began publishing worried notices about declining white fertility rates compared with those of blacks; about threats to the "preservation of the species" if white, New England women were less fecund; and about the higher ratio of births to "foreign parents, principally in the lower walks of life."[52] Although abortion affected all groups, it did not affect them equally.

One can recognize a derivative Malthusian logic, then, in the American Medical Association's (AMA) first "Report on Criminal Abortion," of 1859, which formalized the organization's commitment to a national antiabortion campaign:

> [Abortion's] frequency—among all classes of society, rich and poor, sin-
> gle and married—most physicians have been led to suspect; very many,
> from their own experience of its deplorable results, have known. Were
> any doubt, however, entertained upon this point, it is at once removed by
> comparisons of the present with our past rates of increase in population,
> the size of our families, the statistics of our fœtal deaths, by themselves
> considered, and relatively to the births and the general mortality. The
> evidence from these sources is too constant and too overwhelming to be
> explained on the ground that pregnancies are merely prevented; or on any
> other supposition than that of fearfully extended crime.

Comparative analysis of fertility and mortality highlighted a "generalized de-
moralization" of the country based on the deduced ubiquity of a specific vice.[53]

Versions of this assessment appear throughout the literature—especially
from the late 1860s to the early 1870s, when the medical crusade was peaking—
but the most elaborate appropriation of Malthusian analytics came in one of the
few documents to engage Malthus explicitly, Horatio Storer's 1860 monograph,
On Criminal Abortion in America. The book, which reflects his research that
informed the AMA's Committee on Criminal Abortion and the thinking that
went into the 1859 "Report," was originally published in serial fashion in the
North American Medico-Chirurgical Review throughout 1859.[54] The work was
presented as a "contribution to medical jurisprudence," primarily devoted to the
contention that abortion should be criminalized on grounds that the fetus is
alive at conception and that law based on the quickening doctrine was ineffective
and immoral. Yet with his second chapter Storer committed over twenty pages
to determining the extent of abortion in the United States in comparison with
European nations, France most of all, by way of available data for New York
City and Massachusetts, Boston especially. He analyzed reported stillbirths, induced abortions, and maternal mortality from abortion, as well as census data
on fertility rates, numbers of judicial cases filed under existing abortion law,
and doctors' personal observations on its frequency.[55] These pages are nearly
overwhelmed by disjointed data points, but the trend is clear. New York had
much greater fetal mortality than Europe, nearly double, and Massachusetts
was no better. "In this description of New York, we have the country."[56] As part
of his analysis, Storer compared the fecundity of native-born New Englanders
versus the rates of "'those of *recent foreign origin*'" and of poor versus well-to-do
women, arguing that the only increases to be seen in overall population came
from recent immigrants.[57]

The data were not uniform or consistent, as Storer noted,[58] so he was unable to produce a specific estimate on abortion's frequency, but he did conclude, after considering other reasons for a declining population, "not merely that criminal abortion is of alarming frequency among us, but that its frequency is rapidly increasing."[59] He reasoned directly from Malthusian theory, mostly as explained by John Stuart Mill.[60] Storer deduced that the U.S. population, like that of France, was in decline as a result of criminal abortion, a formulation that he averred was a "perfectly legitimate" application of Malthusian logic. Malthus had allowed for, but neo-Malthusians such as Mill would not acknowledge, abortion as a positive check on population. Storer quotes from Mill: "'The retardation of increase results either from mortality or prudence; from Mr. Malthus's positive, or from his preventive check; and one or the other of these must and does exist, and very powerfully too, in all old societies. Wherever population is not kept down by the prudence of individual or of the State, it is kept down by starvation or disease.'"[61] Storer contended that the decrease in France could *not* "only be ow[ed] to 'prudence' on the part of the community," accusing Mill of silence on the real cause. Abortion, Storer wrote, was common to ancient Greeks, Romans, and Christians, to Europe throughout the Middle Ages, to "Mohamedians, Chinese, Japanese, Hindoos, and most of the nations of Africa and Polynesia, to such an extent that we may well doubt whether more have ever perished in those countries by plague, by famine, and the sword."[62]

In other words, Storer argued that Malthus and his readers were essentially correct *in theory* but that they dramatically underestimated abortion's role in the political economy of populations. Storer then offered a revised principle of population: "It is evident, therefore, that the actual and proportionate increase of still-births, and, by induction, setting aside all probable cases of infanticide, of abortion, and the comparative increase of a population reciprocally influence and govern each other so completely, that from the one it may in any given case be almost foreseen what the other must prove."[63] It is worth pausing to contemplate his new calculus. Disease, war, and starvation are erased, as are miscarriages or restraint in procreative sex, for that matter. The only ratio left is fertility over stillbirths, such that changes in population and changes in still-births predict one another "completely." Any substantial decline in population is therefore the result of abortion or infanticide (the latter being minimal, he argued). In a work founded on the moral proposition that terminating a pregnancy was a crime against the unborn, Storer tailored the Malthusian doctrine to suit abortion and little else; population management predicted civility and barbarity, but all measures of the balance between life and death, other than abortion or, to a lesser degree, infanticide, disappeared. Storer reprised his Malthusian analysis and expanded his legal one in 1868 with *Criminal Abortion: Its Nature, Its Evidence, and Its Law*, but he did not alter his thesis.[64]

Storer was an *anti*-Malthusian, however. Whereas Malthus, Mill, and other political economists saw smaller families as progress, Storer saw the opposite. He was hardly the first physician to explicitly contest Malthus, as Roy Porter pointed out. Physicians in Britain had leveled critiques from the left and the right.[65] Storer definitely fell to the right as he blamed Malthus and his heirs for the pestilence of abortion:

> In asserting that the doctrines of leading political economists for the last half century are accountable for much of the prevalence and increase of the crime, ignorant or careless as these writers all seem of the dire means that would be resorted to for the attainment of their ends, I have in no way exaggerated. Malthus remarks in his well-known Essay on Population, that "in the average state of a well-peopled territory, there cannot well be a worse sign than a large proportion of births, nor can there well be a better sign than a small proportion."[66]

Conscious of the dispersion of neo-Malthusian advice and advocacy, Storer blamed the political-economic clerisy, not the people. Taking up Malthusian reasoning, Storer elaborated a curious inversion of it. It is wrong, then, to understand anti-Malthusian biopolitics as opposed to Malthus root and stem.

The point of reversal rested on the idea of perfectability and the understanding of Providence. Nathan Allen, a physician from Lowell, Massachusetts, would be the one to reconcile this seemingly contradictory endorsement and rejection of Malthus. Reading Allen, it is clear that what differentiates Hodge from Malthus, and what made U.S. antiabortionists in the medical community *anti*-Malthusian, is that abortion was caused not by necessity driven by overpopulation but by ignorance of a true moral physiology (emphatically *not* the moral physiology described by Robert Dale Owen). In April 1868, Allen published "The Law of Human Increase; or Population Based on Physiology and Psychology" in the *Quarterly Journal of Psychological Medicine and Medical Jurisprudence*. He also read a shorter, revised version of the essay in November that year to the Western Social Science Association. The revised version was published as a pamphlet in 1870 as *Population: Its Law of Increase*.[67] The versions are entirely consistent, but some valuable language is unique to each.

Allen rejected Malthus's description of Providence: "There are certain features of Malthus' doctrine of population that have always been revolting to the moral sense of mankind." Instead, he argued that the true law of population was consistent with God's mandate "to be fruitful and multiply, and replenish the earth and subdue it."[68] The error, Allen felt, lay in the material basis for Malthus's law: "To establish a general law which is to have the greatest possible agency in developing the nature of a body and controlling its very existence, the presumption is that such a law must be evolved, in some way, from the designs had in the creation of that body." And so "the most important law of all, the law the shapes its life, character, and destiny, it would seem, must have its seat somewhere in the body itself." Yet when one looks to Malthusians, "the laws that they lay down for [life's] increase have been controlled generally by agents or objects entirely external to the body, and some of them hold only remote or indirect relations to it."[69] Instead of looking to external factors such as inadequate housing, limited income, numbers of children, or prospects for a stable marriage, one needed to look at physiology to decide how many children are necessary to a good society.[70]

This shift in the material origin of the "law of human increase" is decisive because it replaces a contextual, imperfect rubric for making sexual decisions with a purportedly timeless, perfected one. The consequences of Allen's substitution exceed the use of biological determinism to justify patriarchal ideology; Allen laid a conservative moral physiology over where Malthus had enshrined a permanent state of trial. "The principles or laws of physiology, when rightly interpreted, are a part of the will and government of God in this world. The law of increase, as here based on physiology, explains the free agency of man [sic] and human accountability as in perfect harmony with the divine government."[71] For Malthus, Providence was a jumble of constraints that drove people to prudential sex practices; in his view there was no prospect of ultimate harmony, only striving. For neo-Malthusians such as Owen, harmony was possible, given a high degree of sexual restraint. But for Allen and other anti-Malthusians, Providence banned restraint among married couples, commanding humans to fill the earth with God's children. Theirs was an inverted form of Malthusianism in which balance was achieved only when humans conformed to the dictates of moral physiology as defined from the body out, not from society in. The matrix of political economy was a healthy, highly active womb, with female physiology as the Lawgiver's living text of Creation, so physiology should tower over worldly governance so as to harmonize human conduct with God's will.[72]

Governing Life on Earth

Allen did not originate the pivot on perfectability any more than Storer originated anti-Malthusianism, but their views were nevertheless high-proof distil-
lations of a long-fermenting rhetoric. Against Malthus, neo-Malthusians and
anti-Malthusians alike endorsed the perfectability of society through reproductive practices; utopian birth controllers sought perfection through mastering
nature, where anti-Malthusians among American physicians sought perfection
through obedience to nature. Anti-Malthusians in England *had* made scriptural arguments like Allen's early in the century (and Carlyle was pressed to decide which was more dreary, Malthus or anti-Malthusians "quoting their Bible
against palpable facts" and making an "unpleasant spectacle").[73] Allen, however,
exemplifies the medicalized investiture of physiology itself as the plan of Providence made flesh. The discourse of the crusade is impossible without this investiture, although the major writers tended to assume rather than to explain
their biopolitics. Together with biopolitical histories such as Storer rehearsed,
the two precepts of the anti-Malthusians' inverted political economy become
clear: first, God's law organizes the *oikonomia* of life purely from procreative
sexual practices as dictated by reproductive physiology (which produces a perfect world if obeyed); second, by extension, abortion is an unnatural practice
that tells us how far we have strayed from Providence.

In *The Kingdom and the Glory*, Agamben writes of Christian theologians'
centuries-long debate over the relation of a general and a special Providence,
wherein Providence comprises the essential relation between divinity and world-
liness. *General Providence* refers to God's plan (theology), and *special Providence*
refers to the carrying out of that plan on Earth (the *oikonomia* of life).[74] Central
to the dispute was whether God ruled actively by intervening in the everyday, or
designed Creation but left its management to humans. If general, transcendent
Providence was not separate from special, immanent Providence; if they were
redundant, there would be no free will, since all decisions would, in effect, be
God's. Anti-Malthusian physicians did not debate the finer points of this question. Rather, they assumed a Providential model that supposed "the freedom of
those who are governed, which manifests itself through the works" of human
beings on earth, as suggested by Allen's recognition of human agency regarding
physiology and his warning of accountability for that freedom as well.[75] Women
were at liberty to violate God's mandates, if at our collective peril. Yet God was
not extraneous either; divine law was embedded in the body's mechanisms, a

law that reflects a model of Providence wherein divinity is never "separate from the world" but exists "always in relation to immanence."[76] The concept of moral physiology was a medicalized reconciliation of "a God who is foreign to the world and a God that governs."[77] Because God does not make women bear children (which would render morality irrelevant), divine mandates are immanent to the body but nevertheless govern through mediation.[78] The aim of worldly government, then, is to suture an earthly order with a celestial order, as guided by physiological knowledge of moral purpose.

Many notable works evidence the anti-Malthusians' Providential model. For example, David Humphreys Storer, Horatio Storer's father, argued in an 1855 introductory lecture to Harvard medical students that uterine disease was a function of natural law having been violated by abortion or contraception, which led to untold harm.[79] Horatio Storer, in an 1866 essay written to women titled *Why Not? A Book for Every Woman*, compared women to animals and fish in order to demonstrate a physiological imperative to reproduce in accordance with God's law; he closed by discussing the need of the state to replenish itself after the Civil War.[80] Hodges, Hale, and Allen certainly shared this common view of God's government on earth.[81]

The understanding of Providence that organizes anti-Malthusian physicians' discourse is clearly derived from evangelical Protestantism, which thrived during and after the Second Great Awakening (1790s–1840s) on the strength of tent revivals, the evangelical press, and its influence in educational institutions.[82] Mark Noll argues that predominant evangelical thinking in the United States was "much more concerned with human limitation than with human potential" and exhibited a "preoccupation with theological problems as defined by the Puritans' Calvinistic tradition."[83] Nevertheless, no single sectarian theology motivated antiabortionists, as they had diverse backgrounds. For instance, before medical school Hugh Hodge attended Princeton, which was then the most Calvinist institution of higher learning in the United States.[84] Horatio Storer, on the other hand, was raised Unitarian but later converted to Episcopalian.[85]

However, concern among physicians for embryonic life at conception *was not* derived from dominant theological opinion. When Storer initiated his crusade, "he was able to cite only one specific endorsement from a prominent religious spokesman, Bishop Fitzpatrick of Boston."[86] The first ban of abortion at any stage was England's secular Ellenborough Act of 1803, whereas Protestant churches of the time imitated Catholic doctrine, which held that life began *at quickening* and not at conception, as is often assumed. In fact, Mohr documents early medical antiabortionists castigating Protestant clergy for moral failure on the issue, creating antagonism between physicians and religious leaders.[87] Storer was himself critical of Protestants' tolerance of abortion, although he was more moderate than others.[88] As Gordon notes, the "Catholic Church was a follower, not a leader, in restricting abortion," only forbidding it pre-quickening in 1869, when most U.S. states had already criminalized the practice.[89] Dating at least from Hodges, U.S. physicians began to adopt the new English legal point of view, couched in scriptural terms but grounded in physiology. Storer's concern for fetal life, which was highly influential, was informed by his studies in biology, including zoology and botany and his experiences dissecting embryos, not to mention his father's opposition to abortion, which was shaped by his father's research as a naturalist.[90] Both D. H. and H. R. Storer called abortion a grave sin but explained that sin through biological processes of reproduction. Indeed, H. R. specifically praised the blending of science and Christian theology.[91]

The second "Report on Criminal Abortion," tendered by O'Donnell and Atlee to the AMA in 1871, offers perhaps the best window onto physicians' synthesis of a governing mentality from a generalized evangelical view of Providence and physiology. Significantly, it appears toward the tail end of the physicians' crusade, indicating a mature discourse. The authors carefully stipulate that good government is defined by its ability to reconcile a divine order manifested in physiology with the moral choices made in regard to pregnancy: "It is a remarkable fact that the further we advance in civilization, and what the world calls refinement, of the present day, the further do we recede from the main object which should be the end and aim of the institution of all good governments—the well-being of the human family and the preservation of human life."[92] They establish woman's purpose as "propagating the human family," which marriage codifies. However, if a woman "becomes a participant in the destruction of her own offspring" she "becomes unmindful of the course marked out for her by Providence."[93] The authors recapitulate Allen's Malthusian history of declining fertility among "better classes" of white New Englanders and quote from Allen on the divine perfection of physiological law and the inheritance of disease from its violation, such that "the human family is most likely to be propagated in its fullest perfection" when maximally fertile.[94] Further, they hold that God "creates and breathes life into the product of that conception a living soul."[95] From these physiological predicates, they judge the spread of abortion and contraception over the "the last fifty, perhaps a hundred years" to be an evil greater than the deaths of the Civil War, "which lasted for a few years," and more "destructive to human life than ten British Armies."[96] The impact of these practices is felt in population levels and also in the health of the population, since abortion necessarily damaged women (who acted in contravention to nature) and such harm was seen as inheritable: "the effects of such weakness or disease must descend to their children and to their children's children (if they have any) *ad infinitum*."[97]

Every element of the rhetoric runs fully extended, at a gallop through this essay, finishing with a characterization of abortion as worse than the plague: "The plague, though dangerous and fatal in its course, had certain limits assigned to its extension, but the evil with which we have to deal is not confined to a city or to any particular district of country; its march is onward, its increase is progressive with the increase of population, its boundaries marked only by the limits of this hemisphere, and, if not checked soon, time alone can tell the extent of ruin which must result to the human family."[98] The real disease was indifference to moral physiology, which cannot be quarantined, and the measure of a good nation was vigilance in fighting its spread. The authors went so far as to bracket their medico-political economy *within a war to defend society*. They open the essay quoting from Job 7:1, "'The life of man on earth is a warfare,'" immediately placing the tireless effort to beat back disease as part of their mission—"the life of the *physician* on earth is *indeed* a warfare."[99] They conclude by setting the objective: "We have no foreign enemy to contend with, but we have a domestic enemy, and that enemy is in our midst; it surrounds us; yes, we have an unprincipled, an insidious, and unmitigated foe to deal with, an enemy to the human family, as dark and as malignant as the spirit that sent it, and it now becomes us to do our part faithfully towards God in this matter, to crush the monster, and to place the profession right before the public."[100] The doctor was not a soldier, though, but a caretaker, who, "as far as his [*sic*] practice extends, should feel that in his professional department he is the shepherd of his flock, and it becomes his duty to see that these wolves in sheep's clothing should not make any inroads among them."[101]

It would be a mistake to brush off O'Donnell and Atlee as hyperventilating Victorians. The 1871 "Report" culminates early U.S. physicians' anti-Malthusianism and is a striking case of metaphors of war, medicine, and disease converging into the political critique of culture. Foucault noticed this same convergence among French historians of the eighteenth century as war shifted its relationship to history in their writing. The historical consciousness they exhibited would become characteristic of biopower among modern, liberal nation-states, and it fits the early U.S. biopolitics on abortion precisely. War fell inward in modernity, spilling over from external conflicts "between one mass and another mass" in the name of a monarch or God and into "a generalized war that permeates the entire social body and the entire history of the social body."[102] War as an organizing construct of history made "society intelligible" as unending conflict between nationalities, religious groups, classes, races, ethnicities, and genders and *not* exclusively between sovereigns.[103] In other words, a nation could be analyzed in terms of multiple, competitive antagonisms propelled forward not by armed hostility so much as by political conflict "inscribed in society's real struggles."[104] Beyond narratives of war from which nations are born, we begin to see stories about warlike campaigns needed to "protect and preserve society" from itself, particularly its racially diverse self. Hence, "we see the emergence of the idea of an internal war that defends society against threats born of and in its own body."[105] This is precisely the historical consciousness that O'Donnell and Atlee put to use when they name abortion as an implacable domestic enemy of the human family hiding in our midst.

Broadly speaking, the "idea of social war" as endless, vigilant conflict waged against internal enemies marks "a great retreat from the historical to the biological, from the constituent to the medical."[106] Internal threats are not limited to armed insurgencies; they include biopolitical risks to well-being such as disease, insecure food, practices that increase mortality, and so on. These were not epidemics, or "temporary disasters" that "swooped down on life," as Foucault put it, but "endemics" that are "something permanent, something that slips into life, perpetually gnaws at it, diminishes it and weakens it."[107] Lauren Berlant calls such endemics "slow death."[108] The 1871 "Report" is quite ordinary in the respect that it calls for war against the slow death of society from abortion. When governance focuses on "the power to preserve life" against perceived threats emerging from the collective body, such as a surge in fertility control, warfare becomes the struggle to inoculate society from such threats.[109] War is a ceaseless battle with death, the "malignant spirit" whose defeat transforms the medical shepherd into the healing warrior. Wars of this sort are not simply battles of opposites, of vitality versus morbidity; rather, they operate under an *immunitary paradigm*, as Roberto Esposito explains: "As in the medical practice of vaccinating the individual body, so the immunization of the political body functions similarly; introducing within it a fragment of the same pathogen from which it wants to protect itself, by blocking and contradicting natural development."[110] In the case of fertility control, this means implementing ways of life that protect us from the threat of too much life, or too much of the wrong kind of life. Malthus saw the deprivation of life, reduced fertility, as an antibody to a *greater* loss of life from starvation, for instance. Anti-Malthusians saw a little knowledge, the right knowledge, of physiology as an antibody to efforts to fully control reproduction.

The mobilization of immunities to internal enemies, deploying morbid aspects of life to counteract greater morbid tendencies, is a more precise way of stating what "fighting through life" means. Governing life on earth is a struggle to protect life from itself. O'Donnell and Atlee's seemingly hypocritical figure of a medical shepherd fighting a war through saving lives is not as confused as it seems. A war to give more life to a certain race over others by immunizing that race against the "disease" of small families, to make white, well-to-do Anglos live *more*, is perfectly comprehensible within an immunitary paradigm. As legal historians N. E. H. Hull and Peter Charles Hoffer describe it, "The state had taken an interest in abortion to protect the future interest of the state in 'the unborn child.'"[111] As we will see, engagement with elective abortion in U.S. medical rhetoric was organized under an immunitary paradigm, the pregnant body being the anchor point for immunization, as practitioners sought protection against the morbid causes and effects of the practice and its management, sometimes for protection against protections that had become morbid themselves, such as the law. Esposito provides a crucial refinement of biopolitical theory for making sense of commonalities that subtend seemingly opposed projects of medical experts.

It should be noted that among early anti-Malthusians, a shared political economics did not mean agreement on the specific nature of threats to be addressed. Contrary to H. R. Storer, Edwin Hale was theologically mainstream and believed that fetal life was not paramount over the life and health of the mother in all cases and that physicians should never speak of patients' abortions publicly.[112] Prestigious obstetricians Charles Meigs and Gunning Bedford clung to the quickening doctrine, too.[113] Further, Storer strenuously opposed women becoming physicians, which was of a piece with his views on the importance of maternity, the rightful place of women in society, and the evils of abortion. Atlee was as conservative about abortion as Storer, working closely with his ideas, but Atlee did not share his feelings about the additional dangers posed by women physicians.[114] The exact character of risks posed by abortion and the manner by which it was linked to other perceived threats to society were openly disputed by early antiabortionists, even though they subscribed broadly to the same governing mentality.

Abortion had become a medically grounded problem of and for governance, turning on medical knowledge of the morbidity of the practice, and in the coming decades reproductive medicine should be understood as the continued refinement of a nationalized biopolitical project of abortion control. That project was decidedly conflicted with two major governing mentalities, anti- and neo-Malthusian, vying for dominance. Regardless of their differences, both mentalities would continue to depend on a scale of civilization as derived from Malthusian political economics. However, a scale of civilization alone is not sufficient in and of itself for this rhetorical capacity. Such a scale assumes, but does not stake, abortion's value as pathognomonic. Physicians needed to be able to demonstrate *how* we learned about internal threats by the fact that some turned to abortion. Physicians needed abortion's morbidity to produce memories of risks and dangers, of biological and cultural hazards and their trends. Therefore, before beginning a genealogy of what later generations of physicians made of abortion's political-economic value, I need to discuss how its morbidity could function *mnestically* to place the present as declining or falling behind.

2

Remembering, Forgetting, and the Secrets of Life

Remembering and forgetting are linked to disclosure and secrecy.
—EDWIN BLACK, "Secrecy and Disclosure as Rhetorical Forms"

To understand the relevance of medicine to rhetoric about abortion, an account is needed of how medical knowledge production is entangled with memory work and biopolitics. The previous chapter established the principal biopolitical mentality of early physicians, subsequent mutations of which will be analyzed in the next chapters. This chapter takes up the relation of remembering and forgetting to the medical research that organizes those analyses. After fleshing out the general conception of memory work that guides my thinking, I discuss how knowledge of abortion is positioned beyond certain horizons of secrecy that condition medicine's memory work on the subject. This process of uncovering hidden knowledge of individuals, groups, and the body was critical for medical experts in estimating morbidity and, thus, situating culture. I then discuss how I operationalize the analysis of remembering and forgetting within material aspects of abortion practices and physicians' treatment of patients. Those material aspects must be understood as active elements within the rhetoric relative to the capacity to address present-day life as afflicted. It matters that improperly conducted abortions can risk women's lives, that embryos develop in a particular way, and that women and their families can afford only limited numbers of children.

Stipulating Mnestic Capacity

To be able to situate the present in time and space is above all a mnestic capacity, resulting from the interaction of remembering and forgetting operating in unison.[1] My deployment of both terms, *mnesis* and *capacity*, relies on two well-established suppositions within memory studies: that mnesis is a process, not a specific thing, and that it operates both nonreflexively and reflexively. In that, "mnestic capacity" contrasts with everyday ideas about memory as the stored impressions of past experience. In the "storehouse model," individual memories are "things" analogous to photographs; and like a photograph, a memory can be clear or fuzzy and can fade over time in the process called forgetting. Augustine famously presented this model of memory in chapter 10 of *Confessions*, wherein he describes memory as a cache of truths tucked away in the gathers of the world, waiting reluctantly to be (re)discovered.[2] For Augustine, memory is independent and unitary; one full, uncontested recollection exists but lies unseen around us and even within us, sealed, waiting to be unlocked if only we could find the key.[3] Forgetting in the storehouse model is a surreptitious force that exists in a binary relation of secrecy and disclosure with memory. Forgetting selectively chips away at the unity of memory, destroying memory piece by piece and retreating into secrecy.[4]

By contrast, my concern is with mnesis as a *figurative* process that manifests a sense of place, not a specific image or representation of the past. Remembering and forgetting operate recursively in this process, iterating contacts between past and present that restrict to whom or what a discourse is addressed (which enables discourse to have focus). There is no unaddressed discourse; the recursive rhythms of remembering and forgetting are a kind of "centripetal" force that centers discourse amid the flow of events. Specifically, as I understand rhetorical recursion, certain events or practices can become points of *inflection* (of stress or contortion) that offer a temporary feeling of place in the passage of time. Inflections sometimes normalize into regular *positions* by which the present moment is recognized as like or different from other times. Such positions may become so privileged as to become points of *inclusion* by which the sum of time's passage is felt relative to a particular event or practice.

Process and Reflexivity

Scholars of memory such as Barbie Zelizer or Jeffrey Olick have spoken to the processual nature of mnesis, treating recollection not as an object of personal, mental reflection but as an effect of collective memory work or, more exactly, as a materialization of the past within present communal activities.[5] In fact, Olick has termed a "pernicious postulate" the idea of memory as an immaterial, self-contained cognition that can be isolated from the processes in which it is embedded. That postulate directs attention to questions of "when memory causes changes or what causes changes in memory." In its place, Olick argues for an idea of memory as an emergent consequence of ordinary engagements with the wider world. Memory is not a thing. Rather, there are *figurations of memory*—developing relations between past and present—where images, contexts, traditions, and interests come together in fluid, though not necessarily harmonious, ways."[6] Paul Connerton makes a similar point, elaborating on the work of Maurice Halbwachs, the great sociologist of collective memory: "Every recollection, however personal it may be, even that of events of which we alone were the witness, even that of thoughts and sentiments that remain unexpressed, exists in an ensemble with a whole of notions which others possess: with persons, places, dates, words, forms of language, that is to say with the whole material and moral life of societies of which we are part or which we have been a part."[7] The place of our institutions, our cultures, and our selves in time emerges in cooperation with the environments in which we dwell, not from just ideas about those environments. For my purposes, the term *memory* refers not to a shared image of the past but to the relations between past and present that are manifested conjointly in ways of life. It is in this way that the production of medical knowledge, as one broad form of interaction between humans and their world, actualizes memory work.

Forgetting, although usually treated as antithetical to remembrance, is not the opposite of remembering; it is the condition of memory.[8] When understood as the ceaseless outflow of memory, forgetting is critical to the very idea of recollection as a process. If memory did not fade there would be no process at all. The past would simply accumulate, never actually becoming "past," but remaining ever present, leaving no need for remembrance. If memory were full and total, if forgetfulness were vanquished, memory would no longer *be* memory. In fact, "most of the time, when we speak of forgetting, we are speaking of displacement (or replacement) of one version of the past by another."[9] This never-finished process of displacement is the indissoluble quality of remembering and forgetting at work. As represented in the Greek myth of Mnemosyne and her counterpart, Lesmosyne, no full and definitive memory can be appealed to and forgetfulness catalyzes some recollections over others.[10] Memory exists only in transit, continually disappearing and reappearing, and lethe is what instigates its transience.[11]

As a result, remembrance cannot be understood as a preservative against the depredations of forgetting. Memory emerges within ongoing fields of interaction as a partial, limited figuration of the present in relation to the past. Michel de Certeau wrote that the "life of a culture and of a society is made of an endless ebb and flow between realities, representations, and their memories."[12] Such figurations are embodied not only in textual objects such as news items, photographs, commemorations, and research but also in wordless material factors of our interactions, from architecture, tools, life cycles of flora and fauna, tides, the movements of stars, the physiological "facts of life," and certainly behaviors as basic as speaking or gesturing in contextually appropriate ways.[13] "This multi-form presence of memory can be found everywhere, even in our most ostensibly theoretical inquiries: thus the interest in astronomy or in the life of the species."[14] A combined ebb and flow within these interactions is what I mean by mnesis: *one* figuration gives way to another, not *the* complete figuration to an incomplete one.

Mnesis is active whether or not we are aware of it, ubiquitous and inexorable. Marcel Proust notably distinguished voluntary from involuntary memory in the individual,[15] but this separation is somewhat misleading.[16] We can and do put great effort into recollection, but unnoticed events of remembering and forgetting cannot be segregated from premeditated acts of memory.[17] Even in a memorial rite, practices that enable the invocation of the past *in support of that memorialization* are not necessarily conscious. Regulations and procedures governing assembly at monuments organize observance and contain the possibility of future observances.[18] They do not invoke a particular event but they make it possible to remember, managing the ebb and flow of ways of life. Further, highly crafted practices not usually understood in terms of remembering and forgetting have become paradigmatic mnestic arrangements.[19] To take up de Certeau's example, evolutionary science is arguably a world-changing reorganization of mnesis, even though it is not usually viewed as a form of recollection. Empirical data, discoveries, metaphors, and logics derived from evolutionary science have radically affected our sense of when, where, and what we are.[20] Memories and amnesias of human societies are now tethered to the lives of viruses, for instance; viral mutation is linked to antiviral practices and human history is shaped by epidemiology. Evolution is not a specific memory but a multidisciplinary discourse that, in describing the persistence and mutation of life, puts to work a dynamic array of practices that bring the past into the present.[21] Attending only to those memorists whose purpose is to conserve or release memory, one misses figurations of mnesis such as evolutionary science.

Recognizing nonreflexive memory work within enterprises such as medical practice and research has consequences for rhetorical analysis. Remembering and forgetting cannot be confined to the work of specific discursive genres but must be understood as constituent functions that enable discourse of every sort to operate *as* a discourse.[22] Sites and ceremonies of commemoration, autobiographies and biographies, eulogies and reminiscences are all powerful, well-formed traditions of rhetoric whose central purposes revolve around the interpretive, frequently divisive, labor of recollecting an "event, figure, or symbol."[23] There are organized traditions of public forgetting as well, as Tzvetan Todorov notes of South African truth and reconciliation committees after apartheid,[24] or in Bradford Vivian's studies of desired, productive amnesias in *Public Forgetting*: "Public forgetting arises from uncommonly pivotal moments in the evolution of communal time, history, and memory, during which either a single agent or collective body initiates such forgetting." Emphasis on memorial or lethean *projects* typically focuses our attention on genres of rhetoric and leaves aside "ordinary and often unnoticed patterns of selective interpretation or partial recollection."[25] To understand how mnesis operates within medical discourse, however, requires resisting the temptation to see one genre through another (as if, say, biography were a metaphor for gynecology).

To understand mnesis as a *strategy* puts a premium on formal discursive features and pushes analysis toward genres, in other words. If instead mnesis is understood as a *capacity*, the concern shifts to what particular figurations enable discourse to accomplish, thus highlighting rhetorical possibilities. At its most general level, mnesis enacts the persistent, yet changing, relationship of the present to the past (and by implication, the future). It is about how a rhetoric inhabits time in order that its discourses may address the world, embodying a sense of what has come before, the state of affairs now, and what could or should be. In that regard, mnesis is a process of "meaning-making in time rather than the production of static objects."[26] The meaning being made is not the referential significance of image, word, gesture, or monument. It is the diffused inference of place, of feeling located. In the case of medical rhetoric of abortion, emplacement was afforded by damage, whether precipitant, immediate, or subsequent to the act.

Recursivity

To investigate mnestic capacity for rhetoric, then, requires attention to the repetitive, variable materializations of the present as a feeling of place in time. In this study, the function of recursion as a concept is to name the figurative dynamism that produces a feeling of emplacement. The value of recursivity for describing the mnestic capacity of rhetoric is implicit in the term's necessary and dependent relationship with discursivity, as seen in the etymologies of the words. *Recursion* derives from the Latin *recurro,* or "to run back," and *discourse* from *discursus,* or "running to and fro." Discourse ranges about, pursuing limitless ends. It moves out, forward, on. It disseminates. Echoing Aristotle, philosopher George Campbell stated that rhetoric was the adaptation of discourse to its end;[27] rhetoric is thus the labor of addressivity (the direction that discourse "runs," either toward, for, or against *something*).[28] Yet to have an end, discourse must have a beginning, and "all beginnings contain an element of memory."[29] A sense of the present as emplaced is thus an orientational prerequisite of discourse; to be adapted to the present, discourse must recur to the past. As often as not, that sense of the present is produced simply through the manner in which the past is acted on in the present; place is frequently unannounced, occupied without fanfare.

An additional value of recursion is that it contrasts with a common understanding of memory as fundamentally a copy. As metaphor, the copy supposes that recollection proceeds through a series of representational likenesses that always move away from an original moment or from preceding iterations, becoming finite points on an infinite line of similar points, each posited as "separable minima."[30] Instead, Gilles Deleuze described the emplacement of the present as a kind of flexion, such that the *"present itself is only the most contracted level of the past."*[31] Recursivity posits remembering and forgetting as a process of *folding* one time and place into another virtually,[32] not as *copying* one moment in the next. Ordinary practices contract the past into the present, in anticipation of the future, by looping back again and again to particular objects, practices, or events. No person or event secrets memories within these various elements. The sepsis that took so many women's lives was not a "fold" in the sense of storing hidden memories; rather, recurrent sepsis "folded" events together in a way that supported orientation of the present relative to other times and places: contemporary life was marked by women increasingly killing themselves by accident while trying to avoid having children.

The folding metaphor describes the dependence of discourse on recursive dynamics more precisely. The movement of cyclical contact may be circulatory but the structure "matches an infolding with an exfoliation."[33] The mainspring for placing the present—infolding the past—drives discursive expansion; dilation occurs *through* contraction. Edward Casey remarks of remembering that "the contractive power of encapsulment is matched only by the distending power of expansion."[34] It is easy to imagine a two-staged process, first tension and then release, aimlessly repeating itself. Discourse, however, is always in the middle of itself and working toward particular ends. There is no prediscursive space outside events in which the present contracts a past before giving itself over to discourse. Furthermore, discourse does not simply repeat; it mutates. Consequently, discourse as the *unfolding* of rhetorical potential is not "the contrary of the fold" that produced that potential "but the continuation or the extension of its act."[35] The present moment unfolds, for example, develops, directly *within* its continuous encapsulation of the past. Against a model of memory as representational copies of past events, the recursive model I adopt understands mnesis as an ongoing, figurative event that locates the present as a distinct moment "born in flux."[36]

Inflection, Position, Inclusion

Conceiving of the present as a place where the past folds into the future does not in itself explain how certain modes of recursion become more important than others and active drivers within discourses such as those about abortion. Recursion curves the passage of time this way and that through three interrelated operations: *inflection, position,* and *inclusion.*[37] An event or practice becomes a point of *inflection* when it modulates the relation of "then," "now," and "later." For a patient who self-induces abortion, but suffers an incomplete evacuation, becomes septic, and nearly dies, the experience can function as a point at which the present bends toward *and* away from the past. She or someone else could easily organize her life as before and after such an experience. Moments like these can so disturb the ordinary flow of events that long arcs of the past and future, which often lie obscured amid the immediacy of "now," become tangible as turning on such a moment (building up to and following from it). The accumulation of similar instances in a population can similarly become communal inflections, with the difference that no one instant creates the stress. Persistent activities and occasions can become distinctive stressors that mark a turn in the present. By the time Edwin Hale bemoaned modern women's lost connection with traditional maternity in the 1860s, as mentioned in the introduction, the rise of induced abortion had inflected the life of the nation.[38] Inflections, then, are events or practices that provide a feeling of the present *as in* flux.

Inflections become *positions* when a particular event or kind of event moves from being one point among others to being a normative way of occupying time. For physicians, induced abortion moved from inflection to position when a political economy devoted to its control emerged. A scale of civilization tailored to abortion was the by-product of a changed recursive status. The forces that elect a particular kind of event to a normative position must be attended to. Mnestic figuration is always partial and selective, and the sorts of practices that become habitual dramatically affect the rhetorical potential of discourses.[39] A dominant manner of circling about the past *secures* the place from which a rhetoric addresses its discourse. The character of discourse about abortion control is decisively altered when the physiology of abortion becomes the ground for positioning present-day culture as sick, rather than an indicator of the socioeconomics of family limitation. Paradigms for recursion empower discourses by giving them a foundation. Such paradigms emerge from ecologies of power for the purposes of exercising power, namely, the coveted power to promise the future, and they continually disintegrate as they are contested or surpassed.[40]

A paradigmatic position for recursion may become a point of *inclusion* by which the present situates itself generally, wholly encapsulating the past and future through particular balances of memory and amnesia. Time's passage seems fully retrievable through *this* inflection, from *this* position. In 1933, William Robinson argued that the march of history was punctuated by transitions from infanticide, to abortion, to birth control.[41] Availing himself of a rudimentary sociology of medicine, he recurred to the transition to and from induced abortion across all known societies. The fate of billions of anonymous pregnancies modulated the United States' place in world progress for Robinson. Points of inclusion show particular figurations of mnesis to be more than ways to locate contemporary life; they are mechanisms for organizing all times and places in relation to each other. "For an experienced event is finite—at any rate, confined to one sphere of experience," said Walter Benjamin; "a remembered event is infinite, because it is only a key to everything that happened before and after it."[42] When a distinctive sense of place in time becomes a generalized method of inhabiting all times, it effectively constitutes the present as the "'place of all places.'"[43] Abortion becomes a point of inclusion when its existence encapsulates that state of any people through time.

Secrecy: Remembering and Forgetting Through Abortion

Figurations of mnesis are not all created equal. The recursive inflections, positions, and inclusions that characterize one may be completely different from another and with those differences come distinct rhetorical capacities. More simply, differing senses of when and where the present resides in the scheme of things radically alter which sorts of propositions entertain meaningful responses.[44] Without a certain minimally shared orientation to time and place among those addressing or being addressed, rhetorical interaction becomes nearly impossible.[45] Even variations on the same figuration, such as those developed by anti- and neo-Malthusian physicians, are distinct from one another in ways important to what those discourses are designed to accomplish. Within the abortion debate, the common experience of feeling that a person from the "other side" seems to be from another planet is a simple, germane example. A recognizable "now" must be manifest within a discourse if it is to function as rhetoric. Thus, a general processual model of remembering and forgetting is not sufficient. A genealogist of recursivity must adapt to the peculiar topography of the discourses in question. In regard to abortion, secrecy is a cardinal feature of the landscape.

"The secret offers, so to speak, the possibility of a second world alongside the manifest world; and the latter is decisively influenced by the former."[46] Contemplating Georg Simmel's observation, it is unsurprising that secrecy is crucial to medical rhetoric on abortion. In the United States and elsewhere, abortion has consistently held the oxymoronic status of an open secret, hidden in the shadows of everyday life. Before the Roe v. Wade decision, millions experienced the underground every year, whether personally seeking an abortion or being involved in its procurement, support, or policing. Jane, the storied Chicago collective that provided abortions from the late 1960s until the Roe decision, served thousands of women; the semi-clandestine network in which Jane operated included people in the medical community and law enforcement as well as other abortion providers.[47] Reports of abortion networks routinely flared up in local and national coverage, such as with the Chicago Examiner's exposés at the end of World War I, or in the 1930s when papers reported on the Pacific Coast abortion ring that involved physicians and state officials from California to Washington State, or the sensationalized raids of abortionists' offices in Portland, Oregon, in 1951.[48] More frequently, local news or magazines such as Woman's Day ran cautionary tales of women who had died or of a lone abortionist on trial.[49] Today, abortion is no longer underground, but it is not an open practice; enormous regulatory obstacles, harassment, domestic terrorism, and assassinations have encouraged women seeking abortions and their providers to proceed with caution.[50] Access to abortion has dwindled such that fewer than one in ten counties in the United States has an abortion provider. Declining access has produced a new, largely overlooked practice of self-induced abortions that some journalists have dubbed do-it-yourself or "DIY" abortions.[51] Susan Wiklund, an ob-gyn, writes vividly of the tenuous state of abortion provision in her aptly named memoir, *This Common Secret*.[52]

Issues of secrecy associated with terminating pregnancies have powerfully shaped the contours of discourse about the subject. For medical observers pre-*Roe*, the entire judgment that abortion was a sign of pathology within the social body rested on the understanding that abortion's secret world was decisively shaped by morbid influences at work in the manifest world. Indeed, medicine's intensive investment in abortion as an open secret epitomizes the basic story line of Foucault's first volume of *The History of Sexuality*: "What is peculiar to modern societies, in fact, is not that they consigned sex to a shadow existence, but that they dedicated themselves to speaking of it *ad infinitum*, while exploiting it as *the* secret."[53] The apparent admonition against frank talk about sex that developed in Western modernity was in fact part of a complex demand to know the truth of sex, which incited "a proliferation of discourses" such that "in the areas of the economy, pedagogy, medicine, and justice . . . an immense verbosity is what our civilization has required and organized."[54] Medical and legal discourse on abortion in the United States matches this pattern; it ignited at the same moment when abortion became a political economic problem in and of the population of white well-to-do people.

The kind of secret typically identified with abortion before *Roe* is that of the *private subject* operating clandestinely. The mind leaps to testimony from women like "Ann." She had two abortions in the late 1950s, one in Germany while she was on a trip in Europe, the other in New York. In both countries, physicians performed the procedure, but in Germany the pretense that Ann was bleeding provided cover for the abortion to occur in a hospital with professional care. In New York, she encountered an arranged time, a code language, and no anesthesia.[55] Or maybe one thinks of more terrifying stories like Caroline's—at college in 1963 in Cleveland, she was forced to turn to a bookie/abortionist in Youngstown. After a saline injection, she began "at least twelve hours of labor," alone in her dormitory. Then came extensive bleeding and the traumatizing necessity of flushing the fetus down a shower room toilet. She bled for weeks until, after confiding in another student, she was referred to an Episcopalian rector who arranged for a doctor. After five pints of blood and a dilation and curettage, the physician kept her secret and the church paid her bill.[56] One might also think of abortion providers' stories as recounted in an oral history like Carol

Joffe's *Doctors of Conscience*, a memoir like Edward Keemer's *Confessions of a Prolife Abortionist*, or a biography like Rickie Solinger's account of Ruth Barnett in *The Abortionist*.[57] These stories tell of sub rosa, isolated people and events that nonetheless braid a "common secret" of wild luck and cruel fate, dense fear and brittle trust. Together they evoke the claustrophobic atmosphere of a criminalized subculture.

However, the secret of abortion is not just *one* kind of secret; instead, different kinds of secrecy percolate around its conduct. A contrast with the confessional disclosure of secrets such as those just mentioned makes this clear. When Foucault discussed sexual secrecy, he was arguing that eroticism was not consigned to a shadow existence. He used an anonymous, eleven-volume Victorian sex diary, *My Secret Life*, and the story of a "simple-minded" laborer, Jouy, near the village of Lapcourt in 1867, as the extremes of the modern injunction to expose the secrets of sex. The former is a catalog of the author's every sexual pleasure down to the most trifling,[58] while the latter is a medico-legal case in which a mentally challenged man was subject to anatomical analysis for signs of degeneracy after he encouraged a young girl to arouse him.[59] Compare these stories with Caroline's, just mentioned. They are crucially alike and different. All are stories of a person caught in a system of power intent on normalizing his or her conduct. The secrets of the autosexnographer, the unconvicted sex criminal, and the postabortion college student share the same horizon of the private subject.[60] The key difference is that abortion is not about sex qua sex.

The general project of abortion control requires secrets of a different sort; confessions alone will not do. Make no mistake; regulation of abortion directly affects reproductive sex and talk about sex. Through abortion, women's sexual conduct has been subject to severe scrutiny, judgment, and punishment.[61] But in itself, the story of a woman who survived a botched abortion is not the same as stories of inspection, by self or other, of sexual behavior. Caroline's story is grounded in the physiological dimensions of a terminated pregnancy and the network of people involved. It includes secrets about what happened to her body, not just about her erotic life, and about how bodies like hers were treated within the community. The medico-political problems posed by the fruits of sex are not reducible to the sort of sex that bore fruit. In addition to secrets of the private subject, secrets of *body* and of the *population* have been indispensable to the governance of abortion. Accordingly, when abortion was a crime, it was never a sex crime. Interestingly, when the American Law Institute, founded in 1923, undertook its first attempt in the 1950s to produce a model penal code for the United States, it classified abortion as a crime against the family.[62] It is customary to read Foucault's concept of biopower in terms of either sexuality or life politics, but as Penelope Deutscher notes, they are overlapping aspects whose conjunctures become readily apparent around issues of reproductive sex and its control.[63]

These other horizons of secrecy immediately seized the attention of medicine as reproductive control emerged a biopolitical problem in modernity. Foucault wrote, "It was necessary to analyze the birth rate, the age of marriage, the legitimate and illegitimate births, the precocity and frequency of sexual relations, the ways of making them fertile or sterile, the effect of unmarried life or of the prohibitions, the impact of contraceptive practices—of those notorious 'deadly secrets' which demographers on the eve of the Revolution knew were already familiar to the inhabitants of the countryside."[64] He could just as well be elaborating on Malthus's prospectus for political economic histories hinted at in the *Essay on the Principle of Population*. The furtive nod to abortion, one of those "deadly secrets," is ironically Victorian; nonetheless, even as Foucault evocatively claimed that the social body's blood was its sex, he recounted a dark labyrinth of secrets not fully explained by confessions of eroticism. In his lectures, he went further, noting the centrality of problems such as public hygiene, grain transportation, and social insurance for governance organized through biopower. Researches on governmentality have since radically expanded our understanding of the kinds of somatic and communal secrets that captivate efforts to know life so as to manage life.[65] Foucault's initial interest in the confession was narrower than the range of secrets the exercise of biopower encompasses and demands. For medicine, *secrets of the body* refers to the biological dynamics to be deciphered in order to determine how human life is born, lives, and dies. *Secrets of the population* refers to the socioeconomic conditions and cultural patterns that enhance or depress individual and communal life.

These other horizons offer different prospects for creating recursive capacity by virtue of the kind of secret that must be disclosed. Jodi Dean observes that a "secret designates that which is desired to be known, that which impels its own discovery but which hasn't yet been disclosed."[66] Secrets direct curiosity and practices of inquiry by virtue of being on the wrong side of knowledge. Secrecy is a matter of position, not content. Simmel recognized as much and posited a certain quantum of secrecy required by sociality: "The secret is a form which constantly receives and releases contents: what originally was manifest becomes secret, and what once was hidden later sheds its concealment. One could, therefore, entertain the paradoxical idea that under otherwise identical circumstances, human collective life requires a certain measure of secrecy which merely changes its topics: while leaving one of them, social life seizes upon another, and in all this alternation it preserves an unchanged quantity of secrecy."[67] Secrecy is ever full of secrets. Abortion's "open secret" is marked by specific varieties of endless revelation. As such, the practice of abortion became a discrete "second world" for physicians that impelled incessant disclosure—who aborts, how often, by whose hand, and to what effect—in order to determine how that practice morbidly shaped (and was shaped by) the manifest world so as to control its practice.

These endless revelations are, on the one hand, what institutional and professional policies are made of. On the other hand, they are what situate the present irrespective of the politics of those policies. As Edwin Black noted, remembering and forgetting are synonymous with the "disclosing and secreting of past events."[68] Disclosure and secrecy are necessarily figurations of remembering and forgetting:

- *Secrets of the private subject* require recursive acts of confession such that individuals are made to remember themselves under the judgment and evaluation of different kinds of authorities.[69] The past is contracted into the present through repeated recollections of individuals to confessors (e.g., clerical, judicial, or medical). This kind of memory work produces autobiographical and biographical senses of the present such as in patient case histories. Physicians might see contemporary women as estranged from the expectation of maternity because mothers like a Mrs. N. or R. state that they have abortions to limit their family size. We think of these recollections as *personal memories*, but to pronatalists they are simultaneously statements of individual women *forgetting* their duty.
- *Secrets of the body* require recursive contact between bodies and body "critics" (e.g., medical, scientific, and artistic interpreters of the body).[70] The sense of the present produced in this manner is felt as a bodily event "confessed" by the body itself. The relaxed, gravid uterus is liable to tear when probed or curetted, for instance; antiabortionists took this fact as a reminder that the womb was never intended to undergo such manipulations. The resulting harm can operate as an impersonal, *biotic memory* of reproductive purpose, but it can simultaneously demonstrate *moral amnesia*.
- *Secrets of the population* require the recursive aggregation of behaviors and events across large numbers of people. The present is felt as an average or an abnormal moment in a distribution, as "confessed" by the numbers. The

Planned Parenthood conference in 1955 produced a statistical analysis of criminal abortion frequency that dominated discussion until the late 1960s. The resulting frequency supported a *statistical memory* of culture and society, but it also produced an *amalgamated forgetting* of specific people and moments that renders abortion numerically faceless.

These different modes of figuration operate in integrated ways. As Deutscher argues, a "procreative hinge" links the body, personally and somatically, with the population in regimes of biopower.[71] One way that procreation has integrated body and population is through the tireless excavation of secrets about abortion. For instance, a patient's case history will include a record of her testimony about what has happened to her and what she has done. But it will also include detailed descriptions of her body, which tell the caregiver about her condition. And, as medicine developed, both the personal and biotic memories of her situation were increasingly mediated by a statistical analysis of likely causes and consequences. In this genealogy, however, my intent is not to "read" specific U.S. medical texts for the manner in which each juggles these different figurations of mnesis. It is to see how the different figurations derived from and adapted to changing material conditions surrounding the provision and treatment of abortion. Those shifting arrangements were critical to substantiating terminated pregnancies as a sign of pathology and, hence, were critical to the ability to fight through over abortion about how we ought to live.

Calling the private subject, the body, and the population "horizons" of secrecy emphasizes that there are no finite blocks of knowledge waiting to be disinterred. Consistent with the view that remembering and forgetting are an unending process, these kinds of secrets are treated as lures—"that which is desired to be known"—that draw intense scrutiny.[72] People's words, their bodies, and their collective actions became footholds in the unknown that promised continued disclosure. A cloud of activity formed around these horizons as practices of inquiry, dedicated to the disenchantment of abortion's secrets, channeled potentially chaotic and disparate events into specific flows of memory and forgetting.[73] Dean describes this relationship, whereby modes of inquiry ceaselessly unveil cryptic knowledge, as a "matrix" of publicity and secrecy. The unearthing of secrets does not drain the matrix of force—there is no last secret to tell. Rather, the matrix is self-constituting: "All the facts can never be known; the very process of searching for them generates new ones."[74] In the case of abortion, its practice was seen as a hidden danger that commanded ongoing revelation; it thus functioned as a *perpetually* open secret, making disclosure ad infinitum the basic form of recursion.

Medical abortion rhetoric exemplifies the broader point that processes of remembering and forgetting are embedded in biopolitical fixations on life's secrets.[75] The forms of knowledge that authorize biopolitical projects generate extraordinary amounts of data necessary for regulation to find purchase. The secrets of populations' bodies and conduct are unveiled, organized, and publicized, often exceeding, even frustrating, the needs of governance by creating a deluge of conflicted, ambiguous information.[76] Data on abortion pre-*Roe* were always contested and unclear on key points, for instance. However, the distinction of abortion rhetoric was the manner in which it drew from a bottomless well of dangerous secrets.

Identifying Mnesis Enacted

It is a crucial if simple fact that women seek abortions for a great many reasons and have been injured or killed because of abortions gone awry in equally diverse ways. Only by recurrence to morbidity does the present become a place inflected by pathological risk taking. The corresponding questions—why women abort and what abortion procedures, whether successful or bungled, do to bodies— are the major features through which the secrets of abortion materialize in discourse. The following chapters consider the manner in which abortion-related suffering was mobilized into a general memory of secret afflictions enervating the communal body. And, moreover, how the materialization of hidden pathogenic forces provided anti- and neo-Malthusians with a spatial and temporal location from which to orient biopolitical struggles about better and worse forms of life. Or, how was trauma from abortion "*loaded* into discourse" such that the where and the when of civilization became tangible?[77]

The analytical issue, then, is to recognize the ways in which the United States' historical moment could be staked by, for example, the severe headaches, violent abdominal pains, and gastrointestinal burning of a woman in the 1870s dying from an overdose of savine oil (from *Juniperus sabina*)?[78] How is this hypothetical case of a piece with Mrs. R., who in the 1890s was separated from her husband and living with a physician? She became pregnant, he punctured her uterus while attempting an abortion that was never completed, and she developed septic peritonitis (infected inflammation of the abdominal lining).[79] What links their circumstances together with the many women in the mid-twentieth century who mistakenly believed potassium permanganate tablets, applied to the cervix, would lead to abortion? The pills chemically burn a crater, causing bleeding and scarring, and only very occasionally excite expulsion of the embryo.[80] Furthermore, how did these diverse situations fall into a menu of causative conditions such as order of pregnancy, fetal development, infection, age of the mother, and extrinsic factors such as personal trauma or socioeconomics?[81]

My analysis hovers between the practices and care of induced abortion and what medical experts said about it, inspecting the *tropes* that organize a flow of memory and amnesia from a succession of impaired and ruined bodies. Because as Olick notes, the figuration of mnesis is material (arising from medical practice in this case), I read the *figures within practice* that allowed recurrent morbid events to become a way of inhabiting the memory of civilization. I understand figures to be embodied by the tropes inherent to messy articulations of human-nonhuman engagements. Such an analysis assumes that the "world of meaning and the world of being are one and the same world, that of translation, substitution, delegation, passing," as Latour put it.[82] Tropes are typically thought of as stylistic devices, but they are fundamentally relationships—metaphors are substitutions, for example. Synecdoches are part-to-whole relationships; amplifying tropes are extensions and intensifications. In the history of rhetoric, the great forest of tropes that have been identified (literally hundreds) principally map relations in the arrangements of words, but also of images, sounds, and gestures; nothing prevents tropological analysis of medical knowledge practices.[83] When physicians touch, listen to, and look at bodies, and when the structures, processes, and entities of and in those bodies act with "trajectories, propensities, or tendencies of their own,"[84] they enact tropological relations *together*, relations such as inversions (turning the body inside out) or interruptions (interposing foreign material into gestational development).[85]

Attention to collectively embodied tropes operationalizes the concept-metaphor of *folding* discussed earlier. These tropological relationships *"allow nonhumans to participate in the discussions of humans"* because without the damaged bodies of women as reminders, and all the many ways that women fell in harm's way when ending pregnancy, the memory work could not begin.[86] There would be nothing to recur to, no curve toward or away from the past within abortion rhetoric, without the material factors that incited risk taking and threatened vitality. Hence, the tropes I look for fall between Mrs. R.'s body, the circumstances that made abortion thinkable for her, the tool that perforated her, and the physician who determined how she died.

My purpose is not, however, to produce an endless ledger of minute figurative turns in case after case, to catalog every fold among folds, but to attend to recursive regularities. A genealogy of what I call mnesis studies the descent of modes of performative interaction with the past, looking for when those modes emerge within struggles over *how* to discourse.[87] In the case of morbidity from interrupted pregnancy, the struggle was over *which* secrets of our collective life were disclosed and how we measured our progress by them, not *if* such secrets were disclosed. As Georges Canguilhem observed, one is healthy or not "relative to the fluctuations in his [sic] environment," which means that undesirable changes in an organism are precipitated by changed relationships between that organism and the pathogenic agents in its milieu.[88] That abortion implicated the broad environment of the national body was never in question. As such, I attend to paradigmatic tropes of biotic and statistical memory work, noting the similarities and differences by which anti- and neo-Malthusian discourse folded the past into the present and the ways that discourse on therapeutic abortion drew from and accentuated the recursive dynamics found in discourse on illegal abortion. This way I am able to describe the manner by which loss of life and suffering associated with abortion *inflected* the course of civilization within medical rhetoric, *positioned* present-day life as endemically afflicted, and *included* the passage of civilization's progress within the fate of women secretly taking steps to limit their fertility.

Part 2

3

"White Man's Plague" | Anti-Malthusian Memory Work at the Fin de Siècle

The history of the world is a series of consecutive repetitions. In the early days of the people fertility is characteristic. As the type of civilization becomes more cultured, and as wealth increases, we find this characteristic to decrease. . . . Any civilization tending contrary to the laws of nature is an infamous one.

—Editorial, *Colorado Medical Journal*, 1903

From the 1880s through the first decade of the twentieth century, U.S. medical rhetoric on abortion enacted a spare, unimaginative declension of the previous generation's rhetoric that nonetheless is invaluable for understanding anti-Malthusianism. Faced with the failure of law to curtail abortion, this generation of physicians clung to increasingly worn tropes, reusing existing modalities rather than cultivating new ones. Where the discourse lacked much of the originality and innovation on display in early crusaders' polemics, the historical value of the moment lay in the fact that recursive patterns set in the first days of public opposition to abortion did not weaken. Increasingly threadbare writings exposed a resilient dynamic of remembering and forgetting that empowered biopolitical critique.[1] This chapter begins the analysis of how major discourses within U.S. medical rhetoric operationalized abortion's dangers as a means to situate the nation as at risk and uncivilized.

As far as the textual corpus is concerned, antiabortion writing of this period was unusually dispersed, lacking grand works or a canon for minor texts to imitate, except for the occasional reference to an archetypal broadside from the earlier anti-Malthusians.[2] Articles, textbooks, and monographs operated on the same level of significance, actualizing a rhetoric as compulsive as it was exhausted.[3] In any given year a handful to a dozen or so articles on abortion might be published, among them case reports, sociocultural commentaries, medicolegal assessments, and the occasional moral tract from a theologian. Also published were special journal forums devoted to abortion, such as in the *Colorado*

Medical Journal and Western Medical and Surgical Gazette in 1903, the *Illinois Medical Journal* in 1905, and *Northwest Medicine* in 1907. But no monograph-length texts devoted to criminal abortion had been written since 1870, although T. Gaillard Thomas, a well-known New York obstetrician, did publish a set of lectures on abortion generally in 1896 that included some discussion of criminal abortion.[4] Gynecological textbooks typically contained a few pages on abortion, maybe something about criminal abortion;[5] marital advice books might contain a section. It is important to stress that these texts are understood as evidence of practices, not only as rhetorical acts themselves. The practices of abortion, what led to the choice to abort, the factors that contributed to a procedure's risks, and the relations between these and medical knowledge are critical to the rhetorical dynamic in question.

Regarding the act of interrupting pregnancy and its consequences, abortion remained a sign of cultural pathology, equally a threat to and an index of modernity, which could risk the very existence of, if not species life, then at least white Christian life. That women seemed no longer to know about maternal duty was evident in the morbidity of abortion; progress had induced amnesia regarding natural and divine law. The new, modern regime of reproduction—the Malthusian couple of the white privileged classes that favored smaller families—courted the death of those very classes. Concerned physicians set themselves to building immunity to such amnesia within women themselves, not just to improving treatment of abortion. Although many remedies were bandied about, the most fundamental and consistently forwarded was to teach women the laws of nature that governed their own and unborn bodies. It was exactly this emphasis on a biotic memory of reproductive physiology that makes fin de siècle anti-Malthusianism so disclosive about abortion rhetoric. The *physiology* of harm to women and the unborn became the impingement that signaled a diseased turning point in civilization, promoted above a position of general significance to a nidus that enveloped the unfolding sickness of the world. Physiology was also the remedy for the amnesiac, nonprocreative ways among the more civilized classes.

Inflection: Morbidity as a Sign of Pathological Amnesia

Physicians of the era were nearly uniform in insisting that abortion was in defiance of nature and certain to bring misfortune and possibly social collapse. Taken collectively, the sequelae from procedures constituted an inflection point that demonstrated the dangerous conjuncture of changes in how people lived, connecting events to one another within a framework of risk. The act itself of ending pregnancy embodied a trope of deviant interruption. *Interruptio* (or *aposiopesis* in the Greek) is to become silent, to break off an address midstream from an inability to continue. Anti-Malthusians derived an embattled sense of place from Progress silencing Nature. The morbidity of abortion was more than clinical; it was a morbidly perverse corruption within ways of living of the very purpose in living. Biopolitical criticism of modern women and their families could be leveraged *through* abortion's morbidity because multiplication of the act demonstrated the "slow death" of a people so confused by new moralities and exigencies that they believed halting pregnancy could improve life.[6]

In 1903, W. J. Fernald, a member of the Champaign County Medical Society of Illinois, published one of the most fully elaborated versions of abortion as the interruption of the natural-social order, "A Sociological View of Criminal Abortion." Fernald, like his peers, placed the heteronormative family at the center of human history: "The unit upon which society and the state is based is the family. All sociological and political structures designed or evolved for the advantage of the individual have this unit for their base. And the evolution of these structures from savagery to civilization has been coincidental with the evolution of the family." Societies evolved through "promiscuity of intercourse, polyandry, polygamy to monogamy," and the morality of governments mirrored this evolution. Thus, sex both held the promise of, and was a threat to, everything. "As the foundation of the state is found in the family, so the foundation of the family exists in the biological structure of the race." Marriage as a religious institution had purified and disciplined the sexual instinct, "animal passion," to conform to natural law, which, as it happened, mandated a sexually complementary, highly fecund, nuclear family. The proof lay in the "startling fact . . . that Nature by the inviolable constitution of things is just even to death; that the judgment is not postponed but is written here and now in the constitutions of him [*sic*] who violates the law."[7] The physical punishments Nature visited on its scofflaws reminded us of reproductive truth. Thus, the risk posed to civilization was its corruption in modernity by the doctrine of Voluntary Motherhood.[8] "The real social disease then, being the desire for small families . . . we may expect to see its diabolical effects in the individual, the family, society, and the state."[9]

Fernald's essay is a thick tangle of Spencerian Darwinism, moral physiology, and biopolitical hyperbole. Fernald patched together a wide assortment of coarse materials used variously by his contemporaries to fashion their own jeremiads against abortion. Many observers shared the belief that birth control and abortion were variations of the same disease of wanting fewer children,[10] but the sheer act of abortion indicated a more acute, endemic pathology. It betrayed a moral cancer, an abomination, a poison.[11] Doctors agreed almost without exception that the etiology of this disease, abortion specifically, was traceable to ignorance, willful or innocent, of physiological law, that biological structure upon which, for Fernald, society is founded. Abortion indicated the presence of a cultivated forgetfulness about the female body's purpose. Mary Dixon-Jones's 1894 turn at explaining abortion's cause is typical: "Girls are ignorant and uneducated, and thousands are led into evil and every-day violation of the most ordinary laws of health as well as of morality, for want of knowledge, or because they have not been properly trained and instructed."[12] Observers had repeated for decades that this ignorance afflicted not just the laboring classes or immigrants but, more perversely ironic in their eyes, also the educated or "better classes."[13] Women were not unlike the slave in Plato's *Meno*, unable to recognize simple truths buried within themselves but in possession of truth if only guided to it. So commonly was the ignorant girl or woman invoked that she became an embodied grammar, in Kenneth Burke's sense of *grammar*, for the literature well into the twentieth century. She was simultaneously the scene of a crime, the agency by which civilization advanced, and the agent toward which acts of reform should be directed; her reproductive purpose was a moral good unto itself.[14]

Acts of abortion were ignorance incarnate, caused by desires to maximize income, to preserve one's appearance, to avoid the unpleasantness of birthing, and similar other reasons that led women to take sometimes drastic steps to limit their families. In 1885 H. C. Ghent took the unusual step of surveying his peers in the Texas State Medical Association in writing, asking why women were having abortions. In addition to the aforementioned reasons, the responses included associating with foreigners such as the French, lack of space, pleasure seeking, selfishness, shame, greed, and many more.[15] The list of justifications, whether posited by physicians or given to them by would-be aborters, numbered in the "dozens," but these reasons counted only as a "category of excuses" for a wrong act (similar to Edwin Hale's list in *The Great Crime of the Nineteenth Century*).[16] These reasons were abetted by advertisements and word of mouth that told women it was all right to abort, that it was normal.[17] Ernest Crutcher's 1903 dictum, "Babies are not fashionable," epitomized anti-Malthusian writers' contempt for limited childbearing. "Besides," Crutcher remarked, "it is easy to find a Pharisaic physician who, for a consideration, will rid the gravid womb of its inmate," even on the northern Great Plains where he practiced.[18] Whatever the professed justification, the underlying cause of abortion was regarded as a "great," "utter," "thoughtless" ignorance of natural law.[19]

The "ignorant woman" shifted focus from the interruption of pregnancy to the interruption of maternity exemplified by the bourgeois matron and later the New Woman. The bourgeois matron of the later nineteenth century rejected the pronatal ideology of antebellum True Womanhood, with its emphasis on submissive and fecund white domesticity, in favor of Voluntary Motherhood; the New Woman of the turn of the century questioned marriage and pregnancy altogether.[20] Both threatened the cult of motherhood that was the crux of the family unit that antiabortionists placed at the core of civilization. Fernald is instructive once more, penning a perfumed ode to maternity:

> That passion which, through marriage, has been sanctified through time by the stainless innocence of babyhood; that passion, the flower of which poet, artist and romancist [sic] have tried in vain through all these years to tell the story of; which has filled the earth with lullabys, [sic]; transformed bare walls into homes and made home a heaven; people it with baby forms more beautiful than seraphs; whose innocent prattle over childhood joys is music sweeter far than the tenderest chords that shall yet be struck by angel hands from golden strings around the great white throne; that passion that has given to language its sweetest word—mother; has transfigured each woman crowned with maternal joy into a real Madonna, kindling in her face a light as radiantly beautiful as the halo that shone round the head of Mary as she bore the Christ child on her enraptured bosom; that passion need no apology from us who mention it, nor from you who listen.[21]

That any woman—bourgeois matron, New Woman, or otherwise—thought she could spurn this ideal proved she was in fact ignorant. There was only one True Woman and women who knew that truth obeyed it. Again the Platonist overtones are powerful. No knowing qualification or rejection of maternity was recognizable to anti-Malthusians, only fraudulent performances of the female sex. For their rhetoric, forgetting was embodied "as an act of misrecognition" by women of their sexual responsibilities.[22] Hence, immunity from abortion and its causes would require women to once again recognize themselves as morally bound, reproductive agents.

The danger of modern women being recklessly unmindful of nature's design was reinforced by the subterfuge that erased their acts from public view. Referring to criminal abortion, New York's E. H. F. Pirkner wrote in 1909, "The enemy is the *habit* of the plurality of American Women, married or not, to interrupt a beginning, or try to interfere with a supposed or dreaded pregnancy, the most dangerous of its allies being the *secrecy* with which that habit is practiced and condoned."[23] Abortion was an anonymous problem because it was kept anonymous, even by those who opposed it. Women and their providers did not talk openly about abortion for a host of reasons, many self-evident. The consequences to the woman were not limited to public scorn. She might lose her family, be subject to abuse, be hiding the evidence of abuse, implicate a friend or loved one, and more still. If a patient was confronted with incontrovertible evidence such as a punctured uterus she might admit to an attempted abortion, but she might not. Regardless, physicians tended to keep patient confidentiality. Sometimes, facing immanent death, a woman might be asked to give a dying declaration, but even then she might not tell her story.[24] Providers or those who made referrals did not tend to out their associates, either, despite calls to expose abortionists among medical societies.

Even among self-titled crusaders, the open secret of abortion remained largely anonymous. Pirkner is a curious case in point. He claimed to have gone undercover for several years, of his own volition and at his own expense, to learn about the "underworld" of abortion. He investigated New York and surrounding states with an assistant who helped him locate abortionists, even hiring detectives at one point. Yet he did not name names. He did not name locations. He did not actually lift the shroud of secrecy he worked so hard to peer beneath. J. Henry Barbat followed a practice similar to Pirkner's, hiring two female detectives in San Francisco to expose abortionists by answering their ads. He noted two examples of abortionists who changed their names to continue advertising, but these were just illustrations. He did not systematically expose providers.[25] In general, reformers aided the public in keeping the secret of abortion from itself—an extraordinary exercise in ad hoc, collective, purposeful forgetting.[26]

Unlike diseases such as polio or muscular dystrophy, whose pathologies are, respectively, infectious and hereditary, the pathology indexed by induced abortion was amnestic. The disease of wanting small families did not harm us through bloodstreams or gene mutations, but it did so through failed memory, a moral disease spread by forgotten knowledge, by lethe. Thus, physicians' indictment of the Malthusian couple's abortion habit alleged two forms of amnesia, bound together in a dangerous disregard for nature's law: the ignorance of women, confused by materialistic society, who could not recall the truth of maternal destiny inhabiting their very bodies, and the strategic forgetfulness of women and their attendants, dedicated to avoiding detection, who conducted abortions in anonymity. The former amnesia was of a subject estranged from self-knowledge, the latter of a public deprived of self-knowledge. Forgotten secrets of the body and carefully hidden secrets of the private subject complemented each other in aiding the spread of modernity's corruption. As a symptom of life gone wrong, abortion was the "language of action," an expression "in its manifest state" of a sick desire to reduce fertility.[27]

However, medical observers saw in abortion not just a symptom but also a sign of the totality of Malthusian lethe. Where each case of abortion and its specificities was symptomatic of interrupting the nature of one life, physicians perceived in abortion the full measure of the civilized pathology to ignore procreative laws, the gesture of a dying society. Physicians turned "symptoms into memories" of forgetting, ironically making Malthusian lethe memorable. Wounds and deaths made the sweeping loss of moral physiological knowledge palpable to anti-Malthusians, and it was as the embodiment of a disappearing society that abortion became, for them, a sign of pathological amnesia.[28] As Foucault remarked of pre-clinical medical perception, "The sign is the symptom itself, but in its original truth." Reminiscent of pre-clinical, eighteenth-century modes of perception, medical observers combined the principle that symptoms are embodied *signs* of pathology with the notion of a *social* pathology. This afforded them "the possibility of an exhaustive, clear, and complete reading" of the order of disease as the order of society. An open-ended signaling relationship between the female body and society enabled physicians to modulate between the past and the present by virtue of the widespread incidence of interrupted pregnancies, providing awareness of the contemporary moment as being in flux from a healthier time to an afflicted one. Such a reading was not only "devoted to totality and to memory" but "calculating as well," thereby substantiating biopolitical critiques of fertility control through the estimation of danger.[29] This flexible sign logic turned birth control of the last resort into the inflection point that powered anti-Malthusians' "argument for social reform."[30]

Given that the signaling ability of abortion was necessarily tethered to its danger, the level of hazard that abortion indexed was critical to the scope of critiques afforded by it. To many observers of the time, abortion's danger was unrivaled; the very occurrence of the practice impeded a reproductive regime and the norms that justified it. In its mildest form, abortion was a public health threat, far more serious than but still a cognate of other biopolitical issues associated with urbanized and industrialized nations, as Washington, D.C., practitioner Joseph Taber Johnson explained in 1896 in the pages of the *American Journal of Obstetrics*: "Questions of drainage, sewerage, quarantine, vaccination, antiseptics are all important in the preventions of disease," yet "more lives are annually sacrificed by the unnecessary and intentional destruction of the human fetus than are saved by all the above mentioned agencies combined." However, the full potency of the threat was imagined through the phantasm of race suicide brought on by lost fetal and maternal life. Johnson continued, "Vital statistics might be quoted to show that in the true American stock in some parts of our country the ratio of deaths over the births has steadily increased. The published number of maternal deaths from this malpractice does not appear to be decreasing."[31] He succinctly located abortion as a problem for biopower, as a hygienic threat to the security of the nation akin to other disease vectors. Thus, halting the danger would require strategic intervention into the circulation of its causes, just as the flow of "germs" and sewage needed to be governed.[32]

Others' warnings were more melodramatic. "We are here confronted with another 'white man's plague,'" cautioned Pirkner, "as sad and of as tremendous proportions and importance as were the ravages of tuberculosis until only twenty years ago."[33] One observer claimed that "countless millions of human lives" had been lost.[34] Yet another wrote of "a holocaust—a great army of little children are destroyed."[35] Amid waves of new immigrants and a surging white nationalism, turn-of-the-century physicians turned to immigration to specify the risk of lost "native" fecundity.[36] For example, Walter B. Dorsett, then chair of the American Medical Association, asked in a 1908 address to the obstetrical-gynecological division, "With feticide among our best element, and with a constant increasing influx of degenerates from foreign countries, what can be expected of us as a nation a few generations hence?"[37] The more significant reference, however, was France's much-noted drop in its birthrate. Since before H. R. Storer made a scandal of it, physicians had pointed across the Atlantic, where reports of a precipitous drop in the ratio of births to deaths confirmed the dangers of Voluntary Motherhood.[38] A study claiming a doubling or tripling of abortion rates in Paris between 1897 and 1905[39] only cemented France's place as Exhibit A in the case against the Malthusian couple; France was expiring. "It is up to the physician not only by example, but by precept, to stem the tide, or the extinction of this great American race is as near as that of France."[40]

If birth control was a sign of collective suicide, abortion was the more obscene sign of murder-suicide.

Turning against the self by interrupting pregnancy meant turning back in time. As one physician noted, the slope to barbarism for America's privileged was slippery and steep: "The more highly civilized the people become, the more [abortion] is resorted to; consequently the better class of people ceased to produce; consequently the lower element will take possession of government, and consequently government falls."[41] And although most medical commentators were worried only over the fate of the white Anglo bourgeoisie, some were more ecumenical. Sigmund Zeisler, for instance, took *race suicide* in the most expansive way, voicing sadness at the thought of "the total annihilation of the human race."[42] Despite the odd comment like Zeisler's, the threat of abortion was relative to national health, seizing on hygienic insecurity from abortion as a racial disease that society must be defended from, not in the sense of fighting racial others but as fortifying white Christian Anglos against moral degeneration.[43] Anti-Malthusians desired what Roberto Esposito described as "religious immunization," which involves, "on the one hand, leading the community back into the organic form of the body; and on the other, normatively subjugating it to transcendental principle in order to guarantee its survival in time."[44]

However, physicians were undecided on whether the ubiquity of abortion meant the nation's turn against nature was from being too civilized or not civilized enough, a difference that reflects the contradiction between state laws and abortion's prevalence. That abortion was criminal and everywhere decried was presumably the measure of enlightened times; and yet the practice was extremely common. Writing from Louisville, Frank Green encapsulated the paradox in his essay "Feticide": "Human life is the most sacred thing in the world. So deeply is this fact grounded in our very being or nature that all civilized nations have enacted stringent laws protecting human life, and prescribing severe punishments for those who destroy it.... All the thus far obtainable [evidences] suggest the inevitable tendency of modern ultra-civilization toward gradual race extinction through intentional abortion."[45] Human life is consecrated by nature's very being, yet even as civilized nations act on nature to protect life, their inevitable tendency is to gradually kill themselves. This contradiction produced two contrasting theses on civilization's pathology—either abortion was unique to civilization or it was a sign that civilization was regressing to barbarism—which converged on the same conclusion: the United States, even modernity itself, was engaged in slow motion self-destruction.

The less common thesis was that abortion was unique to civilization. E. F. Fish wrote that abortion "travels hand in hand with civilization. One never hears of it among the savages, the barbarian, and semi-civilized races. One never hears of it among the densely ignorant peoples. It finds its hot bed in America, the United States, with its private and public school system, universities and medical colleges."[46] A backhanded compliment to "savages," to be sure; modern custom had placed Americans so far from nature that even the rude and untamed knew better.

More commonly, abortion was seen as a return to a brutality that supposedly had been transcended as modernity regressed to a primitive state. The regression thesis held that a gradual ethical movement toward human life as sacred defined civilization, such that protection of the unborn became a principal indicator of national health. Denver physician Edmund J. A. Rogers provided a concise précis of this view: "Abortion has been common among almost all uncivilized and semi-civilized people of whose custom we have any record. It is only with the advance of civilization that the idea of the sanctity of human life comes to be grasped and appreciated. Indeed, the standard of any people's civilization may be judged by the degree in which they recognize the right of each individual to life, liberty and happiness."[47] The end of the nineteenth century was a special moment in global history when, at last, the true value of human life was being recognized, or as fellow Coloradan Minnie C. T. Love said, when "science demonstrated, social economics demanded, and religion exhorted" that life began at conception, and nations did away with "any distinction in the matter of the period of gestation."[48] How in the moment of moral triumph could abortion become so widespread?

The answer accepted both sides of the paradox as true; the United States was both ultra- *and* undercivilized. On the one hand, civilization brought with it enlightenment, which allowed the full truth of nature to be visible as never before; on the other hand, it cultivated wanton ignorance of nature among the materialistic classes, who sought to avoid natural law in order to reinforce their privileges. At the very hour of history that the truth of reproduction could be known not just morally but also scientifically, the most important audience was not listening. In an address to the Nebraska State Medical Association in 1904, William B. Ely explained that regression was a function of selfishness born of privilege: "The ethic of egoism is retrogressive; it is destructive to the moral development of society. The tendency of such a code is to carry the individual backward toward the primitive savage state."[49]

Isolating perpetual, hidden threats is requisite in the medicalized rhetorics of biopolitics,[50] but the consequences exceed the development of law and policy to meet the perils uncovered. That abortion reduced overall fertility was menacing to white medical experts and spurred enthusiasm for criminalization. But beyond that, for rhetoric critical of changes in society, abortion materialized a loss of traditional mores. As Canguilhem explained, disease is a different, erroneous way of life. It matters not just *what* this symptomatic morbidity signaled but also that it *could* signal. For anti-Malthusians, the interruption of maternity heralded societal afflictions such that its occurrence folded different societies together in comparative, regressive decline, such as in the United States and France falling backward into primitivism and death.

Position: The Visibility of Natural Law

Given that abortion was a barometer for a disease of failed moral physiological memory, the therapy proposed was to institute a different anamnestic system, "memory being precisely what enables one to pass from ignorance to non-ignorance," as Foucault observed.[51] Remembered by the consequences of pathogenic ignorance, biotic memory is an antibody that produces immunity.[52] Biotic memory as a source of protection is consistent with progress-as-pathology rhetoric, which assumes the more true to nature, the better; thus, the truth of nature (as revealed by its corruption) holds the key to treatment.[53] Accordingly, physicians argued that exposing the secrets of the body was the only remedy for combating a social disease whose secreted expression demonstrated that the public, women especially, had lost the ability to care for themselves.[54] Doing so, physicians made the iniquity of abortion a source of revitalization for morality; in Esposito's terms, they fashioned "the positive *of* a negative" by enlisting abortion's morbidity as the antigen to activate an "antibody that protects the Christian body from what threatens it."[55] The cure was to acquaint women with the laws of reproduction made visible *by their violation.*

In any case, nothing else seemed to be working. Institutions of law, religion, and medicine had been wholly ineffective in bringing privileged American women back to their proper place at the foundation of civilization for anti-Malthusians. N. E. H. Hull and Peter Charles Hoffer argue that after 1870 prosecutions and convictions were common,[56] but medico-legal commentators of the time noted with increasing pique the confusing futility of state law. They remarked that abortion laws were hard to adjudicate because their language was poorly drafted, witnesses would not testify, juries tended not to convict, and judges often suspended sentences. Even a dying declaration was no guarantee of a conviction. The law was essentially a "dead letter" for them.[57] Religion had also proved unsatisfactory, as the pastoral power of churches was neither effective nor much evident to physicians. Antiabortion doctors asked where the church was and wrote of themselves as needing to act as clergy.[58] Worst of all, the profession on the whole was unmoved or simply afraid to break confidence with patients or colleagues about abortion.

The emphasis on remembering what the body teaches us elevated the human toll from abortion from an inflection point to a normalized manner of positioning the present as a moment of high risk. It paired an outflowing of knowledge and life with a regularized mode of recovery. Essentially, antiabortion physicians took the opportunity to do more than punctuate the passage of time by noting the relative commonality of abortion. They used abortion as a sick turn in civilized life to position a politics of life *against* the present. They tied critiques of the emergent small family to a deluge of harmed bodies, such that revisiting the harm was fundamentally generative of their discourse. A return to the broken body, an inspection of the forms of breakage, was requisite in talking about abortion. Physicians had recognized the rhetorical capacity presaged by Nathan Allen's internalized, corporeal political economy as medical rhetoric came to depend overwhelmingly on the gruesome aspects of abortion. They needed the body's participation in extremis to demonstrate what Nature itself wanted life to be.

Return to the Broken Body

After Allen inverted Malthus's principle of population from social to physiological law in 1870, statistical thinking largely faded from the literature.[59] Despite H. R. Storer's influential use of vital statistics a decade before, the unreliability of data contributed to physiology's becoming the key site of memory work.[60] As T. Gaillard Thomas noted, "Statistics showing the frequency of criminal abortion never have been, and never will be written, for the crime creeps stealthily beneath the scrutiny of society."[61] The lack of reliable data was a direct consequence of the collective, strategic amnesia that protected the underground. The incentive was to misrepresent and it showed in the variability of the data. In 1881 the Michigan Board of Health commissioned a nationwide study, which contended that approximately one hundred thousand abortions were criminally induced per year with at least six thousand deaths resulting.[62] Also available were some city estimates, depending largely on extrapolations from hospital data. For instance, New York was estimated at eighty thousand criminal abortions per year with six thousand deaths at minimum, and Chicago at six thousand to ten thousand abortions per year, but the estimates were inconsistent across studies.[63] One cannot reconcile the turn-of-the-century New York City estimate with Michigan's national estimate from 1881, for instance, or the incredible discrepancy between New York and Chicago, given that Chicago's 1900 population was 1.7 million and New York's was a little over 2 million.[64] Despite efforts to quantify abortion, Frederick Taussig observed that "the only accurate statistics are those obtained through the patient's anamnesis [patient history]. The evidence thus far at hand from [clinics] is very insufficient."[65] Bolstered by experience, patient testimony, and inconsistent but suggestive data, antiabortionists nevertheless were satisfied that the danger was great, given declining white fertility rates and unchecked terminations.

If institutions could not or would not numerically bring abortion practice into the light of day so as to cleanse America of its dangerous ignorance, then reacquainting women with the truth of their own bodies was the best (and only) program. In this way, physicians treated "memory as a process through which origins are retrieved," a process that could restore wisdom.[66] Such anamnestic therapy meant identifying flows of biotic memory as well as developing practices that could usefully channel those currents to make Nature's law apparent regarding reproduction. Like earlier antiabortionists, turn-of-the-century doctors contended that physiological laws remembered nature's highest mandate through the consequences to those who defied them. Thomas explained that "the workings of nature in [reproduction], as in all other physiological processes, are too perfect, too accurately and delicately adjusted, not to be interfered with materially by the clumsy and inappropriate measure adopted to frustrate them."[67] C. C. Mapes laid this out simply: "Any violation of Nature's laws must necessarily produce its effect upon the economy."[68] For Dixon-Jones, as for others, this meant, if not death, then the loss of fertility: "To interrupt these processes is a shock—a shock to the whole being, the nutritive, nervous, and mental systems; it does violence to the procreative organs, and renders them incapable of ever as efficiently performing their special functions."[69] This might be the result of sepsis or organ damage, but the outcome was that women who induced, if they did not die, became sterile or at least faced greater risks of spontaneous abortion in the future. At the same time that the flow of the dead and the injured produced by abortion made moral lethe visible it offered the body's wordless anamnesis of truth.

The bodies of women such as Mrs. S. of Chicago, who died early on Monday, July 11, 1904, thus became recursive agents, with each fatality, each poisoning securing the moment that physicians addressed as dangerously stricken by ignorance. A mother of two in her fourth month, she had by her own admission consulted Mrs. A., a midwife, who used a tampon-and-tent method to induce abortion.[70] It was still conventional to anonymize patients by using the initial of their last name. Dr. J. V. Fowler was summoned at 3:00 A.M. on the eighth because Mrs. S. had severe abdominal pain. She developed endometritis, an inflammation of the uterine lining, and a septic embolism in her brain, possibly the result of a blood vessel being blocked by infected tissue from the endometritis. The cerebral infection caused notable muscular and linguistic impairment, not long after which she died. Fowler used standard diagnostic methods, taking her history, pulse, and temperature; employing visual and manual inspection of her body; and taking a bacterial culture. Upon death, her body was submitted to autopsy.

These methods, aspects of the "clinical gaze" Foucault that described in his history of medical perception, worked with Mrs. S.'s body to enable its tissues, fluids, cells, and temperatures to become rhetorically salient. Clinical methods articulated a living memory of purpose through "*sensorial triangulation*" of hearing, touch, and sight. The odor, the pulse rate, the pre- and postmortem condition of her uterus, the colon bacilli from the lab culture, and the embolism from observations of her body became expressions of natural law by her body.[71] However, antiabortionists sought a unifying Providential order in disease, fusing contemporary methods of mapping the body's density with the expectation of a higher purpose for the body. Rudolph Weiner Holmes, a member with Reverend Callaghan of the Committee on Criminal Abortion, appointed by the Chicago Medical Society, reported the case of Mrs. S. as part of that committee's report to the society.[72] Invoking the familiar figure of the ignorant woman, Holmes argued that women like Mrs. S. lacked "proper realization of the heinousness of destroying the unborn child" because of the "nonsensical belief" that the fetus is alive only after it kicks.[73] Nature knew otherwise and said as much through trauma. Before anatomic pathology, the study of disease within organs and tissues that emerged in the eighteenth century, medicine "never ceased to hesitate between a *pathology of phenomena* and a *pathology of cases*."[74] Similarly, fin de siècle antiabortionists generalized from a theo-medical certainty: "That there is a punishment for the guilty is evident from the self-executing laws of nature," as Rev. J. Heiermann put it.[75]

Antiabortionists melded clinical inquiry of divine purpose with a sense of proportional justice derived from Christian moral physiology. "With the advent of Christianity, which imposed more moralized notions of disease," Susan Sontag wrote, "a closer fit between disease and 'victim' evolved. The [ancient] idea of disease as punishment yielded the idea that a disease could be a particularly appropriate punishment."[76] Thus, infertility or death resulting from abortion implied the weighty judgment of Nature holding court on the woman who chose abortion. In 1907, Montgomery Russell described vengeful Nature's expectation of moral obedience:

> Man is not like the tree which, after the growth of hundreds of years, at last falls as a mere log but, as we believe, his physical nature is inseparably correlated with the moral, and while he is yet a dumb and unseen embryo, undergoing a secret growth, he is by degrees being shaped and perfected for the hopes of the loftiest estate of any created thing of which we have knowledge. That this hope should be blighted, and that the precarious life of the defenseless human being should be snapped off by a violent expulsion from its natural place of lodgement [*sic*], is an outrage which disappointed Nature punished by calamities to the mother, both physical and moral, of the most threatening kind.[77]

A cheated Nature gets revenge, and so natural law is evident in its enforcement.

Abortion sequelae were not rigorously delimited within the literature; rather, post facto reasoning ruled such that any negative, postabortal condition could be considered an *intended* consequence of Nature. The law of Nature, remembered by its punishments, folded the past into the present, bringing "now" into contact with "then" by virtue of the character of select people's distress. The meter by which such calamities measured time was simple. As one doctor sanguinely remarked, "Fortunately, nature kills off the woman who shirks motherhood, but, unfortunately, it takes her a generation to do it."[78] Not only was morbidity the body's way to disclose the secrets of life, but expiring bodies joined together set the clock of a moral disease's progression over time. Abortion became a moral antigen *because* it aroused Nature to make itself brutally clear.

Return to the Unborn Body

Although antiabortionists echoed earlier rhetoric by emphasizing harm to women's bodies as the reminder of Natural law, additional emphasis on harm to *fetal* life emerged at this time, auguring what would become the central theme in public pro-life advocacy of the late twentieth century. As Sara Dubow notes in *Ourselves Unborn,* "Antiabortion physicians intensified their efforts to persuade the public that fetal life began at fertilization and to convince women to carry their pregnancies to term."[79] In the 1850s to the 1870s, the loss of unborn life was a significant inflection point for antiabortion memory work but not the primary danger through which medical discourse positioned the present in time. But from the 1880s forward, the threatened embryo increasingly became a site for remembering the truth about ways of life, even though embryology as a field was highly contested. The increasing emphasis on unborn bodies was understood through an undigested composite of theology and cell theory, which gained surpassing status. Antiabortion physicians were unwavering in their theology and in their view that embryology confirmed life at conception; however, where the religious precepts were simple if largely unexplained, the biology was nebulous.[80] The change in medicine was part of what Dubow calls "prenatal culture," which developed around the turn of the twentieth century, wherein the fetus was "a blank slate upon which the mother's feelings, thoughts, and actions inscribe the future of the child, and thus the nation."[81]

With few exceptions, commentators refuted the common law premise of life at quickening with a belief in ensoulment at conception, occasionally claiming a Catholic origin of the doctrine but typically forwarding it as a universal fact of metaphysics devoid of sectarian origin. Scriptural or canonical support almost always was lacking. The largely asserted doctrine of ensoulment functioned as the minor premise to the major, "Thou shalt not kill," to form a religious proof for physicians' critique of culture. There is no better example of how unexplained embryological claims nestled side by side with theology than J. H. Lyons's address as the outgoing president of the Washington State Medical Association in Seattle, in September 1907. Lyons's lecture, "The Moral Qualifications of the Physician," was a call to duty that placed the physician in the role of godly servant who must practice medicine according to higher law.[82] Neither sermon nor scientific paper, it was resolutely an act of professional and cultural critique. He stated, "The physician recognizes a higher law than that of the state, and he directs his course in obedience to his conscience, his duty to society, and his responsibility to his maker. And for this purpose it does not matter whether that conscience be a product of evolution, or a gift fresh from the hand of the Creator; it still remains our highest authority in all matter in the realms of moral ethics." Citing the discretion that state law accorded to physicians to administer abortions, Lyons denounced the lack of moral training for physicians: "There are thousands of innocent lives sacrificed every year, not in wantonness, but in pity, and from the purest though mistaken motives, because the physician does not recognize the application of the higher law which says, 'Thou shalt not kill.'"[83]

In a 1913 article, "Some Moral and Ethical Aspects of Feticide," professor of gynecology E. A. Weiss of the University of Pittsburgh echoed Lyons and encapsulated the mixture of Christian ethics and basic embryology. After noting the decline in religious teaching and the lack of ethical training in medical school, Weiss rejected the Aristotelian doctrine of vitality at quickening: "In this day of advanced thought and enlightenment it should not be necessary to present arguments as to the exact time when the fetus is animated by its own specific principal [sic] of life—its human soul. Modern scientists have demonstrated that from the very moment of conception, the human embryo is animated by the same principal of vitality that animates man."[84] The embryological rationale for ensoulment at conception depended, as it still does for pro-life advocates, on the potential of the zygote. So said Frank Green: "Human life, with all the potentialities of the fully developed human being, begins just as soon as there is a vital union of the male and female generative elements, and the destruction of this life, no matter how lowly the form nor early the stage of development, is just as much the destruction of a human life as it is to kill an infant, a child, or an adult."[85]

Despite such professed certainty, scientific proof based on cell theory was an impressionistic enthymeme in contrast to the plain religious syllogism based on the sixth commandment. After Matthias Schleiden and Theodor Schwann proposed, in 1838 and 1839, respectively, that the cell was the basic unit of life, research gradually demonstrated that conception was the merger of gametes (egg and sperm cells), which then developed into an embryo through mitotic cell division. A number of botanists and zoologists were able to "ultimately resolve the processes of fertilization and cell division" in the late 1870s.[86] However, science certainly had not shown newly conceived zygotes to be invested with a soul of moral equivalence to that of an adult. It was not clear at the time how fertilized ova developed or what the process of development revealed about human nature, with scientists debating whether regions of the ovum were pre-determined to develop into specific organs and systems (preformationism) or whether the first embryonic cells was pluripotent, meaning each cell possessed the "latent potential to produce a complete organism" (epigenesis).[87] Perhaps the greatest debates were about phylogeny recapitulating ontogeny: did the embryo pass through stages of earlier ancestral forms?[88] Moreover, the turn of the century saw descriptive embryology based on detailed inspection of animal specimens give way to experimental embryology.[89]

Any of these debates—and their outcomes were deeply implicated in one another—could have offered grist for arguments contrary to Green or Weiss, had embryologists been interested in the moral status of the human ovum. For example, if under Darwinian embryology, embryos passed through evolutionary stages, could that not offer support for some modernized version of quicken-ing? Embryologists testified in favor of evolution during the Scopes trial, after all.[90] At what point did an embryo reach its human stage? Green's assertion of ensoulment "no matter how lowly the form" seems to admit the need to estab-lish an originary place for the soul within theories of recapitulation, or, turned around, that embryology did not have to presume a divine soul to explain devel-opment.[91] In fact, in her exceptional history *Icons of Life*, Lynn Morgan demon-strates that embryologists did not think of human embryos in terms of souls or the morality of induced abortion.[92]

Most turn-of-the-century U.S. physicians had meager science education, and it is unclear from the literature to what extent a study of embryology by those who did have such education influenced medical opinion on abortion. What is clear is that antiabortionists like Green alluded to cell theory but of-fered no specific arguments derived from it, nor did they acknowledge debates within embryology that might support positions counter to their own. Rather, the authority of science was invoked and this was enough, as Prudence Saur illustrates: "That the embryo is alive and hence quick from the moment of con-ception, modern science has abundantly proven," with no explanation of what exactly constituted that proof.[93] The reason is simple—no secular view of con-ception is apparent among physicians who wrote of it. A soul was *assumed* to enter the body at life's first moment; modern embryology indicated that concep-tion rather than quickening inaugurated an unbroken chain of prenatal devel-opment, so ensoulment must happen at fertilization. Case closed. Science was taken as independent confirmation of theology, but in practice it was only a restatement. Regardless, unborn souls had become significant moral antigens within the rhetoric.

Unfolding Life's Anonymous Memory

The austere quality of the biotic memory enacted by maternal harm and fetal development is worth noting. Wrote one physician, "The primary object of nature in the creation of the sexes is the continuance of the race, and the fulfillment, therefore of a woman's destiny is complete by marriage."[94] The secrets of life unveiled by clinical inspection of damaged female bodies and by embryology acted on the memory of a natural order that required high rates of reproduction. This memory was collective in that it was the same for every conception and every woman. It was anonymous in that it belonged to no one. This was not a memory of unique events, of wars or assassinations or revolutions; it was a memory of an allegedly universal, embodied law. In fact, this memory was indifferent to the peculiarities of events except when the order of nature was defied, in which case punishment followed. Governed by natural law, all women's lives should be essentially the same; more precisely, the past, present, and future of Woman should be the story of all women, and would be if women would only relearn the truth of being Woman. The secrets of life to be remembered held a narrow, unyielding memory of what *ought to be*, not a memory of what *was*.

In addition to the basic inflection of "life interrupting itself," a recursive dynamic within medical practice *secured* physiological harm from abortion as a position for contesting diseased ways of life: direct and postmortem examination channeled streams of biotic memory—brimming with the injuries and infections of women and with unborn lives—to feed the recollection of an anonymous, collective maternal imperative and to remedy a pathological amnesia regarding family and procreation. The recurrence of and recurring to trauma became a touchstone for discourse, yielding to medicine an ability to address the diagnosis and treatment of culture through specific, damaged bodies.[95] Through recursion, physicians fixed a mnestic position for pronatal rhetoric to inhabit.

Barbara Maria Stafford calls practices that unveil corporeal truth *body criticism*: rituals that painstakingly expose and excise the unseen.[96] The tropology is revelatory and in the context of medical abortion rhetoric, body criticism embellishes the basic trope of civilization attacking itself in the womb because physiological revelation attempts to turn a fall into primitivism into a source of protection. Truth is extracted from error, which is of a piece with Georges Canguilhem's observation that normative health proceeds from knowledge of disease and resonant with Esposito's description of immunitary biopolitics. The "immune mechanism functions precisely through the use of what it opposes" by "outflanking and neutralizing" the threat.[97] The antigen is derived from the pathogen. Physicians' body criticism appropriated the pathology of interrupted pregnancies in order to build a "selective memory capable of protecting the system," which it did by discriminating ways of living that did not belong.[98] Those ways that violated natural law were excluded by Nature.

The appropriation of pathology proceeded by *inverting* the invisible to the visible, that is, making the body's interior perceptible, while *converting* morbidity to vitality profaned, turning death into law. Tropically, this is a combination of *chiasmus* and *metonymy*, a structured reversal plus a reductive substitution that not only turns the body inside out, creating a visible parallel to the invisible, but also transforms knowledge *in* the body to knowledge *of* the body in the same motion. A combined trope like this is called *metalepsis* in the Greek, or *transumption*, as Quintilian named it in Latin.[99] It is the means by which tropes that work conjointly, a reversal and substitution in this case, create a passageway from one place to another even though the conceptual distance may seem far. From the interruption of Nature (a woman bleeds to death from an incomplete abortion), we arrive at a moment of crisis in civilization whose remedy lies in the secrets of her body revealed by Nature's anger. The very thing that shows civilization to have stumbled becomes the means of righting itself in the future. As Michel de Certeau remarked, the dynamics of memory afford *"passages into something else* through 'twisted' relations, through successive reversals."[100]

Inclusion: Enveloping History as Pro-life Struggle

The recursive significance of the patient's damaged body and the unborn soul went beyond that of a reminder for a forgotten moral lesson. If the state of abortion was a measure of civilization, as anti-Malthusians had it, then time was punctuated by a series of struggles against forgetting maternity's place in Providence. This imperative to remember the truth of life founded a *"theater* for practical *actions"* around reproductive physiology, and the extent to which a society took appropriate action determined its place on the scale of civilized life.[101] Consequently, treatment for moral amnesia was sited in bringing women to the truth of their bodies, which meant that battle against the enemy within, that malignant spirit, as O'Donnell and Atlee described it in 1871, was to be waged at the level of woman's ethical relation to maternity. Furthermore, woman's relation to her biological self became the envelope of world order, the whole of which could be folded up within her ethicality regarding abortion. Civilizations were intimately related by pragmatic decisions about pregnancy and wars against its willful cessation.

Medical Pastorate and the Advisory Regime

Anti-Malthusians saw medicine's mission as a historic, Christian struggle. The brutality of inept abortion made a biotic memory of reproductive duty apparent, they believed, but how could the gruesome appearance of truth be made effective to decrease the practice?[102] Physicians lacked biopolitical savvy and so they found it difficult to operationalize their preferred leverage point for pressuring wayward women about procreative responsibilities. They were trained to think at the level of the patient's body and did so in moralistic terms, not at the level of the population as a distribution of behaviors and desires. Doctors worked with clients in offices, homes, and hospitals, under a regimen of occasional visits as initiated by the patient. That they did not have constant, direct supervision over their patients made physician-directed disciplinary control impractical. The educational system, despite its structural design assuming girls were future mothers (for those girls fortunate enough to be educated), was not teaching Natural law to girls as physicians imagined it ought or else, so they believed, women would not abort. Maternity homes existed and women were constantly forced to carry to term by a variety of coercive means.[103] Nevertheless, a fail-safe, uniform system of forced parturition did not exist. Anti-Malthusians' legal or regulatory tools to coerce women into childbirth proved blunt.

What remained was to talk to the patient, and in this caregivers' war to defend society from itself, there was really only one battlefield anyway, woman, and one objective: she "must return to the self" with a kind of Christianized, pronatal Stoicism.[104] Ancient Stoicism encouraged, as Foucault put it, that you "'turn your gaze on yourself'" through coming to know the world and your place in it. One form of such early body criticism was the "material analysis of the flesh" in the philosophy of Marcus Aurelius. Individuals were mentored to rigorously ask, "What am I?," pairing "looking and remembering" in order to recall the truth by its evidence in nature, including bodily nature.[105] The self-directed analytics of the Stoics, designed to instantiate a certain ethical relation of self to self, aimed at creating the conditions of freedom through truth, thereby granting the ability to reject "all the false values and all the false dealings in which we are caught up."[106] In a kind of latter-day, scientist Stoicism, anti-Malthusians envisioned themselves as counselors to women, encouraging them to return to the self through knowledge of their flesh. Where Marcus Aurelius advised "penetrating to the heart of things" to gain perspective on the totality of Providence,[107] physicians advised immersion in the womb to see the full order of things both as it is and as it ought to be. Then women might be freed of their false desires to limit fertility. Of course, doctors used a Christian, not a pagan, ethic and vocabulary.

Ethically, Stoics imagined that taking care of the self as they advised would broadly lead to self-finalization; by contrast, the Christian ethic animating anti-Malthusians was directed at self-renunciation. In place of the freedom created by spiritual knowledge of fulfillment, such as Marcus Aurelius might promise, physicians promised that obedience to the demands of Providence would bring a freedom *from* choosing.[108] A classically Stoic ethic would arm a woman through true knowledge of her nature as a living being to make decisions in a world filled with distortions and confusions. She would become the subject of her own life, and specifically of her own reproduction. The evangelical ethic cleaved to by antiabortionists was to remove the woman's agency; she was to sacrifice herself for child and family in accordance with the plan of the divine text pulsing inside her.

Accordingly, antiabortion doctors enunciated their ethic of care of self in the language of *pastoral power* but grounded it in the recursive, material analysis of woman's flesh that they had developed, rather than in scriptural exegesis. Since the opening days of the AMA campaign, physicians had seen themselves as a medical pastorate relative to abortion. H. R. Storer once remarked that the doctor's office was in fact a confessional; his sentiment was not just echoed but also plagiarized over the years.[109] In 1907, the journal of the Washington State Medical Association, *Northwest Medicine*, published proceedings from its annual meeting, which had been thematically devoted to criminal abortion. These publications are as exemplary of anti-Malthusian rhetoric on abortion as Fernald's or Pirkner's essays, and even more so on the question of pastoral power. For instance, C. N. Suttner of Walla Walla, the incoming president of the association, presented a manifesto for a medical pastorate, "A Plea for the Protection of the Unborn," in which he wrote,

> That ever the priest physician became the plain physician, it has been our lot to direct the body along lines of nature's laws, assisted by and assisting the kindly mentor of ethics and morals.

Inasmuch as the physician is nearest the home, the unit of our society system, it behooves us, and it seems opportune, to recognize fairly the ills of our social system, and see if there be a betterment.

The correlation of the various branches of our social system and their mutual inter-dependence, enact the final cause of creation—the propagation of the species; their ulterior perfection by civilization necessitates healthy bodies with healthy minds.[110]

He fused Christian pastoral traditions effortlessly with a medicalized neo-Stoicism.

The shepherd, whether clerical or medical, is "essentially a doctor who has to take responsibility for each soul and for the sickness of each soul."[111] Unlike Christian pastors, however, physicians were not responsible for their patients' salvation as eternal souls, and it is here that they affected a Stoical ethic by way of a materialist spiritual analytic. Physicians were responsible for the persistence and proliferation of souls in the "flock," the propagation of the species, although of course for most, "the species" was confined to the population of native-born, white Anglos.[112] As a shepherd of (white) procreation, the medical pastor also differed from the Christian preacher in that the care was voluntary and circumstantial. Like a follower of Seneca, a patient must seek guidance; she was not compelled to follow. Medicine was not a church to which the patient owed obedience and continual devotion.[113] The doctor was a source of advice, expertise, and care, not obligation.

The need for priestly physicians had only grown more urgent for turn-of-the-century anti-Malthusians because, from Suttner and his colleagues' perspective, churches had not taken up the call against abortion: "how many, what percentage, are nowadays taught these morals by denominational religions, and how effectually?" The time had come for a renewed medical pastorate. "It is not our province, some may say, to get into the realm of the preacher. But it is our province to advise correctly, to direct and suggest effectively."[114] Besides, as one discussant remarked, the clergy were "ignorant of the prevalence of venereal vices, abortions, etc."[115] With devoutness to medical teachings among women or theologians lacking, the pronatal pastorate faced what Foucault called a "revolt of conduct" against Natural law. Like other moments of resistance to forms of pastoral power from the Middle Ages forward, "revolts of conduct are often linked up with the problem of women and their status in society, in civil society or in religious society," and abortion could not have been more antithetical to anti-Malthusians' concept of women's purpose in a good society and God's government on earth.[116]

As moral physiological shepherds, doctors imagined themselves responding to this revolt by individualizing it, directing the flock toward the good, one wayward sheep at a time. In the end, pastoral power avails itself of ethical persuasion "that guides toward an end and functions as an intermediary towards this end" but that is addressed to "all and each in their paradoxical equivalence," to the flock as a individualized multiplicity, "and not as a higher unity formed by the whole."[117] Doctors conceived of guiding each patient toward maternity as treating the one *and* the many; to save her was to save the one and the many. They did not conceive of persuasion in terms of addressing audiences composed of different groups or interests. Such a medical pastorate related to disease as a matter of individual moral deficiency, not as a public health problem in the twentieth-century sense of the term.

Antiabortionists widely shared Edmund Rogers's view that once a "woman realized the full meaning of this act of destruction" that it was unbelievable "she would so often consent to it being committed."[118] The doctor's office, then, was the idealized site of pronatal shepherding where women could be brought back to the truth of their destiny. Modern education did not teach "that such deeds are wrong," and "many mothers, until so instructed, do not consider the destruction of the product of gestation in the early months morally wrong, but look upon the embryo as a cell or combination of cells, having no individuality and no soul, only as a part of her organism, which has no right, legal or moral, prior to hers."[119] Consequently, physicians exhorted one another to impress on women "by facts and threats, to let nature alone."[120] Medical leaders called on rank-and-file members to provide an "adequate conception of the duties which a woman owes to herself and to society as a wife and as a mother,"[121] although if abortion was an open secret, then surely the demand that women bear children was the most open of secrets. Most important, though, "womankind should be instructed in and taught the first principle of feotal development, and taught it so thoroughly that she cannot fail to comprehend that an abortion is the destruction of a living body, the murder of a defenseless life, whether the deed is committed six months or six minutes after conception has taken place."[122]

Some doctors did talk of public education as well, but it always smacked of dream weaving. For instance, Barbat asked in 1911, "What means can we adopt to limit this slaughter of the innocents? First by educating the public along proper lines. Show them that the happiest people in the world are those who have large families."[123] The publicity campaign presumably wrote itself. An equally implausible suggestion from James Foster Scott was to task a federal department with the problem: "I would urge that Congress appoint an additional cabinet minister who would be the director of a National Bureau of Health. . . . A cabinet officer of Health could disseminate knowledge and bring about many much-needed reforms."[124] A Department of Education and Welfare, later to become Health and Human Services, was decades away, and even then, teaching that abortion was wrong would be of less immediate concern. No, the emphasis was on the physician as shepherd to his or her flock, as Rachel Gleason characterized the counseling role of doctors to patients considering abortion: "Physicians should be like ministers—guides to the people, and when their patients want to go wrong, they should lead and hold them to the right."[125]

No one averred that a new, pronatal pastorate was a perfect solution, only that physicians "may control part of the evil, though not by any means banish it," according to Jennie Oreman.[126] By all accounts, many doctors did attempt to act as pronatal shepherds, sharing stories of counseling successes and failures on occasion, even rehearsing their scripts for each other.[127] The quality of ministry was irregular owing to the variance in persuasive skill of physicians. Reported appeals ranged from calls on women's higher sense of duty to a "good scolding for thinking such a thing" to violent language such as comparing abortion to strangling a baby or, in one report, of telling a mother "that she go home and cut the throat of her oldest child and her family would then number the same."[128] In general, the content of the advice seems to have been that abortion is murder and nature will punish you if the law doesn't. There is no indication that an educational discussion of the female body or the embryo featured.

Fundamentally, the belittling concept of a tractable, dutiful female, epitomized by the figure of the ignorant woman, left doctors incapable of developing a more effective means of making the patient recur to the procreative truth of the body as they did. Instead, the new pastorate employed simple belligerent persuasion that relied greatly on the assumed authority of the physician and a naive view of women as inherently placable, timid, and motivated by maternal sacrifice. Not everyone took the idea of tending a flock of sheep so literally, however. Some recognized that the physician had no command over the patient, only a position of authority that must be used intelligently. Holmes noted that "so soon as we present to the woman that she is doing a criminal offense, is breaking a moral law, we arouse her enmity from the suggestions implied that she is immoral or a criminal."[129] Another commentator remarked, "Our opinion carries weight and our advice, if given with tact, sincerity and, supported by appropriate arguments, is very likely to be heeded."[130] Nonetheless, it was inconceivable to most antiabortionists that women and their families would seek to space and reduce the number of their children if they were truly aware that they should not. Nor was it conceivable that fertility control could represent a decision to be a better mother, that it could be an act of maternal care of self and others rather than a failure.

A further limitation to the powers of a pronatal pastorate was the fact that ultimate responsibility lay with women, even among critics who noted the apparent moral ignorance of doctors who performed abortions. For example, Lyons turned his attention to the well-educated but morally ignorant woman after noting the ethical weakness of the profession. She, not the profession, was the focal point of struggle, although in addressing her, the profession addressed itself. There are several reasons for the focus on women's responsibility. First, the properly reproductive woman held anti-Malthusian biopolitics together. Ghent put this simply: "Properly educated, woman, as we have said, holds the key to the situation to a remarkable extent. When she is deficient in all that tends to enlighten, elevate, ennoble and adorn the race, society, to that extent, is debased; when she is morally pure and intellectually enlightened, society will be adorned and elevated in like proportion."[131] The improperly educated woman was the rot at the heart of the Malthusian couple. Second, physicians could not shepherd one another without some of them becoming visible as abortionists. It was easier and less dangerous professionally to put the burden of reform on the unrealistic return of large families. Finally and most abrasively, the misogyny and contempt of many anti-Malthusians was overpowering. The general professional reaction to women who sought abortions was to label them stupid and find ways to intimidate them within a pastoral relationship.

The conflict between a kind of neo-Stoicism and evangelical self-renunciation in anti-Malthusians' ethical project is manifestly evident in the general failure of the medical pastorate to build any greater immunity to the spread of moral physiological amnesia. The abortion underground continued apace. A fully realized mentorship of the patient would teach her how to inspect her own body, to become a lay student of medicine with adequate proficiency in the necessary modes of body criticism.[132] She might then be able to understand herself for herself and incorporate the supposedly self-evident truth of her divine purpose into her decision making. But such an approach would conflict with the conservative evangelical view of most physicians, who wanted the patient to learn the most obvious moral lessons of the body as she was told, not to become self-sufficient in deciding the truth of her body. In order to implant the desired immunity to false and dangerous desires, physicians would have had to trust their patients to learn and remember for themselves. They could not do this precisely because the reality of women's thinking for themselves about reproduction was the very measure of the ignorance anti-Malthusians saw on display in the morbidity of abortion.

Placing Civilization

If woman's relation to self held "the key to the situation," as Ghent put it, then a long arc of civilized struggle to live in accordance with Providence was known through women's relation to their nature and to abortion. Women's collective moral significance to the nation allowed anti-Malthusians to "see the world in its general order, the tiny space we occupy in it, and the short time we remain here."[133] As Radhika Mohanram has written of pronatal nationalism, "Woman 'is' the nation in that her function, literally, is to reproduce it and maintain its boundaries."[134] Physicians' concern about the United States becoming like France illustrates this exactly, with two nations losing their distinctiveness in the way that they were perishing. For anti-Malthusians, each decision not to bring another life into the world had to be weighed against a maternal imperative within the broad scheme of Creation, "grasping ourselves again here where we are, at this point where we exist," which required "placing ourselves within a wholly rational and reassuring world, which is the world of divine Providence."[135]

Thus, the success of this maladroit, semiclerical project was not decided by the failure of early attempts to exploit its rhetorical capacity; rather, the margin of critical potential is what matters most. "Memory mediates spatial transformations," writes de Certeau, by which he means that memory "modifies the local order," producing a rupture or break within the present. Memory provides "recourse to a different world from which can, *must*, come the blow that will change the established order."[136] In Edward Casey's terms, if a thing or event reminds us of a different, alternative state of affairs, we recognize ourselves differently.[137] Anti-Malthusians hoped that a recovered pronatal truth would rupture the established order. But whether or not that rupture occurred, their formulation of induced abortion as a sign of moral decay and historic decline constituted a sweeping ability to generate critical, evaluative discourses. A mnestic figuration of essential sickness has powerful capabilities, illuminating the space of the collective through the relations between self and others and suggesting means of living differently. Disease limns the host whether or not it is curable.[138]

The reach of this capacity, the limit of abortion's morbidity to silently expose our failings, was set by its potential to integrate the state of woman's body, the social body, and the where and the when of the United States as one fact. Integration was accomplished through two broad, simultaneous, and contradictory moves, one contractive and the other expansive. When diverse locales and events are compressed into a "single composite memory," as with physicians' discourse of American decline, Casey observes, there is a concomitant distention. Contraction depends on extension—stretching out and gathering up places, their differences falling away as they compact into one, overstuffed mnestic object.[139] Hence, a final layer of embodied tropes completed the recursive dynamic powering anti-Malthusian discourse. Rendered schematically, the full sequence of tropes involves, first, the diseased interruption of life; second, the transumption of disease into truth; and third, the contrary composition of society as extended from the sexual organism *and* contracted to nothing but the sexual organism. This last relation, a composition of contraries, is called *antitheton* and in this case involves opposed actions that constitute a single, conglomerate entity of white civilization.

Regarding expansion, mapping the inner world of the organism is key to determining the causal relations of a disease and is essentially an expansive project.[140] Although the human organism's volume is finite, as we have refined our abilities to see into the body, human space has grown as the scale of parsing that space has shrunk.[141] In other words, this expansion is not volumetric, but a kind of amplification, *peristasis* specifically, which is the elaboration of circumstances, including location, time, history, behavior, and so on.[142] Socially, abortion as pathognomonic retained an organic seat, the womb and its contents, but the body was collectivized such that the agents causing the sickness were not physically organic but morally amnestic. Whereas with organic disease, the "space of the disease is, without remainder or shift, the very space of the organism," with social disease, the space of the disease is the very space of society.[143] The disease of wanting smaller families exposed a pathological space that crisscrossed the collectivity, passing from the corporeal to the social and back again. When indicting America by way of women like the unfortunate Mrs. S., doctors like Fowler prosecuted by amplification. However, amplification was not simply emphasis created by detail piled on detail. Society itself, in its every aspect, was presumed to be an amplification of "the final cause of creation—the propagation of the species," as Suttner stated. The human geography of Providence was elaborated in the refusal of Providence.

The same move that made society an amplified body also contracted the virtual space of discovery.[144] Individual and national reproductive weaknesses were confined to the thin, anonymous memory of natural law upon which physicians grounded their critique of fertility control. Physicians analyzed the "habit" of abortion by roughly transferring organic *metonyms* to a collective body and with that, blending the universality of female physiology with the homogenizing ideology of Woman. The nation's body was *an* organism, a white, native-born one, made up fundamentally of reproductive mandates. So if reproduction was the base of the family and therefore the nation, as Fernald and Suttner fervently believed, society was primarily a raced sexual organism driven by the laws embedded in its physiology to carry out one primary task.[145] In conjunction with the metonym of reducing female corporeality to an alarm system for pathogenic forces, physicians condensed the social body into the organism, creating telescoping part-to-whole relationships: society into body, body into discourse. The recursive dynamic of anti-Malthusians was a particularly aggressive mode of contraction: national life was made to fit the space of biotic memory retrieved from theologically authored life.[146] In this way, recurrence to tricks of fate that made things like knitting needles or soap accidentally lethal enveloped the United States in a global struggle over life's purpose and ethical management.

If diseases are "other ways of life" that depend on an organism's environment for their development, then when body and society become a composite entity as they did for anti-Malthusian physicians, the body's external environment is folded *into* the organism as an extension of it. Civilization becomes the *unfolding* of a Natural history of reproduction, which is the logical consequence of Allen's physiological inversion of Malthus. Instead of material conditions affecting moral advancement and cultivation, a people's adherence to unyielding moral codes regulates the material prospects of their society. The vitality of prenatal life determines the material ecology for biopolitical survival throughout time.

Antiabortionists' use of racial Others from colonial imperialism to explain regression to primitivism exemplifies the globalizing, contrary action of prenatal amplification and reduction.[147] American physicians did not tend to discuss Western imperialism per se; unlike their counterparts in Europe, they did not see themselves as part of colonial projects. They did, however, see the world through Western imperialist eyes and wore the whited lenses of racial anthropology.[148]

For example, Scott wrote that in "China, Japan, India, and Africa this practice [of abortion] has been, and still is, fearfully prevalent. These benighted peoples, with their teeming and redundant populations, place very little value on human life."[149] It was not that whites were becoming unraced or that the white race was devolving. Rather, abortion was reversion to a pre-Christian whiteness, which in its pagan ways was no better than the benighted and teeming Others of Asia and Africa. "Like divorce, abortion has been a revival by Anglo-Saxon civilization of an ancient pagan practice," Reverend O'Callaghan worried. He served on the committee on criminal abortion appointed by the Chicago Medical Society in 1904.[150] Hardly alone in feeling this way, he voiced the Christianized racial history that buttressed medical fear of race suicide, which Saur summarized in her advice to mothers in *Maternity*: "If we examine the history of abortion, we shall find that this crime, now so commonly practiced as to demand the attention it is receiving from moralists, is of extremely ancient origin, having existed among pagan nations from the earliest times; that the influence of Christianity has ever been to banish the practice, and that in proportion as Christianity become weakened or destroyed, the fearful evil in question reappears and extends."[151]

The general plotline adopted by physicians had Greece and Rome, the great Western antecedents, as foils to modernity's decline. This is unsurprising, as the decline of the West has been a powerful narrative for organizing cultural critique in modernity. In the anti-Malthusians' story, Greece, and especially pre-Christian Rome, tolerated abortion, which became the sign of their civilizations' pathology too. Observers pointed to satire VI from Juvenal, for example, wherein he criticized noble Roman women for aborting, unlike their plebian sisters.[152] They noted Plato's and Aristotle's tolerance of abortion as well as Greek and Roman opinion on human ensoulment at about forty days; ancient medical opinion established the precedent for the concept of quickening recognized by English common law on abortion.[153] Physicians' history was little more than anecdotal, plucking references to abortion such as from Juvenal, possibly Ovid or Seneca, maybe Hippocrates or Galen, and compressing centuries of ancient history into one indistinguishable moment. "But national sins beget national woes, and the Roman empire overrun by Northern hordes perished for want of men," worried William Goodell; "what happened in Rome, what happened to Greece, may yet befall our own beloved country."[154] The United States was reverting to the habits of its pagan forebears, not unlike France, whose "decadence," after all, was "unquestionable."[155]

By some accounts, nations like the United States and France had arrived at the most uncivilized state ever, worse than at any prior moment in history. "A community that will permit this has the elements of decay in it," Scott somberly observed. "There is no darker page in history than this sin. Countless millions of human lives have been thus sacrificed, and probably at no period of the world's history has the slaughter been greater than in our own times." He might have been paraphrasing Dixon-Jones, who lamented, "Uncounted millions of unborn infants have thus perished. There is no darker page in history."[156] In the context of rampant hyperbole about the end of civilization—"The nation is as certain to decline as the night is certain to follow the day"—it is easy to dismiss such comments as overwrought, but that would be an oversight.[157] The dynamic that makes such statements possible was enduring and substantial.

Western history thus became a referendum on reproductive morality, with great expanses of time evaluated by the relative portion of Christian and pagan influence. Insufficient Christianity placed white Western nations at risk of depopulation. The assumption was that the world is a singular space ordered developmentally, composed of places formed around differences inherent to those locations, such as in comments like those of Dixon-Jones. Geographer Doreen Massey explains that the Western, "modern, territorial, conceptualisation [sic] of space" is an "essentialist, billiard-ball view of place" in which "the differences between places exist, and then those different places come into contact."[158] Remarks about savage and civilized peoples exemplify this concept of territory, but so do those about the place of the relation of the pregnant body to the nation. Female and embryonic bodies were essential, preformed places in permanent, formative contact with less stable spaces of reproductive custom. As the order of the world was set by different, preconstituted places, so too was the body a terrain of preconstituted places within that order. Furthermore, "different 'places' were interpreted as different stages in a single temporal development." Contemporaneous, different ways of life—diverse abortion traditions in this case—are "rendered as (reduced to) place in the historical queue."[159] When the United States is assessed as more savage than its peers, pathology becomes location staged on a scale of civilization.

Anti-Malthusian rhetoric at the fin de siècle unknowingly worked the "equation of memory with production and forgetting with negation" to the point of strained exaggeration,[160] where procreation became synonymous with all cultural and biological production, and abortion synonymous with their negation.

Physicians' ability to locate contemporary America so as to critique its culture depended on this figuration, regardless of the superfluity of their warnings. For anti-Malthusians, what brought far-flung moments into contact with one another followed from the same base fold, the starting seam upon which all others depended: the act of abortion as a sign of sickness. Esposito wrote, "By placing the body at the center of politics and disease at the center of the body, it makes sickness, on the one hand, the outer margin from which life must continually distance itself and, on the other, the internal fold which dialectically brings [life] back to itself."[161] Not only did abortion's morbidity provide a means for women to look at themselves and their practices; because of the collapse of the social and maternal body into one, interrupted pregnancies also were a way for society to look at itself. From the primary task of reproduction all institutions were raised and on its failure all institutions fell, as determined in secret by the unseen acts of faceless women.

4

"More Wisdom in Living" | Neo-Malthusian Memory Work at Midcentury

Contraceptives or Abortion—which shall it be?
—MARGARET SANGER, *Woman and the New Race*

For anti-Malthusians, the answer to the question Sanger asks in the above epigraph would be "neither." Contraception could not provide protection from abortion because the disease fundamentally was a desire for small families; birth control indicated the same moral lethe, but in a less dramatic and dangerous way. For neo-Malthusians, the answer to Sanger's question had to be contraceptives, lest it be abortion. Abortion continued as a sign of disordered life to medical reason, but prior to the establishment of the first birth control clinic in the United States, a figuration of remembering and forgetting contrary to anti-Malthusianism began to empower physicians' discourse. In the unending stream of wounds, infections, and fatalities, observers started to recognize a society bruised and rent from living in an outmoded past. During the Great Depression, the new figuration reached dominance as physicians refashioned the harm of botched abortions into a reminder that the United States obstructed, not encouraged, the Malthusian couple. The contrary biopolitical disposition of neo-Malthusians grounded a critique of reproductive culture that was subtler than one might expect. In fact, remembering and forgetting shadowed anti-Malthusian discourse, again placing the nation in a backward drift through history. The difference was that now the greater part of recollection was performed statistically. Neo-Malthusians enacted mnesis differently but maintained the established dynamic.

Algernon Black, executive secretary of the New York Society for Ethical Culture, concisely summed up neo-Malthusian physicians' biopolitics at the 1942 conference "The Abortion Problem," sponsored by the National Committee on Maternal Health (NCMH): "I assume that we all think abortion is evil, and that we all would like to reduce it to a minimum. I assume that we do not want anyone to become pregnant who does not really want to become pregnant. That would require a tremendous amount of education, not only in the purposes of life, but in moving toward those purposes, the development of more wisdom in living—in our own living."[1] Black exposes the common understanding of abortion connecting neo- to anti-Malthusian discourse: it was a slow death endemic to civilization. He also points up the divergence between a diagnosis that was shared and a remedy that was not: all agreed that too little wisdom contributed to this ill state of affairs, yet they differed on exactly what knowledge was missing or what the necessary program to instill proper wisdom was, because they had different views of what sickness was indicated.

For neo-Malthusians, the existence of criminal abortion was a shameful monument to the wreckage left by dated medical and legal orthodoxy. Widespread illegal terminations in the United States indicated that the disease was a lack of professional help for reproductive control caused by backwardness and concomitant restrictions. The extant "remedy" for abortion, criminalization, only prolonged and aggravated disease, trapping the United States in an unscientific and unjust era. Abortion's morbidity still served as an antigen, but it provoked a different immunological response. Where anti-Malthusians rejected smaller families, neo-Malthusians endorsed family limitation and thus contraception, sex education, and more. As antagonistic declensions of Malthus, these discourses were rhetorically similar but abortion's pathognomonic status yielded to each differing secrets about society, which in turn warranted divergent programs to better immunize the nation from its ignorance.[2] To neo-Malthusians, interrupting pregnancy was a less civilized alternative to contraception; it recalled reproductive privation in contrast to moral lethe.

In this chapter, I scrutinize the period in which medical rhetoric on abortion changed its stripes, principally the 1930s until the late 1950s, although the boundaries are porous. Neo-Malthusianism was the major counterdiscourse within medical rhetoric on abortion, but it developed from and oriented its opposition to anti-Malthusianism by redeploying the very same dynamic of recurring to abortion's dangers in order to mark the United States as uncivilized. The manner by which neo-Malthusians preserved but transmuted this dynamic to serve contrary ends demonstrates the extent to which abortion had been rhetorically capacitated to support biopolitical struggle. Unlike in the preceding pastoral period, later literature was much more centrally organized. A small number of writings defined the range of motion of a large set of contributory texts, the bulk of which includes case reports; surveys of patients and clients; and analyses of data from hospitals, clinics, public agencies, and the census. One book and two conference proceedings formed the spinal column of literature on abortion from the Depression onward. A straight line passes through the 1930s publications of St. Louis clinician and professor Frederick J. Taussig, to the 1942 conference on abortion sponsored by the NCMH, to the 1955 conference on abortion sponsored by Planned Parenthood Federation of America (PPFA). The NCMH was crucial to the production all of these texts. Taussig's 1936 masterwork, *Abortion, Spontaneous and Induced,* was supported and published by the NCMH, and his book was the backdrop for the 1942 gathering. Further, the PPFA conference was planned in the image of the NCMH colloquium and included key NCMH members. These publications mark a changing ecology of practice, where socioeconomic stressors, fertility control, and statistics become vital elements of memory work.

The NCMH started as a self-organized group of New York physicians about the time Sanger opened her first clinic in 1916. The group was independent of Sanger and in opposition to her method of lay contraception services but nonetheless similarly influenced by sexology, as shown by the committee's interest in the "social and psychological aspects of sex and reproduction."[3] The membership included dozens of New York physicians, but Robert Latou Dickinson, former president of the American Gynecological Society and a future inspiration to Alfred Kinsey, was the prime mover and leader.[4] The Committee on Maternal Health (CMH) incorporated as a nonprofit entity in March 1923, in response to Sanger's American Birth Control League having in January that year opened a second clinic, the Birth Control Clinic Research Bureau (CRB), later renamed the Margaret Sanger Research Bureau.[5] From 1925 to 1929, Dickinson attempted to merge the CMH with the league's CRB, ostensibly in order to improve research and broaden the available data. The proposed entity, the Maternity Research Council, would have brought Sanger's research clinic under physician direction and purged its activist ethos. Initially, the league agreed, so as to gain financial and institutional clout; but the league eventually rejected Dickinson's proposal in 1929 and formed its own medical board, with doctor Hannah Stone directing. It had become clear that the merger would cost the league control of its mission.[6] In 1930, the CMH adopted the name National Committee on Maternal Health, after which it more actively sponsored research on fertility and reproduction, with principal emphases on sterility, abortion, and sex education.[7]

A number of key studies conducted by hospitals or under the auspices of other research entities branched into Taussig's work and the two conference proceedings; these included statistician Marie Kopp's 1931 study of the first ten thousand cases at the league's CRB, an early 1940s Scripps Foundation survey of Indianapolis couples' contraceptive use and ideal family size, and certainly the 1958 book from Kinsey's Institute for Sex Research (ISR), *Pregnancy, Birth and Abortion*.[8] The ratio of abortions to confinements determined by Kopp's study was central to Taussig's calculation of the frequency of abortion. The preliminary results from the Indianapolis study were a key topic at the NCMH conference. Data culled from the interviews used by the institute for its volume on human female sexuality were crucial to the Statistics Committee's report at the PPFA conference and were later featured in *Pregnancy, Birth and Abortion*.[9] There were other influential books, particularly two by contemporaries of Taussig, A. J. Rongy and William Robinson, but these functioned more as polemical extremities.[10]

There were inklings among turn-of-the-century physicians of the coming change in medical rhetoric, but it awaited the flowering of the birth control movement in the United States. As an organization, the AMA refused to countenance even discussion of contraception until 1935 and opposed the practice until 1937.[11] It did not endorse abortion reform until 1968.[12] Nevertheless, medical progressives gradually developed a procontraception, antiabortion discourse about the professional management of pregnancy. A line of inquiry hesitantly begun by members of the NCMH gathered, spurred, and focused production of knowledge on abortion until the Dwight D. Eisenhower years and shaped central features of the rhetoric through the 1960s.

Inflection: Abortion as a Sign of Pathological Privation

As the new century began, outrage peaked over the supposed moral physiological failures of women, but the rare physician voiced a contrary view, as did I. C. Philbrick in 1905 before the Nebraska State Medical Association, arguing that "a perverted sex relationship brought under the stress of economic necessity" caused abortion, but "economic freedom is opening to women escape from the degradation of such marriage"; as a result, "the family is in a state of reconstruction." Similarly, Rosalie Ladova leveled a Marxist indictment of abortion's economic causes, also in 1905. In the same year, G. M. Hawkins argued against a maternal imperative: "There is not one well-founded fact to prove that woman's sexual nature is simply a maternal instinct, that is, only a desire to have a child."[13] Remarks like these understood pregnancy as a volatile site of economic and somatic risk. They also suggested the impact of feminism, European political economics, and psychology, particularly the sexology of Havelock Ellis, on U.S. physicians' concept of the body. These texts bear the marks of Richard Freiherr von Krafft-Ebing, Karl Marx, and Friedrich Engels, but especially before Alfred Kinsey it was uncommon for writers to cite anyone other than Ellis, if they cited anyone beyond the profession at all. Further, in the United States, the empirical study of healthy sexual reproduction, not psychology per se, was considered most important to the debate.[14]

Even so, years of railing against the danger of abortion exerted the greatest influence, like a great magnet bending everything toward it. The force of danger held physicians close together, despite divergent views on small families and maternity. Neo-Malthusians saw progress as a source of risk to personal and public well-being; progress was inherent to being civilized, but social and economic advancements brought with them reproductive disorders that threatened the very achievements that defined civilization. Like conservative members of the profession, neo-Malthusians viewed abortion as an unnecessary risk, even a perverse one, in Philbrick's words, taken in pursuit of limited fertility. Doctors of every sort wanted fewer abortions, legal and illegal, with progressives often repurposing traditionalist tropes of family as society's base and women as fulfilled by childbearing (if only fewer, healthier children). They parted ways, however, in that neo-Malthusians came to see existing controls on abortion as a sort of autoimmune disorder. Existing law and medical pastoring were not simply ineffective tools in "a losing war against an unstoppable opponent"; as Esposito explains, "rather than a failure, a block, or a flaw in the immune apparatus, they represent[ed] its reversal against itself."[15] Protections against abortion had only spawned a vast underground, increasing the threat to the very civilized advancement supposedly desired.

The dim view of existing protections stemmed from a different understanding of how acts of abortion inflected progress. Neo-Malthusians tended to see abortion as the social evolutionary stage after infanticide and prior to contraception, not as the extreme presentation of systemic moral rot in the family. L. Jacobi remarked in 1912, in a clear, early statement that relied on the new mnestic figuration, "The substitution of abortion for infanticide must be considered chronologically and ethically a step in advance. The motives prompting abortion are in general identical with the causes of infant-murder."[16] The cause of lost lives and damaged bodies was the brutality of inadequate socioeconomic conditions and birth control, not some primitive barbarism unchained by a small family ideology.[17] Quoting from Ellis, Jacobi wrote that "'the adoption of preventive methods of conception follows progress and civilization.'"[18] Rongy was even more specific in 1931 that limited fertility ushered in, not followed, advancement (an axiomatic point to the new biopolitics): "Human progress and the security of civilization are impossible unless means are devised for the affecting of the birth rate."[19] Feminists like Regina Downie understood abortion as evidence that women were resisting suffering, risking death to improve the condition of life, especially in the midst of the 1930s global Depression. As president of Women's Medical College Alumnae in 1939, she argued that "because abortion is the only way out, they take this road to death and illness and disaster. World-wide [sic] abortion is a symptom of the fumbling, awkward stirring of awakening womankind. Women are refusing to bring more and more children into hopeless poverty and they are obeying economic law in the only way they know."[20] Insecure reproduction was still the crucible of life and abortion was an index of that insecurity, yet physicians were rejecting the political economy of physiology that had been so crisply enunciated by Nathan Allen.

Although a pivot in medical rhetoric was well under way before the Depression drove home the stakes of family planning, Frederick Taussig's work became the fulcrum for neo-Malthusian rhetoric in the 1930s.[21] Taussig taught, practiced, and researched medicine at Washington University in St. Louis. He first published against abortion in 1906 with comments that fit neatly into anti-Malthusian discourse. In 1916, however, reflecting on World War I, he maintained that war prompted consideration of birth control as a constitutive element of civilized self-governance, a view shared by many progressives in and out of the profession. According to this assessment, overpopulation with its attendant hardships had incited unprecedented slaughter and would do so again.[22] Nevertheless, Taussig set abortion aside as an inhumane, dangerous method to address excessive fertility, one advocated only by leftists. He remarked that as the "power of orthodox religion" waned, the fate of abortion in "every civilized country" hung in the balance as socialism developed internationally. "One group of socialist women," he warned, "claim they have an absolute right to do as they choose with the products of their body and brook no interference from the state." Perhaps he was referring to advocates like Annette Konikow, a socialist physician who favored legalized abortion. Taussig called this position an "extreme doctrine" that ran "counter to all our ideals of humanity. Its parallel can only be found among the lower animals."[23]

By contrast, Taussig foreshadowed the liberal welfare state biopolitics that would come to dominate medical rhetoric; neither pronatalist nor radical, it rallied around contraception and abhorred abortion for fertility management. He closed by noting that his was the mainstream view of physicians, a result of their experience with impoverished, large families. "They naturally desire such reforms as will lighten the burden of these parents."[24] The liberal state, defined by state-supported, professionally managed pregnancy prevention, was the path to a secure, advanced civilization, whereas a more radical socialist state, defined by abortion on demand, threatened animalistic regression. Indeed, Rosalind Pollack Petchesky contends that the initial criminalization of abortion in the nineteenth century and attempts to regulate fertility were "the early origins of the welfare state."[25]

In 1936, Taussig published *Abortion, Spontaneous and Induced*, and with it the new mnestic dynamics of abortion discourse settled in. The volume culminated several years of research. The first major project had been undertaken when the Hoover administration's Department of Labor, Children's Bureau, tasked a report on maternal mortality, and Taussig was tapped to produce the section on abortion. Based on a survey of fifteen states' data from 1927–28 and published in 1934, this was the first multistate study of reproduction in the United States.[26] He also visited a Moscow "*abortarium*" in 1930 to observe its practice because at that time the Soviet Union was the only place on earth where abortion was legally unrestricted, with organized clinics providing service.[27] Taussig's experiences led Dickinson to ask him to write a comprehensive work on the subject with assistance from members of the NCMH.[28] The result, *Abortion, Spontaneous and Induced*, was unmatched in breadth and rigor, immediately becoming the commanding reference on abortion ("now our Bible" as Dickinson remarked), which it remained for over two decades.[29] The volume comprises twenty-eight chapters with several appendixes. Taussig devoted most of his time to technical aspects of diagnosis and treatment, but he also made crucial forays into the biopolitical terrain of abortion control.

Taussig's significance to medical rhetoric did not derive from fresh insight. He reiterated the notion that abortion's prevalence proved the nation was flagging, arguing that "abortion undermines the physical well-being and moral integrity of the community."[30] As a social disease, terminating pregnancy was even more virulent because of its nonbiological vectors: "I know of no condition in medical practice in which the effort to limit its frequency is so intimately bound up with the social and moral life of the people. To some extent the spread of venereal diseases is influenced by these same factors but their control, owing to their bacteriological origin, is relatively simple compared to the complexities that attend limitation of a procedure like abortion that may be practiced in any home at any time." As a consequence, the practice was "probably the most wasteful of known ills in its expenditure of human life and human health."[31] Taussig demonstrated the shared-threat logic of contraception advocates and their anti-Malthusian peers. Interrupted pregnancies were a pestilent negation of life incumbent on poorly managed progress. Hence, the negation of life's negation persisted as a political premise for immunizing the United States against abortion's symptomatic afflictions.[32]

Although the practice still negatively inflected the course of civilization for Taussig, if abortion is considered an antigen, then fertility control measures were in his view the antibody, not moral admonition. He based his analysis of threats to "well-being and moral integrity" on a calculation of risk from the excess, not the dearth, of fertility. The pathognomonic trope remained morbid interruption (*aposiopesis*), only now interruption was a prompt for recalling the maladies of too many, not too few, pregnancies. His position on contraception was unremarkable, quite similar to the revised position Sanger adopted after she returned from Europe and began to organize lay contraception services, for example.[33] She stated many times that abortion was wrong, and from the day her first clinic opened, she advised clients against it.[34] Rather than breaking new ground, the significance of Taussig sprang from the decisive way in which he synthesized understanding of abortion's overall morbidity and the way in which he aligned *and* juxtaposed anti- and neo-Malthusianism through morbidity's causes.

Taussig's iteration of abortion as a social disease had weighty consequences, although this element of his text passed into conventional wisdom without commentary. His comparison to venereal disease reflected the euphemism of "social disease" for a sexually transmitted illness. Prior to World War I, tuberculosis was typically (but not exclusively) the anchor for metaphoric "social disease," as in Pirkner's previously noted comment that abortion was a "white man's disease" like tuberculosis. During World War I and after, as efforts to control syphilis developed, the term *social disease* became more readily identified with venereal disease.[35] Taussig's vision galvanized physicians to manage abortion through public health mechanisms not unlike antituberculosis and anti-VD campaigns.

He reimagined the early maxim—that moral education of "ignorant women" was the answer—in terms of programs to combat communicable illness.

Not everyone hewed to this refiguration of the disease. For instance, contraception advocate Downie drew a different conclusion from Taussig's data for the Labor Department: "A recent survey by the Children's Bureau tells of another part of the same huge human problem. The number of maternal deaths in this country is shockingly high. Maternity is not a disease—we doctors are being asked why these women die. . . . Too many children are born in too short a space of time."[36] However, her position was uncommon. In 1942, the NCMH conference in New York City extended Taussig's formulation of disease. Nearly four dozen experts attended, mostly physicians but others as well, including sociologists, lawyers, judges, and, notably, Halbert L. Dunn, a statistician who from 1935 to 1960 headed the National Office of Vital Statistics. The conference was divided into four parts. In the fourth, dedicated to "control of the abortion problem," New York's assistant attorney general, John Harlan Amen; its superintendent of insurance, Louis H. Pink; and two MDs, Herman Bundesen of New York and George Cooper of Raleigh, led sessions on the importance of legal, insurance, and public health models for addressing abortion, particularly considered as an "outbreak" of a communicable disease.[37]

The 1955 conference hosted by PPFA was even more emphatic about the formula of abortion as sexually transmitted illness. Mary Steichen Calderone, the new medical director of PPFA, conference organizer, and future founder of the Sexuality Information and Education Council of the United States (SIECUS), stated, in a letter soliciting participation from Christopher Tietze, the leading statistician on abortion, the necessity of considering public health models.[38] She expressed fascination with the attempt by the 1942 conferees to grapple with the extent and control of abortion, which is exactly what attendees of the PPFA gathering continued to do at length. The list of participants was a who's who of abortion authorities, including Alfred Kinsey and Alan Guttmacher, as well as eight participants of the 1942 colloquium. Most endorsed a forceful concluding statement extracted from their debates: "The demonstrated high incidence of terminations of unwanted pregnancies by illegal abortion could be looked upon as a disease of that society, presenting a problem in epidemiology as real and as urgent as did venereal disease three decades ago."[39]

The 1955 proceedings, published in 1958, were widely reviewed, and despite dismissal from *Medical Economics*, reviewers publicized the memory of a secret disease constituted by the findings.[40] For instance, *Scientific American* endorsed the findings: "Nevertheless it is clear, on the basis of a mass of data, than an enormous number of abortions—running into the millions—are performed annually the world over. We are faced, therefore, with a matter of the highest medical and social importance: a disease of society, the more serious because many communities refuse to recognize it and do nothing to eliminate its causes and mitigate its effects."[41] Similarly, *Science* publicized the recommendations, legitimated by the probable memories of anonymous strangers: "The woman who resorts to pregnancy termination is often emotionally disturbed. Family, social, and economic factors may enter into the causation of the pregnancy and its undesirable end. Induced abortions may be traumatic experiences for the individuals involved and do not solve underlying basic problems."[42] Even the magazine *Sexology*, which played to the popular sexual imagination despite its title, framed abortion as a social disease in its review of the conference.[43]

Because neo- and anti-Malthusian rhetoric collocated with abortion as a disease, a shift in terminology taken by itself, from *moral* to *communicable* disorder, does not sufficiently parse the discourse. What matters most is the revised indexical logic between abortion's open secret and its pathology, namely, that the unending stream of deaths and injuries revealed a sickly imbalance between criminality, fertility control, and socioeconomic conditions. On this point Taussig's book is equally decisive, evincing a starkly refashioned rhetoric of "civilization as risk." At the close of the second chapter, "Historical and Racial Aspects," Taussig dismissed theology as a limited mode of reproductive control, reframed the moralistic causal scheme for abortion, and asserted inadequate progress as an equally important contributor to abortion. He noted that Catholic theology had had "some effect," albeit "relatively slight," on numbers of abortions, but that the overall rate had continued to climb for fifty years. Social and economic factors were "largely responsible" for the trend, of which two sets of factors were critical, as follows: "(1) Increasing secularization of thought, increasing hedonism and pleasure philosophy of life, urbanization and the frantic desire to raise the economic standard of life by limiting offspring by any means, however desperate. (2) Cultural lag: the resistance to change, responsible for the slowness in diffusing reliable scientific contraceptive knowledge."[44]

Between the first and second set lies the shift in mnesis I have described. Taussig was in sympathy with anti-Malthusian moralism (we are hedonistic, frantic, and desperate), but he also understood moralism as impeding scientific progress, which would provide a more effective remedy for abortion. No moment in the literature so perfectly announces the change—one can hear a heavy clang as medicine's rhetorical armature swings about. Scientism replaced moralism, as the underlying sentiment shifted from "Thou shalt not abort" to "It is not safe to abort."[45] This upended the assessment of what an endemic interruption of pregnancy said about the nation. The degeneration of reproduction did not arise from material progress outpacing morality; in fact, moralism itself retarded contraceptive practices and so contributed to social blight.[46]

As the memory work that abortion practices contributed to changed, the embodiment of abortion's pathogenesis changed as well. Instead of directing abortion's misery toward a biotic memory of natural law that would supposedly protect white America from racial decline, physicians, with Taussig as the standard bearer, channeled "pregnancy wastage" from abortion into a statistical memory of unacknowledged privation. Employing the enumerating techniques of public health discourse, abortion's morbidity still figured a memory of secrets; only these were the secrets of a population, not a physiology. Speaking at the 1942 NCMH conference, Taussig organized the flow of morbidity into broad channels: "When pregnancy is prematurely interrupted by what we term abortion, the human race suffers loss and damage in 3 ways: First, an infinite number of potential human beings are destroyed before birth. Secondly, abortion carries with it a considerable death rate among expectant mothers. And finally, abortion leaves in its wake a high incidence of pathologic conditions, some of which interfere with the further possibility of reproduction."[47] Channeling abortion in this way hardened existing segmentations between forms of damage: harm to fetal life, maternal life, and overall fertility. However, the emphasis on the measured extent of the damage, its rate and probable outcomes, demonstrates that the rhetoric had modernized. From the 1930s onward, the most important studies turned an administrative, not a clinical, gaze on abortion, reckoning vital and social statistics, expounding abortion's threat across the population, and amplifying general pathological risks developed from clinical practice.[48]

An administrative gaze uses the lenses of spreadsheets and tables to perceive, Bruce Curtis explains, "focusing and extending" attention paid to populations as composite "articulations of equivalent human atoms."[49] Statistics were as much a material factor as was physiology in the new discourse. The particular materiality of data collection, calculation, and correction became a primary embodiment of abortion's damage. Numbers did not dematerialize harm, they transformed it, and the specific challenges of working the data were as important as patient cases as far as concretizing the harm of interrupted pregnancy goes. The rise of an administrative gaze relative to public health was not special to abortion, of course; indeed, if Calderone's 1954 letter to Tietze advocating a public health approach is indicative, its development in regard to abortion was slow in coming.[50] Criminality, which made data collection difficult, and medical ambivalence had much to do with the sluggishness.

In fact, existing law and medical confusion themselves became pathological *because* they impeded treatment. The specter of prosecution impinged on data collection and aggravated the harm, a common complaint that Judge Anna Kross succinctly spelled out for conferees at the 1942 NCMH conference: "Abortion appears to have been widespread in the United States for at least a century and although sound statistics are lacking, we know that it is rife today. . . . Abortion, as a practice, is driven underground instead of being eliminated."[51] Greater control required greater visibility, which the law thwarted. If the law itself had become an autoimmune disorder, then the United States needed protection from its protection against abortion.[52] More than that, better control required that physicians not hide *themselves* behind the law's failure. She continued later the same day: "You have not, even in your own mind, decided what is the evil. . . . If you are not fundamentally decided, once and for all, on whether abortion is essential from a medical standpoint, you will get nowhere"—an unusually blunt and accurate description of medical discourse. Lack of agreement among doctors also inhibited effective management and so contributed to the disease. Kross underscored that "to solve this problem you must go beyond the law to reach the roots," which is exactly what organizers of the 1942 conference wanted to happen.[53]

In a lengthy, handwritten invitation to Taussig, Clair Fulsome, lead organizer and executive director of the NCMH, frankly discussed their purpose: "You will notice that I have omitted the ever entangling problem of abortion indicators in the usual specialty fields, viz: [*sic*] surgical, medical and psychiatric. Dr. Howard Taylor Jr, [*sic*] feels, as do I, that these will be brought out in secondary discussions while the real problem includes social, economic and educational factors in both causes and methods of control of induced abortion."[54] The NCMH aimed to establish an interdisciplinary research agenda that could redirect the discourse of abortion toward a new mode of reproductive governance and thus intervene in its control. Fulsome continued:

> The social scientists must be stimulated to encourage research in social causes and prevention. It would appear that we want to face the larger

portions of the problem, *the common causes*; to martial evidence for and against the interruption of pregnancies on social, economic and more general grounds (domestic relations such as incompatibility, rape, divorce) et al.; to tackle the problems the sacrosanct medical groups (such as the Academy, College of Surgeons, AMA) flinch from for fear of criticism, and lastly to develop from these ideas, obtained at this conference, a large scale research program and, possibly, an education docket to stir up hospitals, medical societies and medical schools.[55]

Fulsome fused research, cultural critique, and biopolitical advocacy into one program.[56]

That medical progressives repurposed, not repudiated, abortion as an inflection point of progress is acutely evident in that the network of etiologic factors leading to abortion remained structurally the same. Physicians like Fulsome still held ignorance to be the efficient cause of abortion and a wide range of nonexclusive conditions to be the material causes: principally, standards of living[57] and the stigma of "illegitimacy";[58] selfishness, vanity, and sexual violence also figured but not centrally.[59] Physicians commonly discussed causes as an admixture of factors, possibly singling out one or another as more important.[60] Moral degeneracy was not among them, nor was a right to choose after 1920.[61] The ultimate source of danger was every pregnant woman who was not properly wary of abortion. A benighted state regarding the procedure's risks and contraceptive alternatives propelled the incidence rate more than did some bleached-out maternal imperative. Women were unaware of how to avoid pregnancy or of the chances they took by aborting.[62] If women did not know the risks, they would not consult their doctors. If reproductive services were not available, most women had no one to consult even if they did know. If the law prevented provision of information and services, then the nation itself was contributing to the disease, needlessly denying itself effective medical care. Such ignorance left them highly susceptible under challenging socioeconomic conditions that health care professionals lacked the tools to combat. Abortion no longer originated in the alienation from instinctual truths but originated in the alienation from conditions necessary for healthy, planned pregnancies. Fewer abortions would signal alleviation of socioeconomic distress, not redemption before an "outraged" Nature, but the crux for developing immunity was still to educate pregnant women about danger.

Position: Making Memories of Privation Visible

Neo-Malthusians clearly took criminal abortion for more than a portent of ailment (Black's comment that we need to develop more wisdom in living is a cue). They, too, leveraged danger from abortion to position themselves against the present; only they inhabited that position quantitatively. With Taussig as the herald of the new medical rhetoric, the NCMH lead the development of statistical memory of abortion wherein the anonymity and unknowns of data ordered the mnestic folds of its discourse. Before Taussig, the anatomical body had been the means to dispel secrecy; people could hide abortion, they could lie about it, but it was hard to suppress the damage it caused. Later physicians like Dickinson, Taylor, and Fulsome set the population as their horizon, and managerial logics coupled with an administrative gaze allowed them to turn the secrecy surrounding abortion into a form of numerable visibility. People did hide abortion, they did lie about it, but not only could researchers anticipate such obfuscations in figuring type and kind, pattern and frequency, they used the anonymity of patient records and research to build an impersonal remembrance of America through abortion that anchored neo-Malthusian critiques of U.S. culture.

The apposite difference between a biotic memory of physiology and a statistical memory of a population is not based on their relative descriptive power.[63] Statistical discourse was not always more accurate than generalizations of frequency based on clinical experience, as Rudolph W. Holmes suggested in 1939 in relation to the rate of procedures: "Statistical study will but intimate the frequency of induced abortion."[64] Rather, the key distinction is that a statistical memory of the population relates secrecy/disclosure to forgetting/remembering in an entirely different way from a biotic memory. In place of a teleological determinism, where physiology was law, neo-Malthusians saw a world governed by contingency that could be revealed through large data sets.[65] Vital and social statistics made millions of unidentified women recognizable as an amalgam. Further, when discussed in terms of rates, percentages, and estimates, the morbidity of abortion attained new rhetorical worth as a subjunctive reminder of luckless, unwanted pregnancy—not as a bodily scar left to remind womankind of Nature's will. The statistics of abortion's harm became a kind of generalized, unavowed memory: medical experts evoked a *likely* past of routine conduct and, thus, a *probable* future.[66]

Probabilistic, nonspecific memory is "at once highly intrusive and completely anonymous, self-scrutinizing and other-directed, familiar and impersonal."[67]

Records suggested that any woman, maybe, would risk her life to maintain control of her life if deprived of adequate resources such as contraception. Further, secrecy and uncertainty surrounding records of abortion became resources for, rather than obstacles to, statistical recollection. Concealments and confusions that twisted the record formed a thick burl of archival amnesias, but that thickness was itself calculable and from it an impersonal memory of unseen risks could be approximated. Moreover, epidemiological estimates were founded on confidential data from patient records and interview subjects—which people aborted, when, and for what reasons—were all anonymous categories. As Edward Casey notes of memory's general limits: "That which is evoked . . . is the remindand, but it is crucial to stress that it is *e-voked*: called forth from obscurity and often still partaking in some of the dark Lethic indistinctness from which it arises."[68] A statistical memory of the social "nature" of abortion's pathology did not just partake of the amnestic indistinctness in the record but was in fact founded on an intensification of strategic amnesia.[69] When viewed from the altitude of populations the sub rosa character of abortion became the hollowed-out substance of memory about it.

Hospital case series, public records, and surveys constituted the new bureaucratic, numerical memory work.[70] Clinical series are aggregates of selective data derived from observations and treatments. Beginning in the 1930s, a number of institutions started to publish case series covering multiple years, usually encompassing several hundred or several thousand patients, such as Kopp's study of the first ten thousand cases from Sanger's Clinical Research Bureau.[71] Public health records include tabulations of death and disease, vital statistics at the municipal, state, and federal levels. Taussig's study of maternal mortality for the Children's Bureau, which relied heavily on vital statistics, is an important example.[72] Surveys also began to appear in the 1930s, largely interviews such as Regine Stix and Dorothy Wiehl's surveys of postabortion patients funded by the Milbank Memorial Fund.[73]

Each of these broad sets of enumerating techniques depended on clinical modes of perception, yet of necessity looked away from the physical body toward community. Where a clinical gaze transforms ante- and postmortem traces of disturbance into an archive of observations, testimony, and tests, an administrative medical gaze organizes such archives into tables of events.[74] Case series and vital statistics mass and partition disparate traumas, turning an immense, disorganized archive of unique incidents into a ledger of risks. This conforms to a shift in the level of abstraction at which danger is assessed; morbidity scales up from patients to populations. Interview-based surveys synthesize stories of specific people into a demographic stranger. In terms of abortion, the stranger's relation to others is fixed by a medical procedure: whether or not she had had one (or more) and if so, whether or not it was sanctioned.[75] Even though confidence in the numbers was low, the "average abortion" replaced the clinical anecdote as the common coin of medical discourse.[76] Better yet, the average abortion *became* the anecdote, the "*figurative and schematical adumbration*" of the abortion problem.[77]

The average abortion was roughly modal, not arithmetic, meaning it reflected the most commonly occurring sorts of abortions. Figuratively, probabilities based on the most common incidences realize the recursive potential of morbidity through a different tropology from the violation of natural law. The latter required inversion of the body, the interior becoming exterior, and the reductive substitution of texts for direct observations. The average abortion too was metonymic, with numbers condensing series of cases, interviews, and so on into quantitative values, but because these data were amalgamated from specific instances, they were metonymies of metonymies. The harm to women and fetuses was still the primary recursive agent in the rhetoric but at a further, more abstracted, remove. *Enumeration* is a wholly different tropological relation from chiastic inversion. Enumeration divides and classifies and is, of course, necessary to calculation. The average abortion revealed no inner truth; it amassed a dispersed, contextual truth about disease-as-error by segmenting the harm from accidents and mistakes and organizing them. To produce discourse critical of the status quo, physicians *transumed* morbidity from the practice into a calculation of civilization, its past and its future, thus turning women's risk profile into a stable position for addressing threats.

Vital Statistics: *Quantifying a Memory of Danger*

The bedeviling ellipses perforating records on abortion became resources of statistical recollection through corrections made for known reliability errors, particularly within rates of incidence and maternal mortality. In 1942, Halbert Dunn, then attached to the Census Bureau, explained to NCMH conference participants why solid data on mortality and incidence was hard to come by. It so happened that despite a century of regulation and a surfeit of indignation, abortion had not meant something medically specific until the International List of Causes of Death (ICD) rationalized its definition in 1938: "the termination of a uterine pregnancy prior to 7 lunar months (28 weeks) of gestation (whether the child was born dead or alive)."[78] The ICD was first adopted in 1900, when twenty-six nations met at a conference hosted by the International Statistical Institute in Paris.[79] Nonseptic abortion went unlisted as a cause of death until 1920 and septic abortion until 1929; even then, many abortions could be subsumed under other classifications.[80] Further, abortion was listed as a primary factor in cases reporting two or more causes of death only after the U.S. Census Bureau revised its *Manual of Joint Causes of Death* in 1939. According to Dunn the revised categories could capture "practically all of the deaths certified as due to abortion," *except* that error, deception, and conflicted definitions assumed by existing data meant that "about an equal number of deaths from abortion [we]re concealed."[81] Indeed, P. K. Whelpton, who directed a Scripps survey of couples' ideal number of children, stated at the same conference: "It seems to me *one of the fundamental things we have to settle is a matter of definition of abortion if we are to secure comparable statistics.*"[82] Records of maternal mortality were based on noncomparable, irregularly reported data, which put consistent tabulation out of reach. The only option was to infer.[83]

Yet inference, which works the seams of fragmentary perception, is not a defeat of recollection any more than snapping photos is. It simply evokes and alludes to memory in a different way. The correction Dunn applied is a simple example of turning a palpable, invisible presence into a visible regularity, a known unknown in which "the already perceived parts of an object suggest to the perceiver the presumptive character of those parts that have not yet been perceived."[84]

Taussig's 1936 estimates, which Dunn was addressing, epitomized a subjunctive memory of abortion pieced together through inference. Quantifying the lethality to women of poorly executed procedures was crucial to materializing a memory of women's privation through morbidity, and Taussig's numbers swiftly became the indispensable statement on the matter. He concluded that approximately seven hundred thousand abortions occurred annually and that about eight thousand maternal deaths resulted, with a probable range of eight thousand to ten thousand. He arrived at these figures by estimating the ratio of abortions relative to births and multiplying the result by the estimated percentage of maternal mortality, which he extrapolated from unrelated studies.[85] His numbers were the most authoritative to date; nonetheless, they were similar in spirit to earlier, less evidenced calculations. The 1881 Michigan study had found one million abortions per year and six thousand maternal deaths, for example.[86] Birth control advocates such as William Robinson, who reckoned one million illegal abortions annually in 1919, or Rongy, who figured 1,250,000 in 1931, offered higher estimates of total abortion numbers. The common understanding was that many thousands of women died, mainly from sepsis.[87]

Two decades after Taussig estimated seven hundred thousand abortions per year, researchers at the PPFA conference unsuccessfully attempted to refine the numbers by reconciling data from Kinsey, various hospitals, surveys, and census figures. The Statistics Committee, lead by Tietze, instead offered a woolly estimate of two hundred thousand to twelve hundred thousand per year.[88] In 1969, Tietze and Sarah Lewit wrote in *Scientific American* that "no information on which a better estimate can be made has been obtained since that time."[89] Depending on how many abortions one assumed, the number of deaths would rise or fall based on estimated mortality rates, ranging from about 1 percent of induced abortions to sometimes more than 2 percent. Such calculations materialized a likely past and projected the future as a gross, per annum collective memory of death. If X number of women had abortions in a year, then Y number of catastrophes struck society. A cascade of loss became a formula of once and future *probable* events, segmented annually.[90]

Virginia Hamilton, a physician and NCMH researcher, confirmed Taussig's centrality, writing that the "estimates of its magnitude as presented conservatively by Taussig are too familiar to be repeated here."[91] They were repeated, though, despite the fact that Dunn argued at the 1942 NCMH symposium that three thousand to four thousand deaths was a better "'guesstimate'" based on recent census data, which would account for 30 to 35 percent of all maternal deaths.[92] Taussig agreed in discussion of Dunn's paper, although he felt five thousand deaths should be the upper limit.[93] In 1948, Tietze revised the mortality estimate downward again to less than two thousand deaths based on a 1944 Special Study by the Census Bureau, which adjusted its mortality data in light of the 1938 ICD.[94] The average abortion was probably less lethal than had been surmised, or it had become less lethal because of improvements in antisepsis and increasing skill among abortionists, yet it was still impossible to say with certainty how many women died every year. A figure of five thousand to ten thousand deaths, roughly based on Taussig's 1936 analysis, maintained its currency into the 1960s, often reiterated and seldom explained, regardless of the revisions Dunn, Taussig, and Tietze had offered.[95] Whatever the estimate, researchers consistently noted botched abortions as the single greatest source of maternal mortality, around a quarter of the deaths per year at minimum, and a significant factor in sterility and chronic illness.[96]

The variability of estimates is distracting in that it invites debate over the fidelity of abortion statistics before *Roe* as a kind of recollection.[97] If measures are weak, then they are not really memory but are in fact its opposite. Accuracy is not the point of remembrance, placement is, and the necessity of inference independent of its rigor reinforced neo-Malthusian countermemories that positioned the United States as slouching into the future. For such a dangerous threat to public health, if we could not see the social body's nature any better than through inconstant, corrected, disputable estimates, then the nation was indeed making itself sick through poor administration of a known risk. For instance, Iago Galdston of the New York Academy of Medicine bemoaned in 1955 that abortion's epidemiology was "corrupted by confusion in the law, by the legalistic shackling of the medical profession, by the morass of superstition that surrounds the subject, etc."[98] That roughly half of abortions went unreported was a sign of a social affliction, as was women's resorting to abortion in the first place for lack of knowledge about its danger. The fact that consistent pathological categories and reporting practices were still being developed in the late 1930s only reinforced countermemories of privation. The indissoluble amnesias haunting statistical study *were* memory, a kind of affirmative disappearance or perceptible absence.

A statistical accounting of fetal life received less and different attention. In 1942, Taussig foregrounded an "infinite" loss of life before birth in regard to vital statistics, but he and other neo-Malthusians weighed risks to embryonic life asymmetrically against risks to maternal life, whether abortion was considered a reluctant necessity, a justifiable homicide, or a religious question more than a medical one. Physicians generally still held that life began at conception but that developing life did not warrant the same rights as adult humans. Here again, Taussig proved definitively conventional. Sounding like Weiss or Green from the earlier era, he stated that "we know from incontrovertible evidence, especially the development of uni-ovular twins, that all the essential factors in the development of the future child are determined at the first union of the two sex cells and that life begins then and there." He assessed two lives of different significance, however, stating, "We cannot weigh in the same balance the life of a two-month embryo and the fully developed life of the young mother. Nevertheless the loss of these embryos occurring by the thousands is a serious handicap to the work of the world. It interrupts the important obligations of the mother to her family, it is a serious financial burden, and often leads to partial or complete disability of the women who have aborted."[99] This line of reasoning updated the developmental logic of quickening by way of cell theory, creating multiple thresholds for in-utero life (a logic featured in arguments over fetal viability).[100] It also melded fetal loss back into maternal harm.

There were others more and less concerned over the loss of fetal life. Among "life at conception" adherents such as Joseph Donnelly, justifications for abortion were sometimes contested by analogy with justifiable homicide.[101] In contrast, William Robinson exclaimed it was "fantastically grotesque and criminally stupid to make such a fuss over the removal of a cluster of inanimate cells," although he did oppose abortion during the last three months of gestation.[102] Generally, though, discussions of fetal life in the medical literature on abortion from the 1930s to the 1960s are minimal in comparison with the pages devoted to morbidity in women. Sara Dubow finds that from the late 1930s, increasing attention was paid to embryology in public discourse;[103] yet when one looks at physicians most concerned with abortion, there is little explicit incorporation of the rapidly developing discourse on prenatal life. Surely physicians were exposed to and thinking through such material, but it did not yet dominate the rhetoric on abortion. Eventually, fetal morbidity would become critical again, but not yet.[104] Among neo-Malthusians up to the early 1960s, however, the harm of abortion that substantiated a memory of privation was based principally on the secret dangers faced by women, not the loss of fetal life.[105]

Social Data: An Impersonal Memory of Risky Subjects

For all the importance of vital statistics and their corrections, anonymous categories of patients and research subjects provided key elements for a counter-memory of privation. Confidentiality turns the secrecy of anonymity into a mode of disclosure, another sort of affirmative disappearance wherein seeing commonality is dependent on masking individuality. For example, if 22 percent of white married women had aborted at least once by the time they were forty-five, that meant that you or your neighbor, your co-worker or your daughter, your aunt or your friend had a one in five chance of being a criminal.[106] This was so for every white married woman and for none in particular. It could have happened yesterday or twenty years ago, in a doctor's office or a home, by drug or surgery or both. Research methods demanded that medical experts abstract individuals' background, motivation, technique, and results into normative categories as a part of data collection and analysis, as well as to protect medical privacy. Beyond their value to inquiry, epidemiological typologies set recursive parameters for enumerating an impersonal memory, further segmenting the annual flow of abortion's danger into branches of descriptive characteristics among women—the ready and familiar metrics of race, age, marital status, class, education, and religion—that could be combined and recombined to describe vectors and pathways, tempos and dispersions of risk. Coupled with statistical inference, anonymity structured remembrance as a litany of imaginable threats by which to "allude to the purely possible," of pathologies in the subjunctive.[107]

As with vital statistics, social data exposed stresses placed on the nation by an outdated order of fertility control. Abortion as a statistical distribution made available to the public a consolidated, faceless version of itself.[108] The PPFA conference held at Arden House and the New York Academy of Medicine is the most salient example of social data's function for recursive positioning within abortion rhetoric. The conference did not pioneer abortion epidemiology, as proved by its dissatisfying revision of Taussig's incidence estimate, but it did establish an up-to-date numerical memory of induced abortion's social profile. Calderone was fully aware that there was "nothing earth-shaking or new about the Conference."[109] Yet the gathering was not redundant; newer pools of data were presented, existing data were synthesized, and psychiatrists aired emerging socioeconomic justifications for therapeutic abortion.[110]

Like earlier, more conservative physicians, authorities at Arden House discussed abortion as primarily a white affliction that differentially affected women depending on their relative needs and advantages. However, the differences between women only demonstrated a variance of risk. All roads led to a rate of illegal procedures "many times the number consistent with sound medical or social practice," according to the conference's concluding statement, which is something of a puzzle because experts have never agreed, then or now, on what an acceptable number might be.[111] In fact, as conferees debated what to say in the concluding statement, Alan Guttmacher remarked, "Of course, to have no induced abortions at all, whether legal or illegal, would be our goal, but that is unattainable, obviously."[112] If abortion is a sign of pathological error, any number of abortions, legal or not, index a backward culture. The threshold of decline is one. Social data provided a means of refining the distribution of risk; hence, abortions among white women were of special interest because their children were valued more culturally and because data suggested that white women would or could turn to abortion more readily if circumstances made pregnancy undesirable.

The hitch was that almost any circumstance could make pregnancy undesirable. Whichever way experts dissected the data, women were risky subjects, white women particularly, because some reason to abort never seemed far away. Which is to say, medical authorities viewed abortion as a communicable illness that one "caught" most of the time by being pregnant and not wanting a (or another) child, for any of a variety of reasons. As Lisa Finn notes, women have been and are increasingly treated as "risky subjects" in medical and health discourses, which assumes that "women are dangerous *because* they are women."[113] Social data presented all manner of women as abortion risks despite their various situations.[114] Hence, the effort to cultivate immunity turned on implanting the necessary resistance to ending pregnancy within women generally.

Consider the two most debated scenarios dating from the early days of antiabortion activism: the unwed primiparous and the married multiparous woman. The stigma of unwed motherhood had been understood as a powerful motive for abortion for some time.[115] Mary Rogers, the first sensationalized victim of abortion in the United States, was an unwed youth from New York City.[116] Physicians frequently shared stories of young women, almost always white, desperate to escape their situation.[117] At Arden House, Kinsey was tasked with presenting a statistical overview of illegal abortion to conferees. He presented the despairing young woman as a quantifiable symptom of racialized cultural hysteria. Based on available data and interviews of nearly eight thousand women for his volume on female sexuality, he reported that the vast majority of white, unmarried college women, 88 to 95 percent, ended pregnancies, whereas "socially lower-level" African American women were typically proud of their unwed pregnancies. He concluded, clearly contrasting whites to African Americans, "That is the product of our education that is not teaching us [whites] to avoid abortions, but to become hysterically disturbed over premarital pregnancy"; attitudes about abortion had hardened since the beginning of the twentieth century, thus magnifying the shame.[118] Kinsey offered a probabilistic countermemory of privation (lack of education) in opposition to the moralism of early antiabortionists, yet he preserved their emphasis on whiteness as a key factor of sickness when combined with higher education and marital status.

Like the stigma of unwed motherhood, family planning among married women with children had long been understood, if reluctantly, as a powerful motive for abortion. The mother who aborted was somewhat unthinkable or considered deranged in the late 1800s.[119] The belief that maternity would convert unenthusiastic young women into mothering angels was compelling both ideologically and sentimentally. After all, if ignorance contributed to abortion, a woman with children must know what motherhood truly is and feel duty bound to carry a pregnancy to term, shouldn't she? That she might end it based on the firsthand wisdom of what it means to have another mouth to feed, another child to raise and to love, was a difficult pill for many physicians to swallow. Within medical discourse, abortion was not seen as the outcome of maternal knowledge, only of the lack of knowledge. However, Kinsey's survey data, like other data from the 1930s onward, demonstrated that a substantial portion of married women had had at least one abortion.[120] Among African Americans, the rate was lower than that of whites for women without a college education, but higher for those with a college education.[121] Either way, abortions among married women made up the lion's share of all inductions. Maternity led to abortion—as some observers had contended many decades before.[122] Why?

Social data provided no clear answers, but studies on the rate among married women required that the etiological thesis of "ignorance as efficient cause" be nuanced. Conferees at Arden House argued that abortions among multiparous women were, not surprisingly, from a failure to use contraception. As to why contraception was not more effective, Calderone summarized Kinsey's presentation of data: "Most failures were not failures in contraceptive method but failure to use the method, either through ignorance, inertia, or carelessness."[123] Beyond a certain quotient of negligence, ignorance had shifted from a lack of knowledge about maternity to a lack of knowledge about contraception. Social data sketched the outline of millions of personal and social failures, a far-flung obstruction of healthy motherhood caused by ignorance of birth control.

Clearly the delineation of abortion rates was not limited to parous and marital status. Religion seemed to be an insignificant factor, whereas education was a powerful one, as illustrated in the above examples. Wealth, too, produced marked differences in rates. The differential rates for services within and across hospitals reported at the PPFA conference indexed the stratification of reproduction by affluence. Data from several New York hospitals indicated that patients in private facilities and those in private wards at voluntary (private, nonprofit) hospitals had a significantly higher ratio of therapeutic abortions compared with general service patients at voluntary hospitals or those at municipal facilities. This pattern tracked with an increasing variety of psychiatric indicators offered as rationales for abortion, while medical indications for abortion had been on the decline for twenty years.[124] From the 1930s onward, affluent women were better able to secure an abortion on mental health grounds. Sophia Kleegman, clinical professor of obstetrics and gynecology at New York

University, contended that the privilege of psychiatric abortions meant that need of and access to abortion was undemocratically and unjustly distributed; this point ended up in the conference's concluding statement.[125] The "average" abortion recalled a society of reproductive haves and have-nots and put it on display. However, this did not mean for physicians that all women should possess the privileges of wealthier women to have such abortions. If abortion was a social disease, the privilege enacted by wealthier, savvier women was not supportable, for it was still a sign of pathology; yet enforced maternity was pathological as well. Greater access to psychiatric abortions was not a policy model as much as a demonstration of the existing, warped landscape.

The one crosscutting factor that *did* differentiate pathological import was race, as abortion remained largely a white problem for the medical establishment. Racial anxiety was less overt among progressives of this period. Concern for the fate of a white race had disappeared from the literature on abortion largely by the 1930s; in fact, the notion of race suicide, on the rare occasion it was mentioned at all, was treated derisively.[126] Still, white pregnancies counted differently. First, abortion's morbidity was almost exclusively divided into white and black racial demographics, operating within a standard U.S. racial dichotomy. Sometimes a hospital in New York would include data broken out for Puerto Rican women, but in general, the chiaroscuro data reinforced amnesia in regard to all other racial groupings, especially in the case of racial hybridity, hence making white risk all the more stark. Second, emphasis placed on white pregnancies among PPFA conference-goers is consonant with Rickie Solinger's conclusions, regarding pregnancy in post–World War II America, that white babies were more important. Solinger details state and institutional policies directed at unwed mothers that pressured unwed white women to carry their pregnancies to term and give them up for adoption to "deserving couples," whereas black women were forced to keep their children as a punishment.[127]

The greatest "tell" of Arden House conferees' racial myopia, over and above comments like Kinsey's reproof of white hysteria, was appendix D, "Demographic Characteristics of Females Interviewed by the Staff of the Institute for Sex Research, Compared with the Urban White Population," prepared by Tietze.[128] Tietze was tasked with assessing the statistical representativeness of the interview data presented by Kinsey in the 1958 Institute for Sex Research (ISR) book, *Pregnancy, Birth and Abortion*, which detailed in full what Kinsey had synopsized in 1955 at Arden House.[129] Tietze carried out his task only in terms of white, urban females, concluding that the data were representative.

But the book included notable and important information on black women of which Tietze made no mention, even though Kinsey himself used racial difference to leverage his concern over white reproductive mores; the data were not of sufficient interest to the editorial team. In that sense, the conference simply updated a constant in the discourse since the 1850s: abortion's epidemiology reminded observers of existential, self-destructive dangers that threatened whiteness.[130] Women were risky subjects, but the risks nonwhite women took were less alarming—not because they were more immune, as Kinsey implied, but because the medical establishment was less concerned about their lives and pregnancies.

Although the language of risk was in its infancy in public health during the period in question, the statistical memory presented a situation wherein abortion placed a pox, hypothetically, on anyone's house.[131] Women were risky subjects because they were women; the metrics categorizing them simply reflected a variable, subjunctive memory of the privations that catalyzed those risks. If a woman was without means or a secure environment, those inadequacies encouraged dangerous behavior. Conversely, if a woman had enough money or station to secure a safe, legal procedure, that advantage also posed a risk because it too encouraged women to thwart maternity for apparently unsupportable reasons. If a woman was not married and was without children, the stigma of being pregnant created risk by putting extraordinary pressure on her to abort. If she had children, the economic and personal cost of additional children created pressure to abort as well. Whatever the case, women without alternatives *and* those with alternatives, women without children *and* those with children, presented risk vectors within the social body because these circumstances could all lead someone to seek abortion. A remedy would be achieved if control mechanisms could activate the social and institutional antibodies necessary to fight *an uninformed decision*. Parallel to the shepherding of a medical pastorate, "permitting the embryo to survive" required neo-Malthusian physicians also to interrupt a woman's choice to interrupt gestation, either by blocking her decision or by convincing her that abortion did not offer protection from greater hardship.[132]

If Mrs. S. of Chicago, who died of an embolism, personified abortion in medical discourse of 1904, then by the late 1930s that emblematic stranger was the white, married mother with too many children who, if she died related to pregnancy, died from a botched abortion more than from any other cause. The "average abortion," then, had not changed the recursive dynamic fundamentally; woman's relation to her pregnant self was still the base fold, the fundamental crease in time around which the past, present, and future could be brought together and positioned evaluatively. The woman who did not seek maternal fulfillment, or who sought it on her own terms despite the unpredictable risks of the underground, still did not exist.[133] Now, however, the woman was visible as an anonymous specter summoned by the data, not by vengeful punishments before nature.[134] The pathogenic nature of her self-relation became a state of misapprehended risk, not obliviousness to ethics.

Inclusion: The New Order of Neo-Malthusian Memory Work

The recursive potential of the average abortion, if it was to capture the whole of progress over time, depended on a highly striated national and global space. It is to be expected that a world imagined on Malthusian terms will be deeply banded by birthrates, death rates, and demographic trends, because biopolitical progress is in the end measured by those in such a world. The very concept of progress seems impossible without lines that give the idea of "moving forward," markers of advancement.[135] Accordingly, medical authorities had successfully turned old distinctions for the spate of damaged bodies into risk vectors. It is significant that the emphasis on statistical memory brought with it an accentuated crosswise, per annum segmentation of danger. Across time, vertically, if you will, annualized striae stabilized comparison on a Malthusian scale of civilization. Across the population, horizontally, the yearly toll of abortion could be partitioned in terms of vitality and demography. Each of these divisions had its own subdivisions, to be sure, such as hemorrhagic or septic death. The flow of disease to and from abortion was now embodied within a richly lined, countable space, as were recommended treatments and the progress associated with them.

Administrative Reason and the New Treatment Regime

In that a countermemory of privation mutated the sickness of abortion from one of individualized, moral alienation to that of collectively ineffectual carrots and sticks, neo-Malthusians founded a new "*theater* for practical *actions*."[136] From an administrative viewpoint, the social body more so than the corporeal became that theater. Typologies of vital and social data, rather than a homogenizing physiology, were the rhetorical *actants* that reached out and gathered together the space of the social body under the sign of abortion's pathology and, concomitantly, defined the space of treatment. As Fulsome wrote to Taussig, "The real problem includes social, economic and educational factors in *both causes* and *methods of control* of induced abortion."[137] A recursive system that spatializes the memory of disease across a population disposes the discourse of potential remedies toward broad cultural and institutional conditions. To that end, neo-Malthusians proposed a slate of reforms that would better calibrate social and economic forces in support of a medically managed, small, nuclear family, thus treating abortion by acting on the culture that spawned it. So doing, neo-Malthusians also used abortion control measures to envelope the whole of civilizing progress through different societies' relative protections from induced abortion. As Canguilhem noted, "The Plan is the modern dress of the idea of Providence."[138]

Treatment regimes are always "regimes of living," or what Stephen Collier and Andrew Lakoff describe as "configurations of normative, technical, and po-litical elements that are brought into alignment in situations that present ethical problems—that is, situations in which the question of how to live is at stake." Medicalized stories about how to live involve "reasoning about and acting with respect to an understanding of the good," inevitably the elastic good of health.[139] In terms of individual patients, *treatment regimes* refers to series of procedures, drug regimens, and so forth. When directed at social diseases, treatment re-gimes become collaborative efforts that often require ways of life to be remade in their "normative, technical and political elements," or correcting the errors within them, in Canguilhem's language. For example, public health campaigns directed at reducing obesity through dietary changes and exercise can be under-stood as treatment regimes for populations; they operate as regimes of living.[140] Such modes of treatment do not follow from diagnosis like a schedule for tak-ing medications; they offer ongoing means of diagnosing the wisdom of various ways of living, of placing the self in relation to generalized notions of sickness and well-being.

In *Abortion, Spontaneous and Induced*, Taussig offered a broad prospectus for a national treatment regime, really a new art of reproductive governance centered on abortion. He set forth a ten-point plan to address abortion that included more study, better training, better facilities, improved home and work conditions, humane indications for abortion, legal reform, education about abortion's danger, improved economic opportunity, sterilization for the unfit, and maternal health clinics.[141] He spoke to apparent causes of, gaps in knowl-edge about, and medical care for abortion. More important, the governmentality of reproduction was inverted relative to birth control advocacy, from contraception as a means of resisting cultural and institutional forces to cultural and institutional forces as means of resisting abortion. The program envisaged a regime of living organized to end social disease, not to implement planned parenthood. A clear distinction between *abortion* control and *birth* control had emerged.[142]

The difference in objects of control is important. Socialist and progressive birth controllers, especially of the early twentieth century, saw contraception as a means of contesting capitalism, lifting up the poor, and exercising self-determination.[143] Each of these perspectives, despite significant differences between them, understood reproductive control as a technology of resistance to, if not of emancipation from, capitalism or patriarchy by way of fewer pregnancies. In contrast, Taussig did not see contraception clinics and public sex education as forms of resistance; rather, they were among a number of tools for the elimination of unnecessary and dangerous abortions, along with more hospital beds for patients with complications, labor laws that prevented businesses from firing expecting mothers, tax policy that favored child-rearing, housing projects for the poor, and liberalized laws allowing abortion for "mental defectives" and in cases of rape or incest.[144] That birth control led to greater reproductive freedom was a supplemental advantage to disease prevention, if greater freedom was a goal at all, but it was not the primary good of the program. Abortion control regimes provided the means to see seemingly disparate social, economic, institutional, and personal conditions as connected pathological conditions and to elaborate new configurations.

Taussig's control model had taken hold immediately. Medical students and faculty at the Women's Medical College in Philadelphia were paraphrasing Taussig as early as 1937, reiterating his program in a reduced form and explaining abortion in terms of sexually transmitted illness, as Margaret Welsh did in her thesis: "As the mask has been lifted from venereal disease in recent times, so it should be lifted from abortion."[145] Participants of the 1942 NCMH conference embraced Taussig's program in its broad outlines if not its particulars, as when Black argued that control of abortion required "the development of more wisdom in living—in our own living."[146] To that end, in the fourth and final session, devoted to abortion control, discussants considered such topics as the limitations of legal remedies, motherhood insurance as a disincentive, improved pregnancy reporting, sex education, contraception clinics, sterilization provision, and pre-pregnancy counseling.[147] The concluding statement from Arden House was more emphatic and included many proposals similar to Taussig's, such as more research, counseling centers, improved availability of contraception, more and better sex education, and more liberal, uniform laws. As one physician aptly put it, "This question has to do with the whole policy of government in our country, the future of which depends to a large extent on how we raise our children and how well it is made possible for us to raise them."[148] Access to the entirety of culture and society could be gained through the factors that contributed to abortion.

More conservative physicians resisted the shift from moral cultivation to conduct management. Although they appreciated the attention to abortion, they found the new emphasis of governmentality troubling. George Kosmak, an avowed anti-Malthusian who chaired the 1942 session on abortion control, objected to the term "control of abortion" because it "confuses the rights and the wrongs of the picture."[149] A neo-Malthusian but observant Catholic, Howard Taylor opposed any significant liberalization of abortion indicators as part of legal reform. In his concluding remarks at the 1942 gathering, he hoped that premarital clinics would teach "the concept that human life is sacred."[150] In a debate thirteen years later over the concluding statement at Arden House, he disapproved of socioeconomic indicators on grounds that they were "completely uncontrollable" and suggested the "health of the mother" instead as the proper legal boundary. He eventually refused to sign that final statement.[151] The change from a medical pastorate to an abortion control regime was unsettling to him, not because the latter was less devoted to ending the practice but because the very mentality of control transformed what interrupted pregnancies signaled about the nation's plagued condition.

The normative, technical, and political problem for neo-Malthusians was to produce a regime of living wherein abortion would become obsolete. Abortion control, therefore, was the tie that bound together a host of related biopolitical projects. Control was not a matter of preventive medicine as much as of aligning institutions and patterns of conduct to preempt the interruption of life. The model first outlined by Taussig did not "have the stability or concrete institutionalization of a political regime." Instead, it was an "abstract congeries of ethical reasoning and practice . . . incited by or reworked" around the problem of abortion, "taking diverse actual forms" as experts and organizations adopted its principles.[152]

Abortion persisted as a point of inclusion but differently. Neo-Malthusians did not depend on elaborate description of damaged bodies (*peristatic* figuration) to place contemporary society in a broader critique of civilization. The average abortion allowed doctors like Taussig to fold time and place through the complexity of decisions about interrupting pregnancy, the past, present, and future encompassed within a unifying matrix of factorable variance. They divided out causal conditions so as to capture the smallest elements of ordinary life within a distribution of risk. The figurative logic of this sort of division is sometimes called *merismus* in the Greek or *distributio* in the Latin, meaning specifically to divide the whole into its constituent parts.[153] It is also a form of amplification, or expansion, like peristasis, except that a distribution is more than the descriptive list of details. Merismic division orders events by their necessary elements. In neo-Malthusian rhetoric, the metonymic and enumerative transumption of harm from abortion into discourse was coupled with a division of a sick culture into constituent risk vectors. The space of society was a changeable mixture of socioeconomic pressure points, not a singular organic system. As a result, new treatment regimes were designed to intervene at those points, attaching themselves to the pathological conditions implicated by abortion such as the cost of housing and employment opportunities. Abortion control consolidated society and culture into a complicated assemblage of interactive parts, such that factors as disparate as tax policy and the availability of hospital beds could be brought together under the same critique of national vitality. It was now possible to contest the entirety of how we regulate our lives, "the whole policy of government," through abortion control.

Re-placing the United States

The physicians I have discussed all imagined contemporary civilization being replaced with a better, more advanced one where abortion was not encouraged. They had ruptured the established order regarding induced abortion and reoriented it away from a sign of moral corruption. However, spatial transformation erases familiar landmarks, and so the new plan to eliminate the old habit of abortion required *re*-placing the United States on a Malthusian scale of civilization.[154] If we were not fading from moral degradation, how did we stack up in the world?

The United States no longer chased a wan and fashionable France into extinction; instead, it trailed a clear-eyed and modern Scandinavia into the future. After a 1934 Inter-Scandinavian Congress of Lawyers recommended reforming the law, one by one its member nations undertook modifications that legalized "social" indicators to varying degrees.[155] As in the United States, the global

Depression had cast abortion in a different light for Scandinavians.[156] Combined with programs of economic support for mothers, contraception education and provision, and clinical research of abortion, Scandinavians were building control regimes broadly similar to those called for by Taussig and others.

These changes took place over thirty years, with an initial surge of activity in the late 1930s and early 1940s. In 1935, Iceland became the second country after the Soviet Union to reform its law, allowing abortions for the life and health of the mother as well as sterilization for women facing risky pregnancies and compelling physicians to offer birth control advice when asked.[157] Sweden passed its law in 1938 (amended in 1941, 1942, and 1946), which allowed for maternal health and humanitarian abortions if approved by two physicians, and eugenic ones too; a special committee of the Royal Medical Board dealt with abortion matters, including all eugenic cases.[158] Denmark legalized "extended medical indications" in 1939, comprising life and health of the mother and "some degree of other conditions of a social nature," but this proved too vague and in 1956 the law was revised to be more specific. Approval for nonmedical reasons came from a regional board of two physicians and a representative of Mother's Aid, a social services organization.[159] From 1930, the Norwegian Medical Association endorsed a law that allowed medical, humanitarian, and eugenic indications.[160] A version was approved in 1960 and went into effect in 1964, under which approval rested with a commission of two physicians and the husband (if the woman was married); socioeconomic indications were not legalized until 1975.[161] Finland adopted a law similar to Sweden's in 1950.[162]

Scandinavian reforms were held up for praise by American observers such as Alexander Simon, who wrote in 1964, "The Scandinavian laws best exemplify a modern liberal statute. Since their indications are well specified, evaluations of over-all results can be precise."[163] Further, the supervision of medical boards in Scandinavia resembled the "therapeutic abortion committees" that many U.S. hospitals began establishing in the 1950s after Guttmacher championed the practice at Mt. Sinai in Baltimore in 1942 (the first review committee was established in Detroit in the late 1930s).[164] The most significant proof of Scandinavia's place in the geography of neo-Malthusians came in the structure and discussion of the PPFA conference. The first major session of the gathering was "Abortion in the Scandinavian Countries." Consideration of abortion in the United States literally occurred in the wake of Norway, Denmark, and Sweden. Participants urged that the United States adopt the advisory systems of these other nations and "follow the lead of our Scandinavian brethren" on the law, because their laws were more honest and, presumably, more effective at reducing the incidence rate. The concluding statement recommended modeling consultation centers "after the Scandinavian centers now in existence" because such consults "help women realize that abortion, whether legal or illegal, may not be the best way or only solution for medical, social, or economic problems." A medical pastorate had thus passed into a system of therapeutic interviews. The closing statement also endorsed a model penal code drafted by the American Law Institute, which included psychiatric, humanitarian, and eugenic indicators, much as Scandinavian laws did.[165]

The contrast with opinion about policy in the Soviet Union and Japan is instructive. Although abortion was legal in the Soviet Union from 1920 to 1936, and relegalized in 1955, the early experiment functioned as a cautionary tale rather than as an ideal. As far back as the 1905 Women's Congress, socialist advocates had called for legalizing abortion in Russia.[166] After the revolution, legal abortion became a reality but the Soviets did not have effective contraceptive support or sex education programs in the 1920s.[167] Abortions had to be performed in hospital clinics and the basic procedure was dilation and curettage.[168] Abortion functioned essentially as the primary mode of birth control for many Soviet women and in that sense the policy was directly counter to American neo-Malthusian biopolitics. The experience provided a wealth of data that demonstrated, in particular, that a properly performed abortion was actually quite safe.[169] However, data also demonstrated that repeated manual abortions, even if performed competently, could risk sterility and other complications.[170] The Soviet approach demonstrated how *not* to reform abortion practices, essentially illustrating Taussig's 1916 concern that abortion on demand was regressive, not progressive.

Japan legalized abortion in 1948 but received far less attention than Scandinavian countries or the Soviet Union. Japanese officials were understood to be responding largely to population growth; they began encouraging contraception as well. Again, this ran counter to American biopolitics because Japan's implementation was perceived as primarily turning abortion into a tool for population control rather than treating it as a social disease that needed to be curbed. Japan was also seen as morally "other" and noncomparable by some, as it was not a Christian culture. In fact, it was discussed among the sociological conditions of "primitive" cultures within the PPFA conference.[171]

Placement of the United States on a scale of civilization still depended on a modernist logic that had different cultures occupying different stages of advancement in a "historical queue," where to share the same space was to be of the same time as well; but the world was queuing up differently.[172] The scene and surroundings determining one's spot in the disorderly global cavalcade had changed.[173] Instead of ignorant women without virtue being vengefully punished, women without knowledge were taking dangerous risks. The surroundings of these two sets of women likewise matched the biopolitics of fearing or favoring small families. The women in the former scenario lived in a world increasingly underpopulated by white Christians, whereas the latter ones lived in a world of social and economic hardship aggravated by too many children. Anti-Malthusians saw the United States as near the lower end of a scale of advancement defined by pronatal virtues relative to its presumed white, European peer group. Neo-Malthusians saw the nation lagging behind on a scale defined by effective fertility management also relative to its white, European peers, but for them, Scandinavia occupied a future space, not a past one. A nation that fosters abortion is sick, agreed the physicians; but how and why it was sick and whether one recurred to physiological trauma or the average abortion would determine the way that that nation remembered itself as it endeavored to heal its ways of living.

5

"The Lesser of Threatened Evils" | Therapeutic Amnesias

If we are to come before the people and the legislators, asking them to unshackle us and to extend our prerogatives in this field, we must affirm our position, making it very clear that *we are not indifferent to anything and everything that is antecedent to, that is involved in, and that follows upon, an abortion;* that we look upon abortion as undesirable, save under given conditions, when it must be considered lesser than, if not the least of, the threatened evils, and that we solicit consent for the free exercise of our judgment *within these commitments.*

—IAGO GALDSTON, "Final Discussion," *Abortion in the United States*

Contrary to conventional wisdom, abortion has always been legal in the United States, although regulation, in law and in practice, has varied widely from minimal to all but banned. To this point I have examined what physicians did and wrote about criminally induced abortions but another discourse on abortion is essential to consider if one is to understand the rhetoric and the full range of its capacity to orient biopolitical struggle. Under common law, abortion before quickening had generally been allowable because the fetus was not yet considered a child, but once states began to restrict the practice, law typically stipulated exceptions for physician-approved abortions, which the medical community called "therapeutic."[1] Not all abortions were bad; some were "good" or, rather, comparatively defensible given the alternatives. However, legal scholars Herbert L. Packer and Ralph J. Gampell noted in 1959, "If there were some general agreement on the precise circumstances under which an induced abortion can be characterized as criminal," the dichotomy between criminal and therapeutic "might be of some use."[2] Penelope Deutscher observes that the exceptions "could, according to the contingencies of individual states, doctors, judges, contexts, and cases, allow for extreme variation in the actual liberality of access to abortion."[3] If interrupted pregnancies are a sign of social disease, then sanctioned abortions that are difficult to distinguish from criminal ones prompt consideration of when disease becomes a therapy and what it treats. When a sickness also alleviates suffering and enhances well-being, it is both harmful and helpful, a poison and a remedy.[4] This chapter addresses the conundrum of the "therapeutic" abortion that existed even before abortion was criminalized and its importance in demonstrating the full rhetorical potential of interrupted pregnancy as pathognomonic.

Medically approved procedures only ever made up a tiny fraction of the overall number of inductions in the United States, but disagreement about the proper conditions for approval took on great significance for professionals. "The ever entangling problem of abortion indicators," as Clair Fulsome described it to Frederick Taussig,[5] became the most difficult, unresolvable issue, because it went right to the heart of medical rhetoric on the subject. In 1950, speaking before the New York Academy of Medicine, William Studdiford, director of obstetrics and gynecology at Bellevue Hospital, began his address on therapeutic procedures by stating that even though "the physician must expand every effort to preserve and prolong life," the practitioner "has always found himself [sic] faced with a dilemma: the problem of the pregnant woman afflicted with a complication which seriously increases her material risks."[6] Deutscher remarks that "the repeated creation of abortion as a state of permanent exceptionality has been one of the essential workings of twentieth- and early-twenty-first century biopolitics concerning women's reproductivity," and I would add the nineteenth century as well.[7] The relief that ending a pregnancy brought to women and their families (if they had families) countered the presumptively morbid signature of the practice, seemingly contradicting the basis on which elective abortion's prevalence assessed progress.

The prospect of a detested practice being used therapeutically highlights an irresolvable paradox at the foundation of this rhetoric: exemptions to the ban sanctioned tolerance for the intolerable. Remedial termination stood on the principle that pregnancy not only was but also should be reversible under limited conditions. As Alan Guttmacher wrote, "The physician who performs a therapeutic abortion is motivated by only one desire, that of correcting the pathologic status of a particular pregnancy."[8] The condition of reversibility was mercy, under which an otherwise abhorrent act became a compassionate one. Such compassion, because it set the danger of parturition *against* the danger of abortion, realized the full figurative potential for memory work based in abortion's materiality. Where criminal abortions were deemed wholly morbid, therapeutic ones switched the polarity, such that interrupting pregnancy became vital and completing it morbid, but without changing the ontological status of abortion. If resort to abortion indicated something amiss in society, then therapeutic indicators also included *pregnancy itself* and anything that made it dangerous. In that, therapeutic abortion shadowed contraception as a site for criticizing unplanned reproduction as harmful. However, authorized terminations were less a legitimate, if extremely variable, zone of reproductive control than a pitiable necessity.[9]

Although standards for therapeutic procedures existed in the West prior to criminalization in the United States, little was said on the topic, because knowledge of the relative risks of pregnancy and abortion was not overly controversial and the sorts of cases thought to warrant termination were very few. Despite significant writings in the previous century and a half, a substantial therapeutic discourse did not develop until the 1930s or flourish until the 1940s and 1950s.[10] I begin by placing abortion-as-remedy within an immunitary paradigm of biopolitics and the memory work that subtends it. Like forms of legal amnesty, therapy operated as a form of strategic amnesia. Then, the greatest share of the chapter is given to the bloom in therapeutic discourse and analysis of the memory work associated with the chief forms of "indicators" for warranted interruption of pregnancy: medical, psychiatric, humanitarian, and eugenic. I close with a consideration of law and regulation as meters of tolerance.

Recursion in Therapeutic Discourse

Therapeutic discourse critiqued pregnancy's risks using the same mnestic dynamics deployed around illegal abortion. It redirected the figurative work of positioning and evaluating national life toward the selective need to prevent undesirable births.[11] The fact that legal interruption of pregnancy was imaginable meant that morbidity associated with the practice inflected the course of national life in not just one but two (albeit contradictory) ways. As an *absolute* measure, abortion's existence marked the level of civilized advancement (with a threshold of one being too many, according to Guttmacher). A good society does not need these things. But as a *relative* measure, abortion was sometimes an act of mercy, so the dangers of *failing* to abort also pegged a failure to advance. A better society considers exemptions, however regretfully. Therapeutic procedures themselves were never taken to indicate that society was advanced, as if a better one would nurture their presence. Yet the *allowance* of therapeutic abortions was understood to signal civilized life by many observers' accounts. The practice of making exceptions was humane, even though the actual need for exceptions was a measure of backwardness.

Compassion required the managed suspension of abortion's absolute mnestic value in favor of its relative value. As the means of that suspension, therapeutic exemptions were strategically amnestic; forgiveness against transgression was operationalized by willfully forgetting the injunction against abortion. This was forgiveness in the sense that Hannah Arendt defined it: "the possible redemption from the predicament of irreversibility," which was not theological or juridical redemption as much as release "from the consequences of what we have done" for our own sake.[12] Therapeutic indicators defined conditions under which the burden of maternity could be forgiven, even at a cost considered extreme. Bradford Vivian remarks that when communities undertake intentional, targeted amnesia as a means of renewal rather than of secrecy, as in suspension of retribution in the wake of war, such lethic projects are typically "judicious responses to the dilemmas of the past in light of exigent cultural, political, or moral circumstances." In the case of abortion, the dilemmas of the past concerned what befell women who, facing similar conditions before, had no choice but to carry a pregnancy to term.[13] Deliberate forgetting of this sort is an effort to let go, to disremember what is otherwise unforgettable. In order to make dangerous pregnancies a thing of the past, then, medicine carved out indeterminate zones of tolerant amnesia, or amnesty, regarding abortion's intolerable nature. It was a sort of "unilateral forgiveness" on society's part, requiring no acknowledgment of wrongdoing by women, no restitution or restoration for harm done to themselves, the unborn, or the community, yet which established society as compassionate by protecting women from unnecessary harm.[14] Women were both victimizer and victim. Therapeutic indicators "regulated aversion," which is Wendy Brown's term for "political deployments of tolerance as historically and culturally specific discourses of power with strong rhetorical functions."[15]

Targeted, intentional forgetting of criminality was a critical component of any immune apparatus for abortion because amnesty organized "the relationship between immunity and tolerance," which had significant implications for memory work.[16] Amnesty did *not* erase abortion's status as a wrong act, as if, relieved of pregnancy, a woman could start over with a clean slate—she was forever marked with an invisible scarlet A. Rather, this kind of amnesia fed the fires of remembrance, because exceptions required more thorough sifting of the diverse circumstances attending pregnancy to determine when a wrongful act of interruption could be a remedy. Therapeutic abortions spurred recollection of the risks that attended childbirth, by intensifying and refining pathogenic analyses of contemporary biological and cultural life so that, ironically, untoward consequences of conception might be more thoughtfully, precisely forgiven.[17] Therapeutic abortion was a limited indulgence, a temporary pass from penalty but not from guilt.[18]

Put differently, by evidencing tolerance of the intolerable, therapeutic exemptions were awkward attempts to absorb and professionalize the risk analysis that was carried out by millions of women who decided whether they could or could not have *this* child *now*. Medically sanctioned procedures acknowledged that they *could* be right; warranted acts affirmed the danger of pregnancy to be true, but only if under medical pardon for a regrettable offense. Women were still risky subjects to be eyed suspiciously.[19] Of course, pregnancy had long been treated as a disease, but even so, pathologizing pregnancy relative to abortion was different because it entailed approaching gravidity *in process* as a dispensable burden. However, if therapeutic exceptions enacted tolerance, then putting otherwise criminal acts into medical practice could be depoliticized. "As communities, dug out of their ghettoized or otherwise anomalous political spaces, are brought under the jurisdiction of the state and into the orbit of mainstream economy and culture," Brown explains, "the belief world from which they hail [must] be excluded from legitimate public discourse."[20] The underground abortionist's barbarism became the doctor's unfortunate obligation. Abortion was legitimized by pity, not by right.[21]

Therapeutics was more than an affective disposition toward politics; it was an indeterminate predicament of the first order. Conditions for when affliction became remedy were materially undecidable in any final sense. All the factors that made reproduction risky—physiological, technical, chemical, economic, legal, instrumental, sociocultural, and practical—participated unpredictably in life politics. Early anti-Malthusians had taken sepsis or peritonitis[22] as unambiguous messages to women to remember why they were on this earth and get right with Nature; but antibiotics like penicillin or simple antisepsis like sterilizing instruments or washing the patient and one's hands countered the rhetorical agency of microbes. Properly applied, mold derivatives, steam heat, and diluted carbolic acid participated in the rhetoric too, it seems, leaving Nature somewhat less clear in its commands. Further, if Nature's supposed mandate to bear children had been the beacon that would guide any rational society to safe harbor, the fact that pregnancy itself manifested dangers showed that light to be treacherous. Biopolitical apostasy was required from time to time, because antireproductive acts were sometimes needed to make life not better but simply less bad.[23] As Roberto Esposito put it, "Tolerance is not non-immunity, a kind of virtuous immune-deficiency; if anything, it is a reverse immunity."[24]

The key fact of abortion's undecidable status is that criminal and therapeutic abortions were isomorphs of each other. When contemplating illegal abortion's history, we tend to think of the "back alley butcher,"[25] but a therapeutic evacuation was not a fundamentally different procedure from an illicit one. Many physicians referred patients to and depended on skilled abortionists such as Josephine Gabler, G. Lotrell Timanus, and Ed Keemer, trained doctors who also operated clandestinely in clinics and offices.[26] By the mid-twentieth century, data suggested that in some locales trained doctors conducted a majority of abortions. Between hospitals of the same era, criteria varied starkly for therapeutic abortion. An abortion by a recognized professional for reasons and by standards that met muster as therapeutic in one hospital might well be criminal in another. "Medical abnormalities requiring therapeutic abortion form an ever changing list," Guttmacher noted, "the components of which vary from decade to decade, institution to institution, and physician to physician."[27] The practical difference between criminal and therapeutic procedures was the raft of untrained, self-taught, or unskilled abortionists in the underground, who undoubtedly accounted for much of the trauma coincident with abortion, but this was a wholly *contingent* difference.[28]

Arendt wrote that people are "unable to forgive what they cannot punish and . . . are unable to punish what has turned out to be unforgivable. This is the true hallmark of those offenses, which, since Kant, we call 'radical evil.' . . . All we know is that we can neither punish nor forgive such offenses and they therefore transcend the realm of human affairs."[29] Abortion was not unforgivable, and so not a radical evil that transcended human affairs.[30] On the contrary, its ethical contingency implicated human affairs, which is why it was such a potent foundation for memory work. Deutscher reflects that when the provision of abortion operates under structures of exception, "there is almost never an illegal abortion, while it's just as true that there is almost never a legal abortion."[31] The same basic act, identical but for whom and when, whipsaws from the unthinkable to the permissible and back again.

The Janus face so evident in abortion's therapeutic applications epitomizes a core incongruity of all political economies that invest in human potential at the level of biological life. Attempts to master life's dangers compel adoption of precarious, mutable metrics because death is a remorseless, inevitable by-product that overflows from the excess of life.[32] In the last full U.S. monograph devoted to abortion of the nineteenth century, T. Gaillard Thomas wrote, "Nature seems to have ordained, not only among plants and lower animals, but also in the human race, that the amount of generative material should be enormous, and also that a large portion of it should be destroyed."[33] Forty years later, Margaret Welsh made a similar observation about abortion *tout court* but more precisely quantified: "Out of every million human beings conceived, between three and four hundred thousand are destroyed by abortion. In the United States alone there are seven hundred thousand abortions each year."[34] Projects devoted to cultivating better ways of life have as their goal to protect life from itself; "progress" endlessly generates new pathologies *because* it fosters new forms of living. Malthusianism is predicated on this fact, dismal in its calculation that a population of otherwise healthy individuals tends toward death. But as Foucault is often noted for saying, "everything is dangerous, which not exactly the same as bad."[35] Death is not the antithesis of life, but a species of it.[36]

Given that what is normally safe can also be harmful, the prevention of life in order to improve life is unavoidable within, yet begs forgiveness under, systems of power devoted to making life live.[37] As Esposito puts it, community, by seeking immunity from itself, "*transforms*—inverts and converts—rather than abolishes the impulses that negatively constitute [it] and which [it] can only reproduce."[38] In the unceasing, unpredictable work to protect life from itself, there arises an array of what Jacques Derrida termed *pharmaka* (Greek for "drugs"), which is to say, practices that "can *equally well* serve the seed of life and the seed of death, childbirth and abortion."[39] When the same practice can both save and kill, it is a *pharmakon* of which the right "dose" will be reproductive (life giving) and the wrong "dose" will be abortive (life taking). Such *pharmaka* are mediators of life's inexorable turn to death and are intrinsic to the search for immunity from within the very thing that harms us.[40] Although he was not addressing biopower per se, Derrida's use of childbirth and abortion as ciphers for life and death writ large is typical, certainly so in medical discourse.[41] Yet as with any aspect of biopower, neither childbirth nor abortion is strictly morbid or strictly vital. They too are implicated in living and dying in reversible ways, which is precisely the political economic conundrum that therapeutic abortion put on the table: "Abortion is often morally justifiable, and sometimes morally imperative," as William Robinson wrote.[42] Childbirth and abortion are part of biopower's pharmacy, as it were; "drugs" that can contribute to *or* ameliorate morbidity.

When bedrock expressions of *bios* and *thanatos* are shown to be convertible, when they themselves are *pharmaka*,[43] the unsettling plasticity in biopower's ethos of "making life live" is exposed.[44] Therapeutic abortion is an archetype for practices of self-negating renewal within regimes of living.

Interruption of pregnancy, as a recursive trope, was also inherently ironic, which made for a robust rhetorical capacity. The resiliency that irony afforded is demonstrated by the fact that deeply conflicted discourses on induced abortion did not unravel its coherence *as* abortion; it remained to medical reason a regrettable practice that always inflected the course of the nation and so enabled critique of society and its institutions. Many criminal abortions were undoubtedly necessary by some criterion, if only the woman seeking an abortion had been able to ask the right person in the right context. Likewise, therapeutic procedures were nearly always criminal if one asked the wrong person in the wrong context. Either way, elective abortion signaled error personally and communally, with accidents of circumstance transumed into reliable measures of vitality within civilizational discourses. Therapeutic abortion was the inverted answer to criminality, a political *antistrophe* that repeated and reversed the same rhetoric.

Shifting Threats: The Evolution of Safe and Necessary Abortion

The history of criminality and therapeutics as a kind of call-and-response within an immunitary paradigm lies in the evolution of safe and sometimes obligatory terminations. The modern story begins in eighteenth-century England, well before the U.S. antiabortion crusade, when abortion-as-therapy emerged after having spent centuries in "intellectual hibernation."[45] After the tenth century there had been no pertinent discussion in Western medicine until 1772, when English physician William Cooper considered the danger to a mother whose pelvis was too small for safe delivery ("contracted pelvis").[46] He argued that the life of the mother balanced against that of the fetus favored abortion over cesarean section in these cases.

Cooper was writing at a time when a common treatment for contracted pelvis, especially in England, was to use forceps to help extract the unborn, a practice introduced in the mid-1700s that could readily cause both the death of the fetus and terrible harm to the mother.[47] William Henry Jones, reviewing the use of forceps in recorded cases, contended in 1767 that "it is preferable to kill in attempting to save," meaning that doctors should try forceps extraction even if the outcome was dire.[48] Cooper simply extended the decision calculus, noting that if a "mature child" could not be safely delivered, "would it not be consistent with reason and conscience" to induce "as soon as it conveniently be done?"[49] It defied medical ethics to force the would-be mother to endure excruciating, hours-long, futile pain on the premise that physicians must battle for life even in a losing cause. The distance between Jones and Cooper seems small but the entirety of abortion's political economy opens up across its span. To Jones's precept that death in the name of life is moral (when life unchecked risks a more terrible death), Cooper added the crucial dimension of preventive action. Termination of a pregnancy can be a better outcome if done well in advance of something worse. With that, induced abortion had become tolerable and entered the pharmacy of modern biopower.

Abortion as *pharmakon* (however restricted) became the common understanding, endorsed by eminent leaders such as Alfred-Armand-Louis-Marie Velpeau, the august Parisian surgeon and professor. In Europe and the United States, indications for a therapeutic procedure gradually expanded, particularly in the later nineteenth century, coming to include "tuberculosis, heart disease, nephritis [kidney infection], and certain forms of psychoses." The twentieth century saw "an increasing tendency to extend the indications to eugenic and socio-economic factors."[50] Under a regime of legal prohibition, Deutscher noted, abortion as remedy not only was highly changeable but also grew. Observers began to recognize the practice as pathognomonic yet not intrinsically pathological. In 1920, as therapeutic indications sat on the cusp of their most dynamic phase, Herman Dekker noted approvingly, "Abortion in the United States is regarded (tacitly, of course) as at the worst ethically neutral and not wrong."[51] By contrast, fellow physician Palmer Findley wrote just two years later, "To interrupt pregnancy prior to the period of viability for any reason other than to safeguard the life of the mother is a moral, ethical and legal crime."[52] However, even among conservative caregivers like Findley, Cooper's eighteenth-century understanding of abortion as *pharmakon* relative to the life of the mother remained in effect. The question to be answered was, When is pregnancy life taking and abortion life supporting?

Safety

Physicians resisted the idea that abortions could be safe, safer than pregnancy especially, for quite some time. The conviction that abortion contradicted the essence of life made it difficult to see it as anything but menacing. With the

caveat that data on incidence rates were no better for therapeutic than for criminal abortion, therapeutic procedures only ever accounted for a few percentage
points of the total number of terminations, as little as 1 percent by some estimates but possibly closer to 3 percent.[53] As hospitals implemented committees through the 1950s and 1960s to police the authorization of procedures, the
already shrinking number of procedures shrank even further for each such institution, sometimes "by one-third to one-half."[54] There were two basic sets of
therapeutic abortions, one where a caregiver completed an unfinished criminal
procedure and one where a patient was authorized for abortion under prevailing
law and institutional or personal policy. The former was uncontroversial, but
the latter was caught in the orbit of criminality such that the induction itself,
regardless of its medical virtue, was routinely described as inherently perilous if
not directly unethical.

The persistence of this view is evident in that the most respected voice of
reform, Frederick Taussig, espoused abortion's inherent danger until his death:
"The immediate danger is a very serious one and the remote harmful sequelae
manifold. Whether the abortion is spontaneous or induced, it is a pathological process that in many instances damages the woman's health for all time."[55]
Joseph Donnelly echoed Taussig at the 1954 meeting of the Medical Society of
New Jersey, warning that "therapeutic abortion is a highly dangerous procedure.
It has a fetal mortality of 100 per cent, and an immediate maternal mortality of
5 per cent."[56] Donnelly was a preeminent anti-Malthusian at midcentury and
medical director at the Margaret Hague Clinic. Taussig and Donnelly were
reiterating in the twentieth-century vernacular of the average abortion the
nineteenth-century principle that interrupting pregnancy violated the natural
order of things.

However, extensive data accumulated that made it more and more difficult to
sustain this older conviction regarding maternal morbidity, and a revolution in
antibiotics greatly affected medical risk overall. A few years before *Roe v. Wade*
was decided, Christopher Tietze and Sarah Lewit noted that "the defenders of
legalized abortion point out that present techniques for the operation, when it is
performed by a competent physician, are so safe that the risk to life is well below
the risk of childbearing itself."[57] In fact, Mary Steichen Calderone declared in
1960, "Abortion is no longer a dangerous procedure."[58] Not surprisingly, much
of the realization of abortion's safety came from investigation of illegal operations, which revealed that criminal and therapeutic procedures were simply
isomorphs of one another and, more important, that illegal practitioners had
the greatest experience with providing safe abortions. Tietze contended in 1948

that abortion was becoming safer for women for several reasons: "(1) Contraceptive methods have been improved and are more generally used than formerly. Fewer women, therefore, resort to illegally induced abortion. (2) Abortionists have become more skillful in avoiding infection. (3) Many lives have been saved by improved methods of treatment, especially by the use of sulfa drugs and penicillin."[59]

One case in point is the data Timanus presented at the 1955 PPFA conference from his twenty-year practice as an abortionist in the Baltimore area. His record of 5,210 patients demonstrated that a professionally conducted procedure was virtually without risk (only two instances of maternal death, or 0.04 percent).[60] Guttmacher had invited Timanus to speak expressly to challenge the orthodoxy that abortion was inherently dangerous.[61] In 1961, Jerome Kummer and Zad Leavy similarly found that "abortion did not result in the ill effects that had been so generally assumed by others" such as "sterility or damage to capacity for achieving orgasm." Further, bodily and psychic sequelae were less common than believed, particularly psychic harms when compared with the frequency of postpartum illness. They speculated, "If the ill effects of induced abortion have been grossly exaggerated, we must ask ourselves why. Might the answer be that this was part of the means of enforcing the taboo?"[62]

Beyond contraceptive availability, Tietze isolated skill and treatments as the two principal determinants of life and death's ductility relative to abortion. Regarding skill, by the 1920s and until the introduction of vacuum aspiration in the late 1960s, dilation and curettage (D&C) was the most common form of surgical abortion under clinical conditions as compared with other common underground methods, three of which were puncturing the amniotic sac, inserting a urethral catheter into the uterus, and filling the womb with soapy water. The D&C, which Timanus used in modified form, is a procedure where the caregiver dilates the cervix, evacuates the uterus, and then carefully scrapes the uterine lining using a curette (a dull scraping tool of which there have been many varieties).[63] As David Zakin, William Godsick, and Benjamin Segal noted, "The experienced abortionist usually resorts to the definitive procedure of dilation and curettage or, in more advanced gestation, to simple dilation and packing of the cervix. The less competent abortionist, or the patient herself, for that matter, may use a variety of other measures, some reasonably likely to succeed and others entirely useless."[64] A proper D&C removes all material, which reduces the chance of infection and avoids the risks of embolism from uterine injections of air or soapy water, or of puncturing the uterus from objects like catheters.

Improvements in methods of treatment, particularly antibiotics, were the other factor making abortion less dangerous. The leading cause of death from abortion, sepsis, was reduced first by the adoption of antiseptic practices across the later nineteenth and the early twentieth century and then, decisively, by the development of "wonder drugs" in the 1930s and 1940s. Of the one-quarter of maternal mortality attributed to abortion, estimates suggest that up to three-quarters of those deaths resulted from septicemia.[65] Physicians combated this hazard with the developing protocols of antisepsis.[66] Concepts of contagion and germ theory radically affected understanding of pathology in the nineteenth century and were followed by the diffusion of handwashing, sterilization, sanitation in clinics, alcohol to clean wounds, and then diluted chemical washes in surgery.[67] The greatest threat posed to maternal life by abortion was microbial and so creating a bacterial dead zone helped preserve the mother's life; antisepsis became standard in gynecology from the mid-1880s to the 1890s.[68]

Antisepsis was crucial to improved safety but it had limits. The chemical cleansers adopted following Joseph Lister's advocacy of carbolic acid in 1867 were often quite stringent and did not necessarily kill the right bacteria, for example.[69] Also, one cannot easily wash the inside of the body. The antibiotic revolution, however, moved the principle of "killing to save" inside the body at the microbial level. The 1930s saw development of sulpha drugs (based on sulphonamide), which prevented bacteria from multiplying, thus letting the immune system destroy unwanted visitors. This drug group was extremely effective against a range of pathogens and quickly went into general use. Similarly, in the early 1940s *penicillium notatum* mold was developed into the first true antibiotic, and it was in heavy use by the end of World War II. Others quickly followed.[70] These drugs completely altered medical treatment.

Fetuses are in no way equivalent to harmful microbes, but in the most general sense therapeutic abortion shares the logic of antibiosis.[71] The unchangeable element in abortion's safety is the embryo—its development must be ended so that a woman's well-being is protected. Donnelly's remark about a 100 percent fetal mortality is an emphatic statement of that fact. Implicitly, and this of course is where most of the contemporary debate dwells, certain fetal mortality weighs against consequences to the woman, which raises questions about the fetus as both a subject and a risk factor.[72] Even among those moderns who insisted on the sanctity of life from conception, there were always doctors who embraced a differential estimation of fetal and maternal life. Hugh Hodge's plea for the unborn life was matched by his exception for contracted pelvis, for instance.[73] Contemporaneous with Hodge, Velpeau wrote in Paris that "I confess I cannot possibly balance the life of a foetus of three, four, five or six months, a being which so far scarcely differs from a plant, and is bound by no ties to the external world, against that of an adult woman whom a thousand social ties engage us to save."[74] He considered only contracted pelvis as a justification for abortion, and his standard of a rigid mathematical impossibility of delivery made him no different from Cooper really, but he enunciated more clearly what was implicit in Cooper's decision calculus. Before the threshold of viability, fetal life is unequal to the woman's, and that difference makes termination potentially tolerable. Even H. R. Storer supported an exception for the life of the mother and one not as narrowly construed as Velpeau's.[75] Other anti-Malthusians such as Edwin Hale advocated abortion as early as possible when advisable.[76] Neo-Malthusians such as like Mary Steichen Calderone, R. L. Dickinson, William Robinson, and A. J. Rongy, not to mention Taussig, felt abortion was justified under a much broader set of circumstances.

If fetal life is treated as developing a claim on existence rather than having an irrevocable one, the window of tolerance opens wider. It is significant that Jones, defending the use of forceps in 1767 for contracted pelvis ("it is preferable to kill in attempting to save"), sounds so similar to Robinson, when advocating in 1933 for the repeal of all laws prohibiting abortion: "Isn't the prevention of life very often in the highest degree preservation of life?"[77] Conservatives and progressives alike felt that weighing one life against another was clear cause to take pity on the expectant mother. Yet the developing status of the fetus allowed physicians to think more generally about the harms of pregnancy and the suffering it could bring to women. As Thomas put it, "Whenever it is felt that prolongation of pregnancy is going to destroy the life or intellect, or to permanently ruin the health of the patient, abortion should be brought on."[78] Beyond immanent death from parturition, granting a therapeutic exemption hinged on estimating what was destructive in pregnancy both to women and to society, which engaged a highly conditional, aspirational politics of pity. Doctors had a professional obligation to analyze prospective suffering and to make exceptions accordingly.[79]

Necessity

Rongy reasoned it would be impossible that so few doctors were prosecuted unless "the profession and the community at large were not agreed, at least *sub rosa*, that abortion is a social necessity."[80] Necessity was a moving target complicated by the fact that pregnancy had also become safer, with many of its complications having been alleviated or found to be have been false threats. The vanishing list of hazards accompanying parturition *and* abortion prodded "two movements running counter to each other" after World War I, Taussig noted. One group held that abortion had been overprescribed and adopted the standard, "'Not a single abortion too many and not a single one too few.'"[81] The other group sought recognition of abortion's advisability in the case of problems other than those afflicting the woman's body, namely, mental health, socioeconomic conditions, and eugenic concerns.[82]

Deciding when an abortion was indicated became so troublesome because calculations of when negating fetal life was on balance life affirming involved too many imponderables. Packer and Gampell listed the many sorts of questions doctors confronted that blurred the lines between life, health, and other considerations:

> Is the procedure limited to cases where its purpose is to avoid shortening the pregnant woman's life? If so, how do we determine whether carrying the child to term will shorten life? If not, what other considerations are relevant? Is a threat to health necessarily a threat to life? Must the threat to life (or health) be on account of a somatic illness? Or is the woman's mental condition also to be considered? If so, is a probability that suicide will ensue a justification, or will the probable precipitation of a debilitating psychosis justify the procedure? Must the psychiatric indication be limited to the immediate effect of bearing the child, or may subsequent effects caused by the strain of the burdens of child-rearing on an already disordered woman also be considered? What about the probability that the child, if born alive, will be defective? Does the defense of necessity require the jury to find that the procedure was necessary (whatever "necessary" means)? Or must the jury merely find that the defendant doctor believed in good faith that the procedure was necessary?[83]

It is unsurprising that "life of the mother," let alone her health, was so hard to define.

These vagaries were why so many hospitals adopted the committee system. Initially, therapeutic boards were set up to regulate eugenic requests, but eventually psychiatric professionals were added to committees, and mental health cases were considered along with humanitarian ones. Packer and Gampell's survey showed that by the late 1950s, depending on the institution, an abortion might be approved in the case of conditions such as heart disease, severe anxiety, psychosis, risk of fetal abnormalities, rape, child onset diabetes, cancer, Rh incompatibility, and poverty. Most institutions seemed to reject cases without clear risks of maternal mortality, but the authors concluded that procedures "that cannot be said to be 'necessary to preserve life' are being authorized for performance in reputable hospitals."[84] Ultimately, searching for the "right" balance between fetal and maternal harm was futile. As Guttmacher once remarked, "What is the proper incidence [of therapeutic abortion]? It is impossible to answer this."[85] Death of the mother is not, and never had been, the sole negative consequence attending childbearing, a realization inherent in Malthusianism and in the decisions by millions of women to forego having a child. Increasing safety forced medical experts to reckon with those other consequences as they attempted to define thresholds of necessary tolerance.

Medical Indicators. The language of "medical" indicators refers strictly to physiological conditions (heart disease, tuberculosis, etc.) and the risk analysis assumed considers the life of the woman as well as her health, as Thomas described. Historically, a suite of systemic, gynecological, and fetal conditions gradually joined the first indicator, contracted pelvis. Systemic conditions included hypertension (particularly hypertensive-renal disease), kidney lesions, pernicious vomiting, cardiac disease, pulmonary disease (tuberculosis mostly), malignancy (cancer), diabetes, hyperthyroidism, and varicose veins. Because of effective treatments and better understanding of the risks posed, by the mid-twentieth century nearly all these conditions seldom if ever called for therapeutic abortion, cancer, hypertensive-renal disease, and some cardiac disease being the exceptions.[86] Gynecological indicators included fibroids and ovarian tumors. Although such tissue masses occasionally gave cause to abort, unless a tumor was cancerous or a fibroid unusually large neither was seen as a strong indicator.[87] Fetal indications were eugenic, referring to abnormalities in the unborn, unless the fetus was dead or certain to die either in delivery or postpartum. I address eugenics separately.

Given the discourse on criminality, if fewer procedures were adjudged medically necessary, presumably both anti- and neo-Malthusians could rejoice in shared moral physiological purpose without dwelling on yesteryear's biomedicine or law, and the United States could be judged ethically *and* scientifically advanced. Yet that did not happen. Instead, a wider spectrum of problems posed by pregnancy gained visibility. Physicians turned to debate the relative threats of pregnancy more intently, always recurring to protection from abortion's morbidity as the struggle for a better world. Neo-Malthusians such as Taussig saw the expansion of therapeutic indicators as a humane and progressive response to pregnancy's inadequate management: "It is fortunate therefore that law in most civilized countries permits therapeutic abortion on the basis not alone of immediate threat to the life, but also of serious danger to the health of the mother."[88] Adoption of an abortion control program such as he outlined in 1936, with its focus on better reproductive care, alleviation of poverty, *and* more tolerant exemptions, addressed the conditions that made pregnancy malignant beyond the immediate threat of death in childbirth. The final statement of the PPFA conference was so insistent about this point that many more conservative attendees would not sign it.[89] Noting that "present laws and mores have not served to control the practice of illegal abortion," the statement read that, "almost no therapeutic abortions performed today are legal, since with the improvement of modern medicine it rarely becomes necessary to perform an abortion to save a life" and that new frameworks should "recognize the mounting approval of psychiatric, humanitarian, and eugenic indications for the legal termination of pregnancy."[90] Higher levels of civilization in the nation tracked with a greater obligation to redress the misfortunes of pregnancy.

In contrast, for anti-Malthusians the expansion of indicators signaled the continued advance of moral amnesia even as they shed maternal morbidity as a primary inflection point in the memory of civilization. In 1955, Donnelly contested the use of "remote" threats to maternal health in decisions about therapeutic procedures: "Such broadening indications for justifiable feticide tend to practical removal of all that is deterrent to this practice. Individual opinion as to the threat to the mother's life may vary in the widest limits. Indeed, it has been suggested that any pregnancy is a risk to the health of the woman and if this risk be considered as a threat to the mother's life, then there would be no bar to the induction of an abortion in any pregnancy."[91] His reason was that abortion is murder; thus, it could be approved only if it met the standard of justifiable homicide where the fetus would "be classified as an aggressor."[92] Medico-legal observers had made this argument back to Storer's day, but it had always been explained in terms of *physiological* law as made apparent in maternal harm (fatality, sterility, etc.).[93] Donnelly did at the last moment claim a doubtfully high (5 percent) mortality rate for therapeutic abortion, but the rest of the article giving this figure defended the safety of childbirth,[94] which left only an updated, even more restrictive version of Cooper's precept for exceptions. Cesareans were by then relatively safe and preferable for an expectant mother with a contracted pelvis who wanted a child. Death from parturition was rare. Doctors like Donnelly thus held justifiable homicide as the correct standard of advanced nations. "The laws of most civilized countries penalize unlawful abortion," J. C. Ayres wrote in 1938, "and define 'unlawful' as one induced for any other purpose than to save the life of the mother."[95] Pregnancy was pathogenic for anti-Malthusians only if the fetus became an accidental assassin, making abortion tolerable only in the case of incompatible vitalities as a mercy to the woman who could not defend herself.

Whether favoring or opposing a given indicator, medical experts used the confused, exceptional responsibility to perform an abortion as a means to separate a better world from a worse one. And it all depended on the comparative analysis of misery, regardless of sea changes in threat evaluation. As attendees of the PPFA conference discussed what to put in their concluding statement, Iago Galdston, abortion conservative and an executive secretary at the New York Academy of Medicine, proposed, "We first ought to commit ourselves to the proposition that abortion, legal as well as illegal, is a mutilating operation, and that we countenance it only as 'the lesser of threatened evils.' This order of stipulation should precede any suggestions as to the changes in the law, and should frame or condition these changes." Guttmacher responded, "I'll buy that!"[96] You'll not find as clear an agreement about abortion as *pharmakon* elsewhere in the literature between physicians of such starkly different opinion. It echoed Robinson's description of abortion as "the lesser of two or three evils" yet resonated with Storer's dictum that induction was allowable "absolutely and only to save a life."[97] Galdston's proposition promised some kind of concordance about professional obligations, too, but for the fact that it accomplished no such thing. It was agreed that abortion was a tolerable and not a radical evil, but nothing more could be agreed—which is precisely what empowered interrupted pregnancy as a recursive trope of biopolitical struggle. Deciding *when* abortion was tolerable was also a decision about *what* was tolerable in ways of life that led women to seek them.

The simple question put by Galdston and traceable from Cooper—is it the lesser of threatened evils?—is the condition on which abortion becomes a remedy and, at the same time, a weapon of biopolitical conflict. It is pathognomonic regardless, but if it is *not* the lesser evil, then it signals that a terrible decision has been made and indicts those who made it along with the factors that eased its making. If it *is* the lesser evil, then it signals that something even worse is afoot in our communities. All this can be agreed to while finding no agreement on what is evil: necessity as formula, never as conclusion.

Psychiatric Indicators. In the 1940s, as medical reasons were on the decline, ending pregnancy became preventive medicine for mental health as psychiatric conditions took the lead among indicators. During the PPFA conference, Carl Erhardt, director of the Bureau of Records and Statistics for the New York City Department of Health, reported that between 1943 and 1947, 13.1 percent of therapeutic abortions in New York City had been for "mental disorders," as compared with 37.8 percent between 1951 and 1953, making psychiatric indicators the largest category.[98] The data were particularly useful because since 1938, the city sanitary code had required reporting of all terminated pregnancies regardless of gestation length. Clinical studies supported the New York City data.[99] By the late 1960s, "mental disorders account[ed] for ⅔ of the abortions done in proprietary hospitals, more than ½ in the private services of voluntary hospitals and only ⅓ in the ward services of voluntary and municipal hospitals."[100]

Despite the increase in number of psychiatric exceptions, the literature on psychiatric indicators is one of disorganized skepticism. If navigating the waters of medical indicators had been hard, conversation on psychiatric indicators was undertaken without a rudder. "Psychiatric indications rarely actually meet the usual legal demand that the pregnancy endanger the life of the mother."[101] As a result, few experts seemed to think psychiatric conditions warranted an abortion. One thing was clear, though: mental health procedures pointed not to women's ignorance but to their emotional instability. Mental health professionals attempted to disclose the hidden costs of coercion and "maternal rejection" by studying the impact of pregnancy on mothers, society, and the children themselves.[102] A desire to abort indexed emotional disturbance one way or another, whether from a regrettable abortion or an unwanted child. The recursive figuration of civilization had shifted to more fully include *psycho*pathologies of progress.

Typologies of patients had little uniformity and were essentially individualized to each practitioner. Nevertheless, the common understanding was that a woman should bear the child if her emotional disturbance was deemed temporary, if she could be made to accept the child with psychotherapy, or possibly if she could give the child up.[103] Theodore Lidz, professor of psychiatry at Yale, described the common scenarios: "The unmarried woman cannot face the disgrace; the wife cannot continue in a disastrous marriage which will be perpetuated if the child is born; or the woman, later in life, feels overwhelmed by the need to raise an infant after other children are grown. The immature mother cannot assume responsibility and care for, instead of being cared for; the obsessive woman is appalled by the need for responsible decision, etc."[104] In most public statements of practitioners, these situations did not warrant termination and in previous decades they might have been chalked up as "excuses" made plausible because of women's lack of knowledge or moral instinct. May E. Romm, a psychoanalyst, described the mental health community's informal criteria consistent with the standard of a lesser threatened evil. Abortion was justifiable based on "(a) the danger of irreversible psychological damage to the mother during the pregnancy, and (b) the effect on her of the postpartum state."[105] This is the psychotherapeutic equivalent in the mid-twentieth century of contracted pelvis in the eighteenth. The woman's life must be undone by severe psychosis; childbirth needed to threaten psychic murder of the mother.

Chronic conditions like manic depression (now called bipolar disorder) and schizophrenia that might become acute postpartum were considered to meet this standard (maybe). Also, if a patient manifested severe psychosis during pregnancy, an abortion could be approved.[106] At the same time, psychiatrists worried that abortion itself might trigger a break with reality, making abortion particularly nettlesome as *pharmakon* for mental illness. Harold Rosen, a clinician at Johns Hopkins and editor of the volume *Therapeutic Abortion*, was of that camp, saying that "in most such patients, the undesired pregnancy merely highlights existent, and usually pronounced, maladjustment" to married life and motherhood. Interestingly, Rosen treated "severe neurotic or psychotic symptoms" as equivalent to separating from the sex partner or husband in demonstrating mental illness.[107] Abortion once again signaled a "revolt of conduct" among women that could result in the loss of their health, only now to their mental health. One does not have to try too hard to hear the refrain of anti-Malthusian recursivity. Women's unconscious minds, not their bodies, were remembering what the women themselves had forgotten. The clinical anecdote shifted from an obstetrical-gynecological register of body criticism to a psychiatric one of psychic criticism, miming the transumption of harm into sociocultural critique. The patient's mind was turned out in its damaged state (*chiasmus*), inverted and reduced to visible, clinical forms (*metonym*). Furthermore, damage to patients mapped systemic pathologies in the community-as-organism. Determining the situational, proximate cause of the abortion request amplified the damage (*peristasis*), expanding the terrain of psychosis into the community. At the same time, the collective was condensed into a set of positive and negative factors affecting psychic health (another metonym).

Clinicians took patients' maladjustment as the base fold, the inflection point for inhabiting time and place. Individual revolts against maternity remembered a biopsychologized Providence through the consequences of refusal. Galdston, also a psychiatrist, stated this mnestic figuration as a corollary when addressing PPFA conferees in 1955: "If and when a so-called adult woman, a responsible female, seeks an abortion, unless the warrant for it is overwhelming—as say in the case of rape or incest—*we are in effect confronted both with a sick person and a sick situation*" and "neither the given person nor the given situation is likely to be remedied by the abortion, *qua abortion*."[108] One wonders that rape and incest did not seem to be signs of a sick situation. In fact, rape and incest were almost entirely absent from postwar psychiatric discussions of abortion.[109] Galdston approvingly parroted the uterine teleology of the ancient Greeks. He declared, "A woman is a uterus surrounded by a supporting organism and a directing personality. I am neither facetious nor deprecatory of womankind, nor superior in masculinity. I am biologically objective."[110] He pressed on: "Is it really possible to interrupt so profound and so extensive a biological process, one of such great constitution and physiological magnitude, and to expect no dire results?" This is little more than reiteration of the longstanding view, initially voiced by Storer, that abortion could drive women insane.[111] Alfred Kinsey questioned whether Galdston drew any distinction between therapeutic and illegal abortion; he said no.[112] Other conferees debated the merits of Galdston's extreme view but ultimately endorsed less chauvinist versions of it.[113] Only Kinsey objected. "I should like to disclaim the implication that biology put a purposive interpretation upon the function of sex," he said, explicitly contesting Aristotelian biology and Darwinistic biological purpose.[114]

All the while, psychiatrists acted on a different sense of the lesser evil, using psychiatry to alleviate socioeconomic stressors, particularly for women under threat of suicide. As Howard Taylor warned, clinicians concerned about long-term consequences from financial or emotional stress over unwanted pregnancy were in effect authorizing illegal abortions. Taylor was supported by Kinsey's research in that interviewees described this very practice. Some practitioners held that if a suicidal threat was credible an abortion was justifiable,[115] but counterevidence cast significant doubt on the possibility. Further, Lawrence Kolb, director of the New York State Psychiatric Institute, declared suicide threats to be intimidation tactics. He cited a 1954 study from Sweden on patients turned down for abortions, of whom none who threatened suicide (sixty-two) acted on her threat.[116] To determine the reality of a threatened psychosis, clinicians had to recall the full context of the woman's life, including "interpersonal relationships" and "cultural, social, economic, and financial considerations, tangible and abstract."[117] That a depressed woman might threaten herself with grave harm made it difficult to separate psychiatric from other problems. How to discern a real from a false threat or weigh the risk?[118] Separating the overall health of the woman and the public from the specific condition of any one pregnancy was impossible.

Humanitarian Indicators. In the nineteenth century, indicators addressing the woman's relationships in the family and in the community as well as her fiscal situation were typically lumped into the broad, condescending category of "fashion"—custom among the ill informed and superficial. By the twentieth century, "fashionable" reasons began to be treated less derisively by some and increasingly were labeled "socioeconomic." In the first decade of the twentieth century some practitioners, Rosalie Ladova, I. C. Philbrick, and G. M. Hawkins among them, named social and economic injustice, degradation, and abuse as legitimate indicators.[119] Hawkins, a Seattle physician, was crystal clear in arguing that "social problems resolve themselves into economic problems" and that "society presents many symptoms of ill-adjustment, signs that somewhere in the body politic reside frictions that are in need of change. Such, and only such, is the desire to pluck the unripe fruit of the uterus that is springing more and more in human minds."[120] In contrast with W. J. Fernald's "Sociological View," which placed the highly procreative family at the foundation of society,[121] Hawkins argued that "only when we reach the stage of civilized man" is woman deemed a passive vessel of reproductive yearning. Were women equal, especially economically, abortion would disappear. Until then, "the everyday slaughter of nature's attempt at the perpetuation of humanity does not speak well of our boasted civilization."[122]

Few doctors in the United States were as openly feminist or Marxist as Hawkins, especially after the first Red Scare and the Bolshevik Revolution, but abortion as resistance persistently featured in the literature. Recognizing resistance through "humanitarian" exceptions, however, blunted the critical edge of remembering, by way of abortion's costs, that society was unjust. As with Brown's observation of tolerance as depoliticizing, ending unwanted pregnancy palliated economic and gender injustice, soothing a sick society, thus making revolt against maternity an object of sympathy.[123]

The earliest and most potent presentation of abortion as a piteous revolt was the remarkable, anonymous 1867 letter by "the wife of a Christian physician" published in that banner carrier for the antiabortion crusade, the *Boston Medical and Surgical Journal*.[124] The letter writer responded to H. R. Storer's book *Why Not? A Book for Every Woman*, which rehearsed the deprecating view of abortion as ignorant fashion. The unknown author countered that a woman aborted for two reasons in full knowledge of what she did. First, childbirth was "certain agony," which argues for voluntary motherhood and against suffering pain you did not willingly accept to bear.[125] Second, "the true and *greatest* cause" was the "degradation of being a mere thing—an appendage."[126] Echoing the free love movement, she called abortion rebellion ("she rebels") against a lack of sexual power in marriage, which entitled men to the "right of abuse."[127] She alluded to coercion, rape, and more generally a sense of inequality in the deflected language of her day. Forcible pregnancy was subjection, yet she did not call for redress, only "sympathy, comfort, and encouragement." If women were loved and respected, she contended, they would happily play their part. She was no radical, although she was bold and adapted brilliantly to her audience of medical men. Storer promptly published *Is It I? A Book for Every Man*, wherein he acknowledged the anonymous letter and advised husbands to love and respect their wives. He did not caution family limitation.[128]

The reasons offered by the anonymous author had everything to do with remembering the actual lives that women lead in a patriarchal world and the costs that world imposes on them: the morbidity that pays for a certain vitality to male dominance. Forcible pregnancy precipitated ethical as well as physical and psychical damage. Rape, incest, and unwed motherhood, all uncomfortably lumped together underneath the word *stigma*, were causes for pity.[129] In particular, the culture of silence around rape (and the lack of a concept of "marital" rape) made sexual violence nearly invisible in the medical literature until the twentieth century.[130] Requiring a woman to carry the child of a rapist to term relegated the violence to a kind of oblivion by erasing it under license of pregnancy. This differs from the strategic amnesia of tolerance, which intentionally recognized acts of abortion but forgave their prohibition. Sexual violence went unacknowledged, not even forgotten in that it seemingly did not exist to be disremembered. An early and pointed commentary on rape quarreled with exactly this mnestic relation. In 1910, O. H. Hammett of Arkansas objected that rape was ignored and asserted that "our laws should be amended that they would deal most severely with the devilish brute that used his moral or physical force to rape her."[131] In

1931, Rongy described the forced birth of a child conceived from incest as "the height of cruelty."[132] Existing law and practice covered over the sexual violence with the innocence of the newborn and the shame of the woman; exceptions for rape and incest would shift amnesia away from obscurity for sex predators to amnesty for victims, thus supporting recollection of men's license.

Inequities in access to abortion relative to ethnicity and class extended the range of pitiable circumstances well beyond violence and abuse. As the Depression wore on and then as psychiatric indicators became more commonly accepted across the 1940s, hospital data showed a distinct difference in who was granted an exception and who was not. White women who could afford private wards in clinics, foreign travel, or psychiatric care were much more likely to secure a therapeutic exemption than poor or nonwhite women.[133] These others were unfortunates in crisis. Writing in 1931, Antoinette Konikow exemplified the politics of pity vis-à-vis poverty:

> As a woman physician, practicing in the poorer districts of the city, I inevitably became interested in Birth Control. The fear of pregnancy, the terror of undesired motherhood, which seemed to occupy the whole life of the married women, was brought to me continually. I knew these women. I knew their husbands, their children, I knew that their health and their economic circumstances absolutely forbade further childbearing. I saw them using the most desperate means to bring about abortions; I saw tears, unhappiness and endless despair. As a woman, I could not send my patients from one self-induced abortion to another. Something had to be done.[134]

Robinson presented abortion in similar if hyperbolic terms, writing at length in language saturated with pathos about a "poor illegitimate mother," Birdie, who was seeking an abortion.[135] Poorer women rebelled against unwanted pregnancy "in the only way they know how," as Regina Downie put it,[136] yet an ethic of tolerance privatized the difference between affluent whites and the rest. A "differential birth rate" between classes and ethnicities highlighted a tolerance deficit that smothered abortion as a kind of revolt of the mothers, rich and poor, white and nonwhite alike, underneath the hypocrisy of an inconsistent, relaxed privilege based on advantage and opportunity.[137]

Sophia Kleegman, clinical professor of obstetrics and gynecology at New York University and medical director for New York Planned Parenthood, was among the most vocal proponents of distributive justice as a reason for compassion. In the 1950s, she marshaled the available evidence to demonstrate that less advantaged women were left to the dangers of criminal abortion because they were unable to gain access to birth control. She advocated concern for the "unmarried girl who is desperate," equality of tolerance for the poor, and "sociological support and understanding for the unmarried, pregnant girl."[138] A contrast with Dekker's reflection on the changing attitudes toward abortion in 1920 is apropos. He took note of the pressures of urbanism with highly concentrated populations, limited housing, high rents, costly necessities, higher standards of living, and escalating costs of child rearing, arguing that "such undoubted facts make for a tolerant attitude toward the practice of abortion" and that "an ever-growing number of persons will feel themselves morally justified in resorting to a 'safe' abortion." However, he saw this trend as a function of burgeoning equality for women: "She demands the same right to play the game of life as men. . . . Controlled births will be one of the means women of today will surely use to achieve a freedom from age old subjection."[139] Neo-Malthusians like Kleegman, Konikow, and Robinson had argued to extend the umbrella of pity, not to replace it with a broad-based right of female bodily control such as Dekker described.[140] Consistent with the neo-Malthusian logic of opposition between abortion control and birth control, humanitarian tolerance generally operated in a liberal individualist discourse of contraceptive privation, not gendered subjection.

"Tolerance discourse masks the role of the state in reproducing the dominance of certain groups and norms, and it does so at a historical moment when popular sensitivity to this role and this dominance is high," Brown explains.[141] As a form of strategic amnesia, tolerance renews power arrangements by deflecting attention from those arrangements even as it acknowledges resistance. As such, women's revolt against mandatory procreation was taken as a chronic spasm of desperation spurred by disadvantageous circumstances—not by a desire for freedom and autonomy. Humanitarian exceptions in particular were linked with the new birth control practices of sex education, contraception, and child spacing as a sort of fertility control of last resort.[142] Humanitarian abortions prompted remembrance of victimage from sexual violence, economic distress, and the burdens of excessive child rearing, replacing harms from rejecting maternity with harms to desperate women.[143]

Eugenic Indicators. The most sensationalized aspect of abortion-as-therapy has been its eugenic applications. Oversimplified, short-term rhetorical advantage so often encumbers discussion (labeling pro-choice advocates as secretly eliminationist, for example) that it is difficult to talk about this subject at all. Eugenics is highly complex and involves a wide variety of reproductive ideologies, more than I can easily summarize. What the contemporary public debate obfuscates is that abortion was never advocated as mainline fertility control in the United States, only as a lesser evil in lieu of better methods of reproductive management.[144] Coincident with eugenic indicators gaining favor among physicians, therapeutic abortions were generally in decline, except for non-eugenic psychiatric instances. That does not mean physicians did not support or oppose abortion for reasons that now seem grotesque to any number of constituencies. The distasteful history of positive and negative eugenics in medical discourse at the end of the nineteenth and into the twentieth century is well known,[145] and one way or another, terminated pregnancies were used to promote certain groups' fertility over others. However, therapeutic abortion was not part and parcel to any given ideology, pro- or antinatalist, so it is misleading to sequester eugenics within one corner of Malthusianism.[146]

Eugenic thinking about abortion was unlike medical, psychiatric, and humanitarian analyses in that eugenics was not really a separate category of necessity on par with the others (even though it was usually listed as such by physicians). Instead, eugenics operated as a metalogic for the necessity of abortion control at "the borderline of medical science and sociology," as Taussig put it, because there was no distinct set of eugenic indicators that were not either physical, psychic, or humanitarian.[147] Eugenics, broadly defined, is about mastering morbidities passed through reproduction within given populations, such that those populations' vitality is enhanced. The term, coined in 1883 by Francis Galton, referred to improvement of humanity through the management of hereditary traits; it rapidly became a master concept in regimes of biopower.[148] Even before Galton's concept was introduced, abortion control had been eyed with broadly eugenic purposes because of the Malthusian political economics that looked on abortion as a social problem.[149] The positive and negative eugenics of physicians were simply varieties of Malthusian positive and preventive checks on fertility, as made articulate through late 1800s hereditary science. Hereditarianism was a redeployment of the immunitary paradigm, not a new strain of biopolitical rhetoric.

Thus, abortion control emerged in the name of eugenics before there was a name for eugenics.[150] U.S. anti-Malthusians in the medical community typically favored a positive eugenics through which white, well-to-do Anglos would out-reproduce the poor, the nonwhite, the non-Christian. It was these antiabortionists who initially set the eugenic necessity of abortion control. As reviewed in earlier chapters, beginning with rising awareness of fertility rates in the mid-nineteenth century, the apex of this fear was in the first decade of the twentieth. By the 1930s, racial anxiety had waned among medical professionals. For example, in *Abortion, Spontaneous and Induced,* Taussig professed a theory of cultural lag contributing to high levels of abortion *and* in the same breath rejected race suicide as nonsense. "It is difficult to find positive evidence that the practice of abortion in the past centuries has led to a serious deterioration of the race, in spite of the many statements to that effect in the books of history. Nor . . . is there irrefragable evidence that any ancient civilizations 'fell'—was their heritage not handed on to us?—because of the frequency or resort to abortion."[151] There was no grand caesura with racial anthropology, no loud parting of ways; only a few other physicians took issue with the idea of race suicide, such as Ira S. Wile, who described it as an "absurdity."[152] But in the decade following publication of Taussig's masterwork, fascism viciously impelled reconsideration of racial eugenics,[153] and physicians quietly abandoned race suicide and racial degeneration as a reason to regulate induced abortion.

Neo-Malthusians typically braided together two different strands of immunitary logic. One strand followed a negative eugenics wherein limited progeny among the "unfit" would safeguard against degenerative pathogens that traveled via heredity, virus, or toxins. "Unfitness" was a highly unstable category that included a broad range of racial, ethnic, disabled, mentally challenged, and poor peoples.[154] Negative Malthusian, profertility control discourse before and through the Depression favored contraception or sterilization for inherited disability and (supposed) criminality. Abraham Jacobi, then president of the AMA, advocated in a groundbreaking 1912 address that "the propagation of [America's] degenerate, and imbecile, and criminal should be prevented."[155] Jacobi did not mention abortion, but he was the first AMA president to broach reproductive control with the membership. Reasoning like Jacobi's reversed the anti-Malthusian's immunity logic, touting a reduced Other rather than an increased Self as the means to greater vitality, but the biologized anxieties were kindred to the positive eugenics of someone like W. J. Fernald, who had prophesied national collapse if white Anglos did not take up the cause of birthing more children. A second, different strand of neo-Malthusianism operated on the assumption that limited fertility would promote the overall well-being of a population by improving the prospects for the Self. Population control furthered public health by reducing physical and economic stresses on the family,

preserving maternal health against too many children and preventing the raising of unwanted children in poverty, which might contribute to social ills such
as delinquency.[156]

The 1930s saw neo-Malthusians' eugenic concern for fetal abnormalities
crest,[157] but nevertheless, considering abortion a fertility control technique
along with sterilization or contraception was considered extreme, even among
physicians who favored sterilization of the so-called unfit. The contrast between A. J. Rongy and William Robinson, both abortion radicals writing in
1933, makes this clear. Rongy insinuated approval of illegal abortionists; unlike
virtually all other neo-Malthusians, he saw abortion as a tool alongside other
methods of fertility control. He advocated professional sterilization and abortion for "defectives" to limit growth of the "feeble-minded" and for population
control to combat starvation and poverty.[158] However, even Rongy considered
both abortion and sterilization "radical" methods and considered sterilization
the superior approach of the two, while preferring contraception to both.[159]
Calling birth control "intelligent control," he argued that "society has a stake in
the lives and energies that is possesses today. It is to the best interests of society that it conserve them."[160] Contraception was imperfect, though, so lifting
restrictions against health, social stigma, economic, and eugenic exceptions was
rational.[161] Like Rongy, Robinson noted that abortion was a bellwether of un-
healthy numbers of children because so many multiparous women resorted to
termination. He too favored sterilization rather than abortion for the mentally
disabled. Robinson took a more extreme position on the law than Rongy, however, demanding its "complete and total abrogation."[162] Even among more stri-
dent decriminalization advocates, abortion was not a preferred fertility control
and eugenics was a limited factor in the procedure's proposed value to society.

Later, as Leslie Reagan explains in her exceptional book, *Dangerous Pregnancies*, the global rubella epidemic of 1963 and the thalidomide debacle of the
early 1960s would galvanize public support for eugenic abortions and motivate
women to activism, including their presenting challenges to state laws, so as to
secure availability to therapeutic procedures and preventive, non-abortive remedies.[163] Rubella, or German measles, is a virus that produces only a mild rash
for most patients, but if a woman contracts the disease in the first few months of
pregnancy, the child may develop a wide range of conditions, from blindness to
spectrum disorders. "German measles and scientific knowledge about its effects
brought the complex moral and legal questions about pregnancy, possible disabilities, and possible abortion to the forefront of American medical, political,

and media culture and public attention."[164] Indeed, access to amniocentesis developed from rubella malpractice suits, and the culture of prenatal testing so familiar today owes much to the public response to this outbreak.[165] Thalidomide was a drug marketed in the late 1950s and early 1960s principally in sleep aids, but other applications too, that could cause severe deformities in the children of some women who used it while pregnant as well as "miscarriages, stillbirths, and early infant deaths." It was never sold in the United States, but Reagan notes that "more than a thousand doctors" gave away samples as part of an experimental release.[166] Images of babies missing arms or legs alarmed the public. Sherri Finkbine, a mother in Arizona known to locals as host of the children's program *Romper Room*, decided in 1962 to seek an abortion in the public eye after finding that she had ingested thalidomide. News media covered her efforts to procure an induction, which ultimately required her to go abroad. Her public act prompted a vigorous debate and raised awareness of abortion, not just the specifics of the thalidomide scare.[167]

Rubella and thalidomide were both *teratogenic*, meaning they were external causes of fetal developmental problems. The risk analysis surrounding these teratogens made powerful use of tolerance discourse based in compassion and pity (strongly mixed with fear).[168] Women and their children were victims of poor medical care or pharmaceutical testing, and so amnesty for abortion provided immunity of the last resort from malpractice, although it was not a preferred solution to the problem. That is why activists fought not only for more lenient exceptions for abortion but also for legal and medical measures that would minimize the risks posed to developing fetuses in the first place, such as more stringent requirements on caregivers to inform pregnant women of prenatal dangers in addition to prenatal testing.[169]

The public response regarding German measles and thalidomide resonated with physicians' existing attitudes toward developmental afflictions but pushed the medical community to alter its method of calculation for compassionate exceptions. Robinson presented a common view among his peers when he argued that abortion was necessary for "life that is a curse to its possessor."[170] However, inheriting a "curselike" disease is a matter of probabilities as well as opinion. Also, for hereditary disease, the closest analog to teratogenic pregnancies, doctors had been very conservative in recommending abortion; they expected a level of statistical satisfaction not unlike that for contracted pelvis. Reflecting on epilepsy, forms of paralysis, and Huntington's disease, Taussig wrote in 1936, "If it could be proved that such diseases were *always* and positively inherited, there could be little argument against therapeutic abortion to prevent the birth of *such unfortunates.*"[171] Mercy for the severely and permanently afflicted warranted abortion, if one was certain there could be no better outcome.

Rongy perfectly captured the tension in physicians' rhetoric between compassion and limits on abortion. Describing the ancient Roman patriarchal right under which a father could kill his child with impunity, he surmised that "compassion is, in the main, a product of civilization. It predicates a relaxing in the struggle for the essentials of existence. It generally arises only in a society that has lifted itself above the level of bare living. Civilized man, overwhelmed with plenty, can afford compassion and moral strictures against abortion. The savage can afford no such luxuries."[172] Compassion and abortion control appear together, linked with affluence and leisure on the scale of civilization. With progress, sympathy grows for the infant and the unborn, as do moral strictures to protect them, as we saw with anti-Malthusians who viewed expanding Christian compassion for the unborn as the long arc of history, and neo-Malthusians who saw abortion as a stage between infanticide and scientifically effective contraception. However, tolerant exemptions for the intolerable always complicated these schema because compassion dictated those as well. To one set of physicians or another, it was a form of cruelty to force a mother to stare down death on the chance of a successful birth, to bear a rapist's child, or to carry a developmentally afflicted embryo to term.

The rarity of eugenic indicators mirrors therapeutic abortion's relation to population control in the United States generally. In *Malthusian Worlds*, Ronald Walter Greene historicizes the twentieth-century emergence of what he terms the "population apparatus" that grew up around demography and concern for the "population bomb."[173] In the United States, abortion was not a central technology within the population apparatus. Occasionally a doctor might make mention of it in passing, as Calderone did in a letter to Tietze in advance of the 1955 PPFA conference.[174] The procedure was not considered an effective means for significantly altering population levels even among classes of people deemed unfit.[175] R. Gordon Douglas, an ob-gyn from Cornell, remarked skeptically to attendees of the PPFA conference that even if all the mentally disabled were either aborted or sterilized there would still be only an insignificant reduction in "mental defectives." He underlined his point: "I do not think that there are very many indications on a fetal basis."[176] Contemporaneous with Douglas, Guttmacher explained that in cases of potential fetal abnormality, "each such case must be submitted to the most searching scrutiny. After such scrutiny, few pregnancies merit interruption."[177] In terms of population overall, U.S. observers were likely to view increasing abortion rates as a sign that a population was growing too fast, an index of desperation that called for better methods of fertility control, and not for more abortion.[178]

To the extent that it protects against pathogenic pregnancies, therapeutic abortion is eugenic in the broadest sense, meaning productive of good births. Historically, "good" birth has meant children were of the desired demographic, safely born, affordable, free of major diseases or disabilities, or conceived in love, not violence. Good births embody visions of the future immunized from threats, collective and individual. In that, eugenic indicators epitomized the recursive dynamic of enfolding history through the practice of abortion. In 1933, Rachelle S. Yarros anticipated hereditary eugenics as a passing stage of fertility control: "We may some day undertake to restrict the reproduction of the unfit, but the more scientific biology and psychology become, the fewer persons will these sciences venture to condemn as unfit and as proper subjects for the sterilization chamber."[179] Further, when Kleegman spoke in favor of abortion for "mental defectives" based on the need "to protect and to enrich future generations," it was as a sad necessity in an imperfect battery of prophylactic institutions, research, technologies, and practices that would make planned parenthood a reality.[180]

Regulating Tolerance

Exceptions to an abortion ban measured progress not by *more* therapeutic practices occurring but by the rationalized affect under which exceptions were granted. To tolerate the intolerable requires either that there is no plausible alternative (such that tolerance is really a kind of making-do or resignation) or that compassion is felt for those people whose actions are otherwise intolerable. It might be argued that since abortion has existed in every culture that we know of, tolerance of abortion is more akin to resignation. However, abortion was often justified within therapeutic discourse as ameliorating cruelty, but never because it was inevitable.[181] Women's requests needed to meet established standards of pity and, so, women had to confirm that their circumstances were worthy of exemption. Legal and regulatory frameworks regarding abortion loosely categorized which circumstances were pitiable and which were not; they established expectations of sufficient danger to justify the occasional biopolitical heresy. To decide if a case met the tolerance threshold required a managed, selective disclosure of patients' conditions by which the morbidities of abortion recognized by prevailing life politics were channeled into limited comparison with the morbidities of pregnancy. Hence, while state laws failed to immunize the nation against interrupted pregnancy, they did not fail as juridical agents of memory work, because determining the legitimacy of exceptions, approved or not, made society's evolving compassion visible.

Recursively, this is enough. Relative to the goal of ending all but sanctioned abortions, few cases came to trial and fewer still were successfully prosecuted.[182] The law need not prevent anything; it could even heighten the very threat that it purportedly protected the community from, effectively becoming an auto-immune disorder, as neo-Malthusians pointed out. The crucial factor is that adequate substance for memory work kept flowing in and out, with measures of death and decay continually culled from an abundance of pregnancies. Law helped stabilize the horizons of secrecy that inquiry into civilization's progress looked to, providing minimal affective consistency to what was in practice a highly inconsistent standard of the lesser evil. Moreover, if standards for thera-peutic procedures demonstrated the elevation of a people's sympathies, then trends in indicators assessed the overall distribution of amnesty. The clear fail-ure of the law and the expansion of indicators meant that pity was being felt too freely and for the wrong reasons among providers. Even radicals felt that too many abortions were approved. With increasing proof that respectable physi-cians referred most abortions (often to well-qualified abortionists), the image of the underground as a mercenary operation from the nineteenth century was joined by one of reckless mercy in the twentieth.[183]

In this light, the creation of hospital abortion committees was an attempt to demonstrate medicine's powers of affective discrimination. The standards that clinics adopted were an indictment of prevailing standards of compassion. With almost no medical indicators remaining, psychiatric, humanitarian, and eugenic dangers seemed doubtfully the greater evil. Under such a calculus one would ex-pect movement toward only the most begrudging, rarified amnesty from parent-hood, guided by the latest science, as the real measure of advanced life, and such was exactly the kind of future sought by the committee system.[184] Robert E. Hall, who helped pass the liberalized 1970 New York statute on abortion, wrote of the hospital committees, "To prove to the world that we are liberal but not lax, we curtail the number of abortions we do at each hospital and we even enunciate arbitrarily acceptable abortion-delivery ratios. . . . Each hospital, in other words, sets it own rules—some compassionate, some academic, all hypocritical."[185]

Constricting compassion through regulated tolerance, which situated the present affectively in relation to shifting threats, was part of how induced abortion was weaponized to contest ways of living, and not just because the committee system was hostile to women's self-determination. Rickie Solinger documents that hospital abortion boards were part of a postwar conservative retrenchment in the United States heralding the emergence of the fetal citizen and a corresponding clampdown on reproduction that reasserted male control over women.[186] Such boards were also a clear attempt to avoid legal trouble in a restrictive climate and so were self-protective on the part of clinics.[187] At the same time, many of the physicians who favored the committee system on the grounds that it was better for patients, such as Guttmacher, who helped pioneer the board system, also advocated for expanded legal recognition of indicators. Hospital abortion boards, Solinger argues, were a shift in the medical community from "a defensive posture" regarding lax enforcement to an "offensive posture toward women," intended to demonstrate scientific rigor and moral sobriety.[188]

However, as we have seen, abortion control had been part of society's wars with itself from the mid-nineteenth century. Hospital committees were further attempts to protect life from itself, in this case from unwarranted pity that put women and the unborn at unnecessary risk. A danger of compassion toward life's miseries is that the society can become too compassionate, thus contributing to even more misery. At every turn, forms of immunity became dangerous in themselves to biological and social life, prompting further attempts at building immunity, protections from our protections.[189] In that regard, the hypocrisy of the boards is rhetorically significant: it speaks of backlash, yes, but it also realizes the outer limit of rhetoric incumbent to immunitary biopolitics and abortion. Two aspects demonstrate this significance.

First, charges of hypocrisy are tangled up with contempt that follows from pity, contempt not just for the object of compassion but also for the one who feels compassion.[190] The parallel between Quinten Scherman's and Hall's indictments of therapeutic abortion practices reveals as much. Scherman presented data on trends in indicators and the current research on their merits, but he blamed approval for all but the most rare cases on a simple "lack of knowledge of recent advances."[191] By appropriating the risk analysis of women seeking abortions—weighing economic hardship against a fourth child, for instance—doctors were simply furthering the moral ignorance that anti-Malthusians had decried. Compassion had made doctors dangerously tolerant. Writing in 1968,

Hall, on the other hand, exercised contempt for a framework of tolerance altogether: "Abortion is a medical issue only because it is the doctor who wields the instrument. He [sic] is no better able to judge who qualifies for an abortion than the patient's minister, the patient's lawyer, or the patient herself." Hall felt the patient should decide with input from her doctor and "concurrence of her husband."[192] He rejected a standard of the lesser evil, effectively rejecting tolerance as a legitimizing discourse: "All this hokum might result in some sort of empirical sense if it were not for the fact that it is so inconsistently and inequitably enforced."[193] He argued for legitimation by right, not by pity, and rejected the entire dynamic of abortion as a sign of pathology, because the practice was safe (contingent on the status of the fetus): "If you regard the fetus as a potential human being and not an actual human being . . . you must, I contend, ultimately reach the conclusion that all voluntary abortion is permissible."[194] Scherman and Hall adopted mirrored, contradictory standpoints on the failure of therapeutic tolerance to protect life from itself.

Second, while endeavoring to tolerate the intolerable, physicians found they could no longer reconcile the overdetermination of harm associated with abortion. In every direction—law, medicine, culture—signs pointed to a society that was afflicted because abortion was so badly managed. To that extent, the hypocrisy and anxiety associated with the therapeutic board system is the ultimate expression of medical rhetoric's unyielding investment in abortion as pathognomonic. The recursive dynamic of the rhetoric had itself become an autoimmune disorder *because* it leveraged critique of anything about a way of life that affected the levels of danger from abortion. Abortion as a sign of pathology was itself a sign of pathology, indexing physicians' inability to resolve how to weigh competing morbidities, let alone what constituted harm. It is fitting that as part of protecting life from itself, a rhetoric whose capacity was so dependent on placing and evaluating community within a matrix of threats would eventually find that very dependency to be one of those threats. Also, that rhetoric about abortion is itself an autoimmune disorder is proof of the extent to which interrupted pregnancy could envelop history in conflicts over how we should live: anything related to its morbidity, including discourses of the same, recurred to civilization's advancement.

The most significant development in the reform of abortion law prior to *Roe v. Wade*, the American Law Institute's (ALI's) model penal code, takes on a different cast when understood within Brown's model of regulated tolerance. The ALI promulgated the code in May 1959, basing its reforms on medical research and on earlier suggested reforms, including Taussig's own model statute. Taussig's statute influenced discussions of legal reform into the 1960s. The ALI code was more concise but followed Taussig's exceptions for life and health of the mother (physical or mental), rape, and "grave physical or mental defects" in the fetus. It also stipulated certification of the decision to be filed with a public prosecutor.[195] After its release, state legislatures began to consider the ALI model, twenty-eight states doing so in 1967, with Colorado being the first to pass a version of the law that year, followed by California and North Carolina, then Maryland and Georgia in 1968.[196] It was the first significant relaxation of the law in a century but, like the law it replaced, it was still medically driven risk management.[197] Interestingly, Governor Nelson Rockefeller tasked the Froessel Commission, headed by Alan Guttmacher, to study effects of ALI-inspired laws as part of reforming New York law. Guttmacher had been in the room when the ALI code was unveiled in 1959, only to hear the venerable Judge Learned Hand call it "'too damned conservative.'"[198] Guttmacher himself thought it was the answer and promoted it up until his research for the commission. He found, though, that once adopted, these laws only aggravated inequities in access and encouraged dubious, inflated uses of psychiatric conditions that ate up psychiatrists' time in public institutions. Guttmacher made a "reluctant" transformation from advocating abortion control to advocating decriminalization. "I reached this conclusion in 1969, 47 years after abortion first came to my medical attention as a third-year medical student."[199]

It is easy to imagine the ALI code and its adoption as a limited, flawed step toward abortion rights, but it is more appropriate to note Guttmacher's considered reaction. The ALI code was in spirit Taussig's code, and Taussig's code was about regulating tolerance. It changed the conditions of pity for misery, not of autonomy for women. The ALI code's requirement of notification, included by all states that adopted the code, made the demonstration of tolerance a legal obligation. These reforms were part of the abortion control regime begun in the nineteenth century. They added reporting mechanisms that would enable more sophisticated recursion to the management of danger, particularly an accounting of dispensations of amnesty (remembering our communal forgiveness). As I have noted, while physicians or lawyers did not *intend* to build a mnestic system for biopolitical conflict around induced abortion, they needed to do so if they were to contest the ways of living implicated by the practice. The ALI code attempted to legally reimmunize the nation against the now dangerous and antiquated laws of the nineteenth century. Seeking that new immunity, the law necessarily drew on and reinforced the same recursive dynamic that had enabled immunitary rhetoric in the first place. The ALI-inspired reforms were a culmination, not a refutation.[200]

Only when Guttmacher saw that greater compassion in control produced more harm did he abandon control as the meta-strategy. However, he did not abandon abortion as pathognomonic: "The only way to truly democratize legal abortion and to reduce illegal abortion markedly is to establish abortion on request, removing abortion from the penal code.... This conclusion has since been reinforced by observation of how well the New York law has functioned, markedly reducing out-of-wedlock and unwanted marital births, cutting sharply the number of dangerous illegal abortions and resultant maternal mortality and morbidity."[201] For Guttmacher, the discourse of choice still depended on recursion to harm to evaluate progress, but trusting women as the better agents of progress, not fearing them as risky subjects. In other words, to the extent that pro-choice discourse availed itself of *medicalized rhetoric*, it relied on the rhetoric of civilization as risk as well, but with a decisive difference of distributing the governmentality of pregnancy among women, supported by knowledge experts and community. This political *oikonomia*, a different attempt to reconcile the general order of a society with the specific order of individual lives, still inhabited the present as at a turning point between the better and the worse, given the extant dangers of abortion.

Conclusion | Seeking Immunity

Abortion is an endemic plague which never has been and never can be legislated away.
—ALAN F. GUTTMACHER, "Social Problems of Gynecology and Obstetrics"

The real open secret of abortion was that women's ultimate control over pregnancy was incurable. As a governing mentality, abortion control proved an enduring failure, but that was its greatest strength rhetorically because incessant contestation was capacitated *through* the very incurability of the practice. An "endemic plague" of criminal and therapeutic acts provided abundant power for political struggle in a nation forever seeking immunity from afflictions within its collective body. Constant pursuit of adequate protection from abortion became a way to inhabit the present as dangerous and therefore an important diagnostic for U.S. life politics: the relative frequency with which people interrupted pregnancy reliably inserted a nation into history as advancing or declining in an unwinnable fight over how to "make life live." If intentional abortion was a form of self-mutilation caused by the moral or scientific ignorance of the community and the patient, then harm to maternal or fetal life suggested invisible, systemic disorders within the general state of affairs—lurking ethical corruption, privation, inequity, abuse. The persistence of wounds, mortal or minor, enabled biopolitical projects to recur to threatening aspects of culture, medicine, and law as primary contact points between the past, present, and future. The morbidity from abortion provided a rhetorical capacity to emplace the present in ways endlessly suitable for contestation.

The indeterminate pathologization of abortion afforded abundant capacity. Anti-Malthusian physicians from the nineteenth through the turn of the twentieth century worked primarily with the physiology of harm accompanying the practice to fashion the pathological value of abortion, which was morally antigenic. The laws of nature, evident in lives lost and bodies damaged, became reminders of a more virtuous place in time that the United States had yet to achieve. It is not simply that these doctors used the language of disease and decline. A steady stream of women in distress helped fashion a sense of place, a place that the nation must escape. More than that, any time and place exhibiting a similar stream of gruesome events was understood as similarly in decline. Without broken bodies as remindands, the capacity to turn moral amnesia into a memory of permanent dislocation would not have been possible. Although the body in trauma was crucial to a biotic memory of the present as "primitive," an additional component was required if abortion as "social disease" was to be tethered to a feeling of progress. A peculiar, inverted scale of civilization derived from Malthus organized a linear sequence of societies founded on the effective management of reproduction wherein terminating a pregnancy was in every instance a sign of life gone wrong, both in that woman's life and in the life of the people she belonged to.

Principally after the birth control movement caught fire, neo-Malthusian physicians in the United States extended and revised this basic capacity, keeping a Malthusian scale of civilization but moving toward aggregated harm as the prime metric for placement and away from a moral physiology of natural law. Injury and death were still reminders of a time that the nation was yet to achieve, but the present now floundered in the wake of a future molded to the latest research because primitiveness was connected to the privations of poor fertility control. It was not Nature angrily reminding us of our collective failure through vicious infections, poisonings, embolisms, and hemorrhages—it was a callous, inadequate system of reproductive regulation making itself evident. Providence was really just a (bad) Plan, which recalled a sense of backwardness, not sinfulness. When the average abortion replaced the dramatic case as the primary modality of recollecting, a statistical memory of frequency and pattern supplanted physiological trauma as the substance of mnestic dynamics. In the process, medical experts successfully turned the strategic amnesia of the underground's subterfuges into a mode of recollection. Advances in the medical use of statistics made a numeric memory of abortion's secret, second world possible. It is particularly noteworthy that neo-Malthusian countermemory treated existing law and medical care, which had been the prevailing mechanisms to enforce recollection of woman's moral duty, as amnestic priorities. Outdated medical practice and law kept the United States trapped in a past that must be forgotten.

In principle, therapeutic abortion should have unraveled the capacity to locate the present in an uncivilized state by virtue of abortion's many traumas. The fact that what reminds us of ignorant primitiveness can also remind us of compassionate advancement seems destined to relax the arbitrary definition of progress as a world without abortion or the absolute indication of social disease from misfortune. Yet the instability of therapeutic abortion was a critical requirement to turn interrupted pregnancy into a mnestic dynamo for biopolitics. Life is not a singular value; it includes death because sometimes taking life is about making life live, so necessary zones of tolerance for the intolerable must be carved out within any biopolitical project. The ability to recall a better, future life through the dangers faced in this one must be suspended on occasion, the relationship of morbidity to place-in-time temporarily forgotten under the cover of amnesty. In this way, every aspect of abortion control, including its many exceptions, worked together to maintain a sense of the present as always inadequate, always in danger, always needing "more wisdom in living." The long, rancorous history of debating which indicators are valid for a therapeutic procedure can be viewed as a necessary side effect of the dynamic presumably tabled by such procedures.

I have described a mnestic dynamism that afforded some bearing to attempts to address perceived failings in current ways of life, which is why I call it a capacity. It enabled specific rhetorical acts, even long-range campaigns, by providing a broad ability to find the present wanting (*find* in the dual sense of "locate" and "judge") if current circumstances, desires, and beliefs encouraged ending pregnancy for all but the rare reason. Drawing a lesson from the body's immune system for biopolitics, Roberto Esposito writes, "Nothing is more inherently dedicated to communication than the immune system. Its quality is not measured by its ability to provide protection from a foreign agent, but from the complexity of the response it provokes."[1] The complex orientations to time, place, and struggle provoked by abortion as a sign of pathology measure its rhetorical quality. This ability to find the present wanting was not inherent in the terms physicians used because the dynamic energized divergent, conflicted vocabularies (that or moral physiology, privation, and therapy). It was not inherent in the specific ideologies of doctors because it supported any of them in their various antagonisms and solidarities. It was not inherent in conditions of poverty, immigration, religiosity, law, or the state of medical science because, as conditions changed and threats came and went, terminated pregnancy persisted and mutated as a measure of life gone wrong. And it was not inherent in human attitudes about reproduction because this ability had emerged and evolved only in the previous two centuries. The pregnant body in extremis and the shifting but constant engagement of medicine with maternity are the primary components.

As a result, I have taken pains to stress the orientational maneuvers embedded within diverse practices over time so that the dynamic can be felt across discourses and not be understood as the strategic goal of any one of them or as the limited consequence of specific circumstances. Abortion as a sign of pathology became a condition of possibility for, not an end state of, biopolitical discourses.

The existence of induced abortion and its dangers, once transformed into an index of societal afflictions, suspended the present between a lingering, benighted past and a tardy, enlightened future. Several interdependent tropes produced this sense of place by "folding" times and places together. First and primary was that induced abortion was an abnormal *interruption* of life, which made it a disorderly inflection point in the normal order of things. The act itself became an embodied trope of life politics. Next, for acts of abortion to position contemporary society as disordered in general, the false turn of interrupting life had to reverberate with false ways of living. It was not a generalizing move per se but one of *transumption*, one event transformed and subsumed within others. A combined trope that allows different moments and scales of being to pass into one another is needed for this task. In the case of the biotic remembrance favored by anti-Malthusians, medical practice made the invisible aspects of abortion's morbidity visible (a *chiastic* inversion of the body from closed to open) and reduced the damage to a consequence of desecrating Natural law (a *metonymic* conversion of morbidity to punishment). It is possible to sense the immoral regression of the nation in a fatal case of sepsis because it is the verdict of Natural justice. The statistical memory cultivated most significantly by neo-Malthusians accomplished the same task differently. Demographic tabulation of mortality and injury also operated by metonymy (converting harm into a map of society by reducing diverse cases to categories) but coupled with *enumeration* (amassing cases into an ordered dispersion). It is possible to sense the deprived backsliding of the nation in a rate of sepsis because it is typical.

Finally, if the broad sickness of interrupting pregnancy without medical sanction is to encapsulate the world in a history of sickness, as it did in the rhetoric examined here, then the present must be related to the entirety of civilizations past and future. The world in its fullness must be made of the present if the present is to be indicative of that world. Anti-Malthusians, relying heavily on the disturbed order of physiology to situate time and place, enacted a composition of contraries (*antitheton*) that collapsed any and all times into the present and, simultaneously, expanded the present to envelope all times and places. Physicians *amplified* propagation, the supposed final cause of womanhood, into a final cause of all civilization, which at the same time *reduced* all human society to a singular reproductive organism. Combined with reducing morbidity to a metric of moral amnesia, anti-Malthusian physicians extended procreation as the teleology of life to encompass the final order of global time, thus enabling highly flexible part-to-whole relations (uterus into nation, nation into civilization, civilization into uterus). Neo-Malthusians, who relied on the average abortion to locate the present on a scale of civilization, amplified the divisions that organized vital and social statistics to organize this or any society (*distributio*). Constituent risk vectors for elective abortion enabled tabular comparison of civilizations.

These complicated figurations provided a compass of sorts for physicians' biopolitical critiques but they are not properly representations of times and places because a host of actions, words, numbers, and events are involved. Consider again just the "base fold," induced abortion as the abnormal interruption of life. This includes (a) any of the implements, successful or not, by which one tries to terminate a pregnancy: catheters, curettes, sponges, abortifacients, soapy water, falls down stairs, knitting needles, and so on; (b) any of the factors that cause one to turn to such methods: poverty, wealth, no birth control, youth, too many children, no one to help raise a child, dangerous home life, and so on; (c) any of the factors that lead to harm: bacteria, unsophisticated methods, lack of skill, inadequate resources, and so on; and (d) any of the epistemological and representational resources used to makes sense of the previous conditions. The melding of diverse elements into a sense of immediate danger to women and to society is requisite to produce discourse critical of contemporary ways of life *because of how abortion expresses itself within those ways of life*. More than that, once different figural patterns are established, they become a ready platform to produce continuous variations of critique because the present can be found wanting in any number of ways. If women are incurably risky subjects susceptible to morbid influences, then abortion as a sign of pathology is a way to inhabit the world as incurably risky.

Induced abortion was hardly the first or only internal threat by which interested parties in the United States have remembered the nation as living through hazardous times. Countless aspects of how people live have been weaponized for internal "social" wars: labor practices, food ways, education—the list is limited only by the material potential of a given rhetoric. However, induced abortion is set apart through the particular vulnerability of pregnancy, but not vulnerability in the sense of "fragile" or "weak" as is so often assumed about gravidity.

Pregnancy is a site and a moment of vulnerability in the sense that power comes with risk and procreation is extraordinarily powerful. Foucault famously argued that where there is power there is resistance.[2] And where there is power, there is also responsiveness. Without mutual responsiveness between the various actors within an ecology of power, power becomes power*less*. If power is generally an ability to produce affects, to matter in the world, then to be productive all the elements involved in the conditions of power's enactment must affect one another as well. Thus, reproductive vitality shares the same material environment as different rhetorics about it: pregnant bodies, personal circumstances, culture, law, *materia medica*, microorganisms, caregivers, medical knowledge, economic conditions, and many more elements still. These factors exist in exquisite, complex forms of vulnerable interconnection and dependency that are necessary to reproductivity, such that nonresponsiveness is the real antithesis of *bio*power (not death as the opposition to life). Disease means vitality in error, a suite of vulnerabilities become powerful in a way deemed dangerous. Pregnancy is not a vector of threats because it is vulnerable. Indeed, the power of pregnancy is contingent on the woman's conscious and corporeal responsiveness to her environment and as part of her environment. Pregnancy is a threat vector when its power redefines vitality. Likewise, rhetoric about pregnancy, whether its termination or otherwise, draws from these vulnerable interconnections for its power as well. Rhetoric about reproduction develops its capacities *within* the conditions of pregnancy. Reproduction and rhetoric about it are mutually vulnerable because they are not separate; each is of and affects the other, which augments the power of each.

The significance of the pregnant body in biopower has everything to do with its formidable, irreplaceable power as a vital force, whether crudely understood in terms of producing numbers of people or subtly in terms of managing pregnancy to influence everything that procreation touches. And procreation eventually is in touch with everything important to humans: it is pivotal in the lives of individuals, families, and communities; it is foundational to sprawling cultural, technical, legal, and economic apparatuses; and it is critical to the biology of life itself. From a communal point of view, the power of pregnancy entails exposure to risk in seemingly endless variations, but that is precisely the meter of its vigor, not its infirmity. New risks inevitably emerge as reproductive vitality is engaged differently in support of new and different ways of life; the dangers change as the ecology of power changes. Since the nineteenth century, emerging risks to life from induced abortion were greeted with medical resistance, intended to either blunt the changes or to shepherd them as best as possible. The predicate that progress produces pathology is an acknowledgment that power comes with risk, stated within immunitary logic.

In sum, induced abortion offered the rhetorical potential of a wound that never heals to political economies of life. Friedrich Nietzsche wrote in the *Genealogy of Morals* of memory work as a promise that humans make: "It's an active *wish* not to be free of the matter again, an ongoing and continuing desire for what one willed at a particular time, a real *memory of one's will*."[3] Abortion's incurability became a material basis through which different, competing regimes of living attempted to keep their promises (they still do). The danger of abortion, whether conceived as inherently murderous or as reckless if poorly done, was a material history that all parties wished never to forget. Its occurrence was anathema but its memory a lodestar, a thing better gone *but not forgotten*, for its recollection was indispensable to gauge our betterment. Consequently, both anti- and neo-Malthusians forged a way to remember the world through danger so that they might eventually produce a world free of that very same danger. Such memory work comparatively emplaces the will to live, this way versus that way, this moment versus that moment, thus localizing danger so that discourse may be effectively addressed to reduce that danger. A memory of a will to live *without abortion's dangers* allows past actions and events to be folded into new ones, such that the promise of immunity to the practice becomes a long chain of unrealized potential.

It is important to emphasize that this dynamic is not limited to specific time-place markers such as when anti-Malthusians invoked Juvenal's satires to compare America to Rome, or when Alan Guttmacher drew on Prohibition to describe the underground. Occasionally writers produced vague sketches of historical moments. More often, they wrote from a sense of the now, invoking a relation between times rather than depicting those times. That feeling of emplacement is what this book has attempted to make palpable; it was not meant as a catalog of medical representations of the past or future. As I have shown, medical rhetoric did not simply oppose memory to forgetfulness but figured a complex mutuality of remembering and forgetting that sustained the understanding of abortion as a wrong act that was granted, always but only, a place of permanent exception in a civilized world. The extraordinary mnestic capacity of induced abortion was that it signaled no specific disease other than a community's inability to optimize pregnancy's vulnerabilities in a life-supporting way—however *life-supporting* might be construed. Because the conduct of abortion invariably inflected the present as a moment of trailing behind if not falling backward, its predictability offered a continuous, mutable basis on which to pledge the future.

At the outset I expressed my hope that readers might develop "an eye" for the dynamism traced in this book, over and above learning about the internal history of abortion in U.S. medical rhetoric up to the 1960s, because although the figurations have mutated, the dynamic is still operative. Nevertheless, I fully recognize how convoluted the different folds are that embody "abortion as sign of pathology" over the long period analyzed, which is why I described my approach as one of sidelong glances. The capacity to create a sense of time and place within a rhetoric does not exist separate from the discourses of that rhetoric. When one tries to determine how the present is *made* present *while* an interested party is *addressing* that present, it is not unlike trying to see the shadows in the corner of one's eye. You turn to look and they move. Here Nietzsche's description of "a memory of one's will" is especially helpful because he provides a way to synthesize my analytical dissection into a critical observational practice that improves one's peripheral vision. As I have only discussed tropes broadly characteristic of medical rhetoric through the 1960s in the United States, to look beyond their example one should not expect to see the same kinds of maneuvers necessarily. Rather, one must first attend to the future being pledged by a particular discourse about abortion, the promise to be kept. Then it is possible to assess the tropes working in the periphery that suspend the present in a state of risk: look for wounding that must be remembered such that the world in which it occurs can be forgotten.

The basic pledge made about abortion in medical rhetoric was to protect life from its errors, to seek immunity from disease. Attempted immunizations to abortion took two principle forms in the nineteenth and into the twentieth century: immunity *for* women to the causes and consequences of the act, and immunity *from* women whose acts threatened the well-being of the community. Immunity *for* women involved first and foremost better medical care. The initial state laws on abortion were directed at protecting the life and very occasionally the health of the mother, because the conduct of abortion had high mortality and injury rates in addition to being morally repugnant to key physicians. The history of therapeutic indicators roughly tracks with efforts to protect women by controlling badly performed or unhygienic procedures. Eventually, improvements in quality of care, at least for those who could afford it, produced relative immunity for women to sloppy practices. The other aspect of immunity *for* women was based in reducing women's purported ignorance. Whether as a disorganized medical pastorate, a regime of clinical consultation, or a hospital board reviewing requests, physicians organized themselves as intermediaries in a woman's decision making as a form of protection for her because she was believed otherwise incapable of the best choice. A crucial part of actualizing pregnancy's power was the vulnerability that comes from necessarily distributed, uneven decision making about when pregnancy itself is ill advised, as well as from inconsistent, crude methods of acting on the desire to end pregnancy. Yet with improved safety came charges that abortion had become too easy, while tighter control on decisions led to indictments from physicians that medical care was discriminatory.

Immunity *from* women involves less a different set of dangers than a different marshaling of the same ones. It is the difference between protecting the patient and protecting society, which are not opposite concerns. Regulatory measures, whether in law or medical policy, were thought to protect the individual woman *from* the forces that drove her to consider aborting; such measures were treated also as a protection *for* her. Such measures were an attempt to immunize society from women, because women were susceptible to moral, economic, cultural, and personal influence. To protect the "ignorant woman," the wise abortion had to be limited strictly to medically approved procedures (and even then, an affirmative decision was treated with great skepticism). To some extent, law and policy that restricted abortion was an effort to limit persuadability under the guise of protecting society from ignorance. The great vulnerability of pregnancy is that human beings may decide its fate, which is the source of its great power as well. We can increase or decrease the number of children born and we can change how we manage pregnancy. A key element of pregnancy's power is the condition of elective abortion's possibility. To that extent, the attempt to build a collective immunity *from* women who abort is an effort to *decrease* the sensitivity of reproductive vitality to its environment *at the point of decision*.

Having isolated promises of immunity, including new promises or variations on those just synopsized, one can begin to identify specific mnestic figurations that stabilize the present as needing immunization. Relative to the immunity promised, attend to the particular *inflection* of the issue at hand, meaning the morbid turn from the future that a community requires protection from and the conditions that contribute to that morbidity. Is it bourgeois aspiration, inadequate birth control, social stigma, and so forth? Then ascertain the *position* of that pathology within the community. How does this pathology map the collective, showing the community a vision of itself through recurrent, self-inflicted wounds? And then note the possible *inclusion* of other communities in a history totalized through pathology. How does this particular pathology bind different communities together in a macrolevel story of biopolitics?[4]

A primary virtue of pursuing a genealogy of a rhetoric's mnestic capacity is that one can observe how the limits of discursive power vary with the emergence of new ways to inhabit time and place. In light of the preceding genealogy, two shifts in the conditions of medically managing abortion are especially notable for having produced ruptures in the discursive capacity of the rhetoric. The first was the emergence of the average abortion with the shift from moral physiology to statistics to explain social pathologies. With the former, anti-Malthusians strongly relied on a Providential sense of time and place such that each embolism, for example, was like every other one in that it spoke of a divergence from God's plan. The world's clock was internalized to the female body, as Nathan Allen diagrammed in "The Law of Human Increase" when he inverted Malthusianism from a law of population inhering in social-economic order to a law of creation that "must have its seat somewhere in the body itself."[5] Anti-Malthusians focused their attention on building immunity to abortion through belligerent "counseling" of individual patients because abortion evidenced moral amnesia adversely inflecting women's relation to childbearing. They existed in a time and place of un-Christian influence, and this shaped not only the discursive course to plot but also the limits of what could be accomplished at the time.

With the later, statistical assessment of time and place, physicians returned to an externally defined Malthusian world. Neo-Malthusians situated the nation as a civilization via inadequate conditions for reproductive management and so directed their efforts toward broad programs of abortion control. Alleviating the economic conditions that made multiparous and single white women abort so often would usher in a better future, for example. Anti-Malthusians adjusted as well, still insisting on a world where harm was caused by moral deficiency, but they used vital and social data to oppose abortion control because such programs could not eliminate the danger. The world's movement now could be felt through changing calculations of morbidity, not through each woman's ethical relation to self.

The second rupture is the emergence of the safe abortion. If the search for immunity to abortion involved a search for immunity *from* women, then emergence of abortion without significant maternal risk prompted, perhaps more than any other event, a major refinement in the immunitary logic associated with abortion. Immunity *from* women became immunity *for* the unborn.[6] No single event marked this particular turn in medicalized abortion rhetoric. Scholars have proposed a range of thresholds for when the fetus became the focal point, from the first sequential visualization of embryological development, to the development of Rh treatments of a fetal patient in the early 1960s, to the public photographic debut of a free-floating fetus in 1965. The origin of fetal individuality has many inception dates. However, one could do worse than date it to the moment when the threat of maternal harm from abortion began to fade, leaving only the harm to the fetus as the damage by which a nation might measure itself against its former selves and other nations too. At the same time as images of the fetus increasingly took hold of public attention, the medical experts' fears that women were killing themselves to avoid motherhood subsided. I explained in the previous chapter that improvements in treatment complicated the therapeutic exception but did not disrupt the rhetoric as much as bring it full circle. I will close the genealogy now by briefly drawing attention to one final proceeding of experts that marks the completion of the rupture caused by safer abortions and then reflect on a greater continuity that has yet to be disturbed.

In 1967, the Joseph P. Kennedy, Jr. Foundation sponsored an international conference on abortion held in Washington, D.C. Over six dozen attendees represented areas of medicine, law, social science, ethics, and government. In 1968 Bantam published a highly edited conference proceedings titled *The Terrible Choice: The Abortion Dilemma*, which featured sixteen pages of black-and-white fetal images by Lennart Nilsson showing developmental stages from four weeks to six months. This was the first conference to put a prominent emphasis on fetal development, let alone to feature images of fetuses as a way of conceptualizing the harm of abortion. The opening chapter of the report, "The Problem," begins by describing abortion as a surgical procedure from the standpoint of its effect on fetal tissue. The next chapter presents five "legitimacy" scenarios— rape, fetal abnormality, unwed motherhood, poverty, too many children—after which came chapters on the biological then the statistical background of abortion, and finally came Nilsson's images. The biological chapter discusses only fetal development, not maternal risk. The statistical chapter recapitulated the commonplaces addressed in previous chapters, notably that maternal risk is a consequence of treatment inequities. In other words, a limited numeric picture of maternal harm was sandwiched between a five-page discussion of fetal development and a sixteen-page photo spread of fetal images. The answer to the question of abortion's legitimacy in cases of rape provided in the biology chapter indicates a decisive fetal presence: "About one week after fertilization the tiny sphere of cells, often called the blastocyst, arrives in the uterus. Now begins a very critical stage in the struggle for survival. The blastocyst has only about seven days to implant itself in the soft spongy lining of the uterus; about a quarter of all blastocysts perish naturally."[7] The danger to embryonic survival, already at risk naturally, was the one and only biological consideration.

This volume was unlike any prior conferences of experts. Later chapters presented social scientific, medical, ethical, and legal perspectives that contained more complex considerations of danger. But with the exception of the social science chapter, the presentation of expert opinion was significantly if not chiefly guided by the dilemma of choosing between the mother and the newly present fetus. Claims of maternal death and risk were still quite common in public advocacy for abortion reform at this time, but as the Kennedy conference demonstrates, fetal harm was an ascendant concern within medically situated discourse. Not since H. R. Storer had made a case for fetal life had the unborn been as significant in a book on abortion, and never before had a symposium of experts privileged fetal life over maternal life. One could and should point to developments in embryology, photography, and fetal treatment as conditions for this moment. But one must also acknowledge that by 1968, *if* a woman had access to competent care, she faced almost no danger from an abortion. The matrix of dangers had fundamentally shifted so that now immunity *from* women's actions necessarily was understood relative to immunity *for* the unborn. In terms of a genealogy of medical rhetoric founded on an eternal wound, the Kennedy conference is a crucial marker attesting that a new declension had emerged for orienting biopolitical discourse through abortion as a regrettable act.

I will not speculate on this new declension at this time except to state the obvious: the ascendance of the fetus has changed things. But it has not brought a revolution in the rhetoric.[8] To discourse on abortion still engages a medicalized rhetoric of life gone wrong. I bracketed the idea from the beginning of rhetoric as two-sided argument aimed at producing resolution, however temporary. In other words, I put aside the idea of disputation as constructive of agreement or at least a mechanism for cooperative relations. To even talk of fetuses and pregnancy requires that one enter discourses of biomedicine, and the history of medical rhetoric on abortion suggests that it is not organized to produce some kind of ideological convergence around knowledge of life, but to situate open-ended social wars against perceived threats to well-being. Independent of the history of medical ethics and practice relative to patient treatment, medicine has made the chaotic material conditions of abortion's morbidity rhetorically capacious for biopolitics. The memory work inherent in abortion as pathogno-monic catalyzes those politics; it does not lead to an escape from them or bring conflicts to some sort of closure.

Such a realization is somewhat mundane if taken on its face, as is the basic idea that abortion is something people wish to avoid. However, to recognize medicine's function in turning the mundane conditions of abortion into a rhe-torical capability has great import for the current state of the "abortion wars" and for biopower, even though the language of "social disease" has all but van-ished. It means first and foremost that because we fight *through* abortion about life politics generally, we should not expect an end to struggles over abortion. As long as immunity is sought from the harms associated with interrupted preg-nancy and the conditions under which it occurs, harms that are undecidable, the rhetorical capacity for struggle developed in the nineteenth century and con-tinually refined since then will be in operation. To an important extent, abortion wars *are* a measure of emplacement—we are in an age of biopower if protection from terminated pregnancies, including protection from the protection, is a ba-rometer of progress.

The idea of perpetual struggle through abortion may be depressing, but the whole subject of abortion is depressing, as many, many interlocutors have noted at the first moment that I tell them what I research. It is not uncommon at the close of a study like this one for the author to advise some sort of remedy, and I have been asked more than once to provide one (as if I had such a talent), but that itself would entail using harm from elective abortion and its control as a metric for progress, in this case harm from the hot and cold wars that flare up around abortion, thus reengaging the very dynamic that supports perpetual struggle. Ironically, anyone who seeks respite from the divisiveness and carnage of the abortion wars recommits to minimizing morbid tendencies in culture as a way to pledge a different future. The pathological damage attending elec-tive abortion shift registers from bodily traumas to rights and public violence. Put differently, in an age of biopower, even in this late age when the relation of labor and capital is completely transformed and medicine has entered a post-genomic era, there is as yet no transcendence from struggle through abortion. There is only refinement of how morbidity is mobilized within the paradigm of immunity.

If there is to be a great disruption to the continuity of rhetoric about abortion and its control, a new era in which the practice is not a weapon to contest ways of living, it will require a rupture far greater than to what constitutes danger or how that danger localizes advancement. It will require a biopolitics without disease.[9] How to treat abortion ethically, how to ensure its safety, how to determine its best management, how to disagree about rights without investing again in a dynamic that makes such issues fronts in broader struggles to change contemporary cultural order? An unregulated approach to abortion is a position no one would endorse (safety at minimum advises otherwise). Yet every configuration of control—on demand, under physician supervision, with limited exceptions, banned, and all their variance—implicates struggling through abortion about regimes of living in general such that we may need it less and under different conditions.[10] To need abortion or to need it and not have safe access it is to know life has gone wrong somehow by someone's measure. We need/want a less combative politics of care, at least many others and I think so, but how to establish a politics that does not fight *through* abortion as a way to immunize a community from some other part of that community? It would be rash and historically obtuse to assume that new paradigms are impossible, but to imagine a politics that frees abortion from its function as a means of contestation brings to mind the opening pages of *The Order of Things*, where Foucault, drawing from Borges, presents a Chinese taxonomy of animals that is incomprehensible to Western eyes, including categories like "(b) embalmed . . . (g) stray dogs . . . (n) that from a long way off look like flies." Faced with the challenge to imagine a biopolitics without disease, "the thing we apprehend in one great leap," as he said of the taxonomy, is "the stark impossibility of thinking *that*."[11]

I cannot offer a solution to the struggles *over* abortion, then, because as this critique has insisted, any such solution would restage those struggles *through* abortion's pathognomonics. Each solution is another potential symptom to someone, another risk vector. However, recognizing this recursive circularity is the objective of my genealogical approach: put the recursive habits that govern discursive practice under inspection. As I stated in the beginning, the conditions of abortion control do not *have* to indicate something is wrong with us collectively, although thinking otherwise is a daunting charge. This critique suggests why it is so difficult to do otherwise, but my own critical, genealogical rhetoric can only problematize that other, medical rhetoric. Such a critique "only exists in relation to something other than itself," as Foucault observed, and the critical purpose that has circumscribed my analytical relation to medicine has been *to question the question of abortion's pathology*. A genealogy of rhetoric cannot yield alternatives to its object, but such a critique *can* yield the conditions needed to let go of the prevailing order, "at least identifying by what and from what [the prevailing order's] disappearance is possible." Identifying the dynamic that encourages an intractable series of conflicts does not conjure another dynamic to replace it but it does allow one to begin to imagine our rhetoric "not being governed that way and at that cost."[12] I have identified a condition (albeit a remote one) under which thriving patterns of rhetoric that have leveraged over 150 years of conflict might atrophy. Agreement on why people abort, what it means, or who decides when it is allowable is not coming, so one must look to the function of those disagreements within the rhetoric for change. What is required is a different capacity to tell one time from another, one place from another, such that harm associated with abortion control regimes does not measure uncivilized ways of living. What is required is a new rhetoric, not a better version of the one that currently orients struggle, and we have no such rhetoric yet.

The risk of being misunderstood is great here so let me restate this last point. Insofar as a release from the conflicted rhetoric of abortion in the United States is desired, the challenge is extraordinary, maybe impossible. This does not mean that struggle to date has been in vain because the rhetoric seems to trap us in more struggles rather than free us. From the standpoint of women's freedom, women's control of their bodies, and the safety of abortion (which is a standpoint I share), struggle most surely has *not* been wasted and much more struggle is needed now in the face of diminishing access and an underground reborn. It also does not mean that it is a wrong act to lay a claim on a better future by continuing to judge the present as backward or dangerous by virtue of contemporary abortion control measures. Until that moment when the overarching continuity collapses that orients internal cultural conflict by virtue of abortion's incurability, there is precious little ground to stand on in regard to biopolitics. Yet any change that leads to a grand break in the rhetoric will emerge from within the broader ecology of biopower, not from anything a rhetorical analyst will say. No discursive stratagem will change the overall rhetoric until what keeps discourses of abortion situated, what puts them in conflict with one another, changes. Fashioning a new rhetoric that allows for disagreement, nurtures improved medical care, yet retires abortion from broad struggle over the order of things is a monumental task, not a matter of different rhetorical *techné*. It is about forgetting that abortion once was used to remember how far a people had come, and that begins when the conditions of ending pregnancy are no longer a sign of pathology.

Notes

Introduction

1. Luker, *Abortion*, 20; Smith-Rosenberg, *Disorderly*, 218.

2. Foucault, *Archaeology*, 216. Also see Petchesky, *Abortion*, 10–11.

3. Poovey, "Abortion," 240–43; Bordo, *Unbearable*, 71–97; Cornell, *Imaginary*, 32–53; Deutscher, "Foucault's."

4. Luker, *Abortion*, 14–15; Riddle, *Contraception*, 20–24, 62–64, 108–12, 140–43. Quickening means the woman perceives fetal movement; viability is survival of the fetus if prematurely delivered.

5. Farrell Brodie, *Contraception*, 281–88.

6. Luker, *Abortion*, 15; Petchesky, *Abortion*, 78–84; Hull and Hoffer, *Roe v. Wade*, 34. For an overview of abortion law, see N. J. Davis, *From*, 41–64.

7. Bitzer, "Rhetorical."

8. Luker, *Abortion*, 11–14.

9. Riddle, *Contraception*, 20–24. Riddle notes that "there was never absolute uniform opinion, however, in Hellenic, Hellenistic, or Roman thought, in Pagan philosophy, Judaism, or Christianity" (21). Also see Petchesky, *Abortion*, 68–69.

10. See Farrell Brodie, *Contraception*, 57–86, 204–41; C. R. McCann, *Birth Control*, 59–97; May, *America*, 24–34.

11. Schiappa, *Protagoras*, 89–102. The concept of *dissoi logoi* is derived from the "two-*logoi* fragment" of Protagoras, the fifth-century B.C.E. Sophist. The fragment is translated variously into English, which Schiappa organizes into the subjective and the Heraclitean interpretation (the latter so named for the pre-Socratic philosopher Heraclitus). The subjective interpretation translates the fragment as stating that there are two "arguments," "speeches," or "sides" of every "issue," "question," or "subject" (90). I refer to this subjective, debaterly tradition. In Foucauldian terms, a subjective "ars disputatio" cannot explain "scientia sexualis" or the internecine divisions of governmentality based on scientia sexualis. See Foucault, *History*, 53–73.

12. Lake, "Metaethical," 479–87. Lake provides an excellent description of how argument becomes intractable based on metaethical commitments of antiabortion advocates.

13. Meckel, *Babies*, particularly 124–77.

14. Ricoeur, *Memory*, 96–120.

15. The differences between collective, social, and public memory are notable depending on who one reads. I specify memory and forgetting particular to this study in chapter 2. For one useful discrimination of categories, see Casey, "Public."

16. Canguilhem, *Normal*, 100; also see 135.

17. Ibid., 88.

18. Ibid., 144, 137. Also see Hacking, *Taming*, 165, 169.

19. Canguilhem, *Normal*, 270.

20. Ibid., 285.

21. Ibid., 242. As Hacking writes, "The normal stands indifferently for what is typical, the unenthusiastic objective average, but it also stands for what has been, good health, and for what shall be, our chosen destiny" (*Taming*, 169).

22. Hodge, "Foeticide," 223. Hodge's lecture was printed years after its delivery.

23. Nowlin, "Criminal," 179.

24. Green, "Feticide," 590.

25. W. J. Robinson, *Law*, 6, 81.

26. Downie, "Interpretation," 31.

27. Guttmacher, "United States," 456.

28. Rosenberg, "Pathologies," 728–29.

29. Sontag, *Illness*, 72.

30. Ibid., 22.

31. Malthus, *Essay*.

32. Brown, *Regulating*, 166.

33. R. Porter, *Greatest*, 390–94. Samuel Hahnemann developed homoeopathy in Germany in the late eighteenth century. It was premised on the law of similars and infinitesimals, which meant that "to cure disease, we must seek medicines that can excite similar symptoms in the healthy human body" and that smaller doses were more effective (Hahnemann quote, ibid., 391). Eclecticism was an offshoot of Thomsonianism, started by Samuel Thomson in the United States in the early nineteenth century as "a people's health movement based on vegetable-based therapies" (ibid., 393). Eclecticism stressed botanical treatments. Homoeopathy and Eclecticism were both popular in the United States and had a number of medical schools (ibid., 530–31).

34. O'Donnell and Atlee, "Report," 247.

35. Dickinson, foreword to *Medical*, xxxi; original emphasis.

36. Calderone, "Illegal," 948.

37. Farrell Brodie, *Contraception*; Hull and Hoffer, *Roe v. Wade*; Joffe, *Doctors*; Mohr, *Abortion*; L. J. Reagan, *When*; Solinger, *Wake Up*; Solinger, *Beggars*; Solinger, *Pregnancy*. Also see Degler, *At Odds*; C. R. McCann, *Birth Control*; Gordon, *Moral*; Dubow, *Ourselves*.

38. Stormer, *Articulating*.

39. Vivian, *Public*, 3.

40. Kerényi, "Mnemosyne," 130; Casey, *Remembering*, 12.

41. I do not use *mneme*, because it means "memory," whereas, as mentioned, *mnesis* means "memory related."

42. Foucault, "Nietzsche," 152. Also see Nietzsche, *Genealogy*, Second Essay.

43. Foucault, "Nietzsche," 147, 144. My approach to genealogy resonates with Hawhee and Olson's description of pan-historiography: attend to "consistencies and ruptures," "keep texture and complexity in the foreground," treat archives as a plurality of materials, and don't lose sight of "that which moves" ("Pan-historiography," 95, 96, 99, 101).

44. Foucault, "Nietzsche," 147, 148. Also see Foucault, "What Is," 64–65.

45. Foucault, "Nietzsche," 148–49, 150.

46. McGee, "Materialist's," 38.

47. Biesecker, "Rethinking," 126, 110.

48. Greene, "Another," 22.

49. Condit, *Decoding*, 44–49, 49.

50. Ibid., 53.

51. R. Reagan, "Abortion."

52. Gold and Nash, "Troubling." Gold and Nash write, "Over the course of 2011, legislators in all 50 states introduced more than 1,100 provisions related to reproductive health and

rights. At the end of it all, states had adopted 135 new reproductive health provisions—a dramatic increase from the 89 enacted in 2010 and the 77 enacted in 2009. Fully 92 of the enacted provisions seek to restrict abortion, shattering the previous record of 34 abortion restrictions enacted in 2005. . . . A striking 68% of the reproductive health provisions from 2011 are abortion restrictions, compared with only 26% the year before."

53. NARAL, "Who Decides?"

54. Rich, "Stag Party." Rich notes that loyal but critical Republican Tanya Melich first coined the term "war on women" in her 1996 memoir, *The Republican War on Women*.

55. "Fear."

56. Abdullaeva, "Abortion."

57. Pollitt, "Prochoice."

58. Saletan and Pollitt, "Is Abortion?"

59. Ibid.

60. "N.C. Rep." Representative Pittman said his "sources" tell him that 75 percent of Planned Parenthood's money comes from abortions (it is only 3 percent) and that to claim Planned Parenthood supports contraception in order to decrease abortion is "like saying a baker would go around trying to get people to stop eating bread."

61. Mohr, *Abortion*, 237–41.

Chapter 1

1. Smith-Rosenberg, *Disorderly*, 218. Also see Mohr, *Abortion*, 86–118; Luker, *Abortion*, 15; Degler, *At Odds*, 227–48; Farrell Brodie, *Contraception*, 9–37; Hartmann, *Reproductive*, 243–67; Gilman Srebnick, *Mysterious*; Solinger, introduction; Lovett, *Conceiving*, 164–71.

2. Smith-Rosenberg, *Disorderly*, 217.

3. Ibid.; Foucault, "Nietzsche," 148–49.

4. Farrell Brodie, *Contraception*, 269–75; Luker, *Abortion*, 27–35; Mohr, *Abortion*, 147–70; Smith-Rosenberg, *Disorderly*, 217–18.

5. Agamben, *Homo Sacer*, 3, 188.

6. Foucault, *History*, 135–59; Foucault, "Society," 239–63; Foucault, *Security*; Foucault, *Biopolitics*; Stoler, *Race*, 19–94.

7. See Haraway, *Simians*, 203–30; Grosz, *Volatile*; Esposito, *Bios*; Agamben, *Homo Sacer*; Agamben, *State*; Agamben, *Kingdom*; Agamben, *Sacrament*.

8. Foucault, *Security*, 227–48.

9. Foucault, *History*, 142, 143.

10. Nadesan, *Governmentality*, 8–9. See Foucault, "Governmentality"; Foucault, *Biopolitics*; Foucault, *History*, 135–59; Foucault, *Security*, 115–226.

11. Agamben, *Kingdom*, 50.

12. Also, in contemporary biomedical discourse, abortion has shaped how stem cell research is talked about. See Franklin, "Stem Cells"; Lynch, "Stem Cells."

13. Smith-Rosenberg, *Disorderly*, 218.

14. Hale, *Great*, 7, 12–13.

15. Burke, *Grammar*, 326–27; McGee, "'Ideograph.'" Also see Barthes, *Mythologies*, 147–71; Deluca, *Image*, 25–44. For a broad discussion of how medicine from the Enlightenment forward has positioned women's bodies as a terrain for conflict and anxiety, see Kukla, *Mass*.

16. Foucault, *Clinic*, xi–xii, xvi–xix, 88–106; Laclau, *Populist*, 67–128.

17. Hull and Hoffer, *Roe v. Wade*, 38–47.

18. Calderone, "Illegal," 948.

19. Foucault, *Power/Knowledge*, 37–62, 134–45, 166–93.

20. Canguilhem, *Normal*, 285.

21. Ibid., 257. For more on the shift to an understanding of normal health in nineteenth-century U.S. medicine, see J. H. Warner, *Therapeutic*, 85–91.

22. Greene, *Malthusian*, 1–55. For an overview of Malthusianism in relation to abortion, see N. J. Davis, *From*, 20–39.

23. Malthus, *Essay*, 13. For extended discussions of Malthus relative to eighteenth- and nineteenth-century political economics and to the concept of population, see Gallagher, *Body*; Greene, *Malthusian*, 17–55.

24. It is well remarked that the first edition was much grimmer that later revisions, the major turn happening in 1803, and that the more explicitly theological chapters were removed. See Young, "Malthus," 102; Poovey, *History*, 284–95.

25. Malthus, *Essay*, 27; also see Binion, "'More.'"

26. Malthus, *Essay*, 48.

27. Ibid., 140.

28. Carlyle, *Chartism*, 107; Gallagher, *Body*, 26–27.

29. Binion, "'More,'" 565–67; Gallagher, *Body*, 9–11; Hecht, "'Fruitful,'" 544, 546; Walzer, "Logic," 3. As Hecht documents, even those whom Malthus criticized, such as Condorcet, believed in forms of birth control, and other "pre-Malthusian" principles were recognized in eighteenth-century France, too; Richard Cantillon, for example, described postponed marriage and celibacy as population checks (542–43, 545). Claude-François-Joseph d'Auxiron was the only "genuine pre-Malthusian in France" (546).

30. Malthus, *Essay*, 146, 147; also see Binion, "'More,'" 568.

31. Malthus, *Essay*, 150. See Poovey, *History*, 284–88.

32. Malthus, *Essay*, 90.

33. Young, "Malthus." Young traces Malthus's religious influences and notes his "strongly corporeal interpretation of humanity" (100).

34. Malthus, *Essay*, 20. For a discussion of Malthus's impact on data and calculating Providence, see Poovey, *History*, 278–95; T. M. Porter, *Rise*, 26–27.

35. Walzer, "Logic," 2. Also see L. A. Hall, "Malthusian."

36. Gordon, *Moral*, 42–44; Greene, *Malthusian*, 29–30.

37. Gordon, *Moral*, 41.

38. Farrell Brodie, *Contraception*, 57–135; also see Gordon, *Moral*, 38–52; Hull and Hoffer, *Roe v. Wade*, 23–27.

39. Gordon, *Moral*, 46, 47.

40. Ibid., 45; also see Farrell Brodie, *Contraception*, 67–79, 92, 94–106, 127–28.

41. Gordon, *Moral*, 50.

42. Hamlin and Gallagher-Kamper, "Malthus," 118–23; R. Porter, "Malthusian." The sluggish reaction from U.S. physicians is not unlike the British reaction. Porter demonstrates, however, that Malthus had some early medical critics in Britain.

43. Hellebore is a flowering plant prescribed from antiquity to induce abortion. In the first century C.E., Discorides wrote in *De Materia Medica* of white or black hellebore in wine as a common abortifacient. See Riddle, *Contraception*, 54–55; Gorney, *Articles*, 42; Hull and Hoffer, *Roe v. Wade*, 20.

44. Mohr, *Abortion*, 43. Also see Hull and Hoffer, *Roe v. Wade*, 17–22.

45. Foucault, *Security*, 108–9; Foucault, "Governmentality."

46. Hamlin and Gallagher-Kamper, "Malthus," 123–33. Hamlin and Gallagher-Kamper note, similarly, that state-level concern motivated physicians to engage with Malthusian

problems relative to fever in Ireland in 1817–19 and to poverty in Scotland in the later 1830s and into the 1840s.

47. Mohr, *Abortion*, 75–76. Also see Petchesky, *Abortion*, 73–74; Hull and Hoffer, *Roe v. Wade*, 22–23; Spengler, "Notes."

48. Hodge, "Foeticide." For more on Hodge, see Hull and Hoffer, *Roe v. Wade*, 28–29.

49. Hodge, "Foeticide."

50. Mohr, *Abortion*, 76. Also see Gigerenzer et al., *Empire*, 46–47.

51. Spengler, "Notes"; Gordon, *Moral*, 87–88; Mohr, *Abortion*, 74–85.

52. Pendleton, "Comparative"; Collins, "Diseases," 477; Anonymous, "Criminal." Pendleton's note was originally published in the *Charleston Medical Journal*. The *BMSJ* editors presented Pendleton as making a racial, not a local, claim: "proof that the whites are not more prolific than the blacks" (365). Collins does not specify white women so much as fret over the "fairest and best of God's creation" becoming "sickly and puny" in contrast to "our New-England mothers." The editors of *BMSJ* reprinted the anonymous letter by way of Walter Channing. Also see Petchesky, *Abortion*, 78–79.

53. H. R. Storer et al., "Report," 75. Committee members reflected a national interest: Massachusetts, New York, Pennsylvania, South Carolina, Alabama, Missouri, Wisconsin, and the District of Columbia. Resolutions unanimously adopted by the AMA in response to the report were appended: publicly stand against abortion, lobby legislatures to amend the laws (Storer drafted a model law, published in H. R. Storer, *Criminal Abortion in America*, 99–100), and call on state medical societies to cooperate. Also see Petchesky, *Abortion*, 79–80.

54. H. R. Storer, *Criminal Abortion in America*. The 1859 series of articles developed from a paper Storer presented in 1858 to the American Academy of Arts and Sciences (AAAS), "Decrease of the Rate of Increase of Population." Dyer provides a time line of manuscripts developed from the AAAS paper, the AMA report, the article series, and the 1860 anthology of the articles (*Champion*, 137–63). Also see Farrell Brodie, *Contraception*, 268.

55. H. R. Storer, *Criminal Abortion in America*, 13–35. Data on European nations varied widely and covered nearly three dozen nations. Data on New York extended back to 1804, dating only to 1850 for Massachusetts, Boston principally.

56. Ibid., 25.

57. Ibid., 26, quoting from Chickering, "Comparative View of the Population of Boston, 1850," City Document no. 60, 44. Also see 23–27, 30–31.

58. H. R. Storer, *Criminal Abortion in America*, 14.

59. Ibid., 32.

60. Mill was a neo-Malthusian.

61. H. R. Storer, *Criminal Abortion in America*, 22, 23.

62. Ibid., 23–24.

63. Ibid., 24. The sentence is hard to read because the third "and," following "abortion," joins the language about stillbirths and population operating in a reciprocal relationship. It reads coherently if awkwardly if the second "and" introduces the subordinate clause about infanticide and abortion.

64. H. R. Storer, *Criminal Abortion: Its Nature*. Also see Mohr, *Abortion*, 158–59; Dyer, *Champion*, 263–66.

65. R. Porter, "Malthusian," 63–67. Storer's opposition to Malthus resonates with that of Thomas Jarrold, an Essex physician of the early nineteenth century.

66. H. R. Storer, *Criminal Abortion in America*, 33.

67. Allen, "Law"; Allen, *Population*. Also see Allen, "Changes in the Population"; Allen, "Changes in New England."

68. Allen, *Population*, 11, 14.

69. Allen, "Law," 210, 210–11, 211.

70. Allen echoes William Putney Alison, a Scottish physician who had criticized Malthusianism for its ignorance of physiology and failure to account for biology. See Hamlin and Gallagher-Kamper, "Malthus," 129.

71. Allen, "Law," 265.

72. Stormer, *Articulating*, 63–88.

73. Carlyle, *Chartism*, 109.

74. Agamben, *Kingdom*, 140. He writes, "[Providence] articulates itself . . . into two different planes or levels: transcendent/immanent, general providence/special providence (or fate), first causes/second causes, eternity/temporality, intellectual knowledge/praxis" (141).

75. Agamben, *Kingdom*, 141. I describe medicalized Providence by way of Agamben's general description of the "Providential machine," which means the economy that conjoins transcendent and immanent order.

76. Ibid., 140.

77. Ibid. A God who is foreign yet governs creates "the paradoxical figure of the immanent government of a world that is and needs to remain extraneous" (ibid.). Providence represents "theology and philosophy" attempting "to come to terms with the splitting of classical ontology into two separate realities: being and praxis, transcendent and immanent good, theology and *oikonomia*. Providence presents itself as a machine aimed at joining back together the two fragments in the *gubernatio dei*, the divine government of the world" (ibid., 139–40).

78. Ibid., 140. Agamben writes, "Transcendence is never given by itself and separate from the world, as in Gnosis, but is always in relation to immanence."

79. D. H. Storer, "Two." Dyer credits D. H. Storer's lecture with precipitating the activist turn that fueled the AMA campaign, despite the redaction of the section devoted to abortion and birth control. In March 1872 the omitted portion was published in his son's journal.

80. H. R. Storer, *Why Not?*, 29–32, 84–85. Published in 1868, the essay was first written for an 1864 contest sponsored by the AMA, a contest that Storer himself had lobbied for. He submitted his essay anonymously, although his father adjudicated the contest (Farrell Brodie, *Contraception*, 269).

81. Hodge decried women who are "utterly regardless" of the "immortal existence lodged within their organs," and claimed that the patient is "responsible to her Creator for the life of the being within her" ("Foeticide"). Hale argued that abortion was a crime against the state because it lowered population; against pregnancy, "which cannot be arrested without calamitous results"; and against morality for breaking the command "Thou shalt not kill" (Hale, *Great*, 5). Hale authored another book that opened with statistics from Storer, concluded with reprinted lectures on abortion jurisprudence, and drew heavily from the first comprehensive U.S. statement about abortion, written by James Whitehead and titled *Causes*. Also see Hale, *Systematic*.

82. Noll, *History*, chap. 9, especially the sections "Mass Communications and Popular Thought" and "Education."

83. Noll, *History*, chap. 9, last paragraph of "Mass Communications and Popular Thought" and second paragraph of "A Flourishing of Protestant Theology" sections.

84. "Hugh L.," University of Pennsylvania Archives. His brother, Charles, became a notable Presbyterian theologian at Princeton. See Noll, *History*, chap. 9, "The Heirs of Calvinism" section.

85. Dyer, *Champion*, 25, 294.

86. Mohr, *Abortion*, 185–86.

87. Ibid., 182–96. Also see Degler, *At Odds*, 239–40; Hull and Hoffer, *Roe v. Wade*, 31–32.

88. H. R. Storer, "Contributions," 423. Also see H. R. Storer, *Why Not?*, 64–65; Mohr, *Abortion*, 185.

89. Gordon, *Moral*, 26. England passed the first secular abortion ban in 1803. Also see Mohr, *Abortion*, 185–88; Petchesky, *Abortion*, 80.

90. H. R. Storer, *Criminal Abortion in America*, 10–12. Also see Dyer, *Champion*, 3–49, particularly 25, 39, 46; Scudder, "David."

91. Dyer, *Champion*, 293. Dyer notes Storer's praise of James Young Simpson, who pioneered uses of chloroform and with whom Storer studied in Edinburgh. Storer approvingly quoted from an editorial about Simpson: "Deeply loving Christianity, [Simpson] never fears, for one instant, that true science will lead anywhere but to the truth, and that the truth is Christianity." This is consistent with Storer's invocations of divine purpose. Luker notes that "the public, the medical profession in general, and the antiabortion physicians in particular were *not* at odds with one another over the facts about what went on during pregnancy" but disagreed over "*a different moral evaluation of the facts*" (*Abortion*, 26–27; original emphasis).

92. O'Donnell and Atlee, "Report," 250.

93. Ibid., 241.

94. Ibid., 245.

95. Ibid., 248.

96. Ibid., 245, 256.

97. Ibid., 246; original emphasis. Many nineteenth-century currents about the body's plasticity, such as Lamarckian genetics, maternal impressions deforming fetuses, and early cell theory, to say nothing of racialized notions of darker Others being more robust, converge in this essay.

98. Ibid., 255–56.

99. Ibid., 239. The Job quote is from the Douay-Rheims translation produced for the Catholic Church around the turn of the seventeenth century and revised in the eighteenth. The King James translation, for example, reads differently: "Is there not an appointed time to man on earth?"

100. Ibid., 256.

101. Ibid., 257.

102. Foucault, "*Society*," 162. Foucault does not explain the causation of this shift, and he is not arguing that Boulanviellers, Montlosier, or Thierry are the originators so much as exemplifying changing senses of war.

103. Ibid., 163. Foucault isolates only three divisions—nations, groups, and classes—but the category "groups" is too broad, and careful attention to power struggles regarding women's rights, for instance, clearly calls for more specificity. Ann Laura Stoler is more exact with a "genealogy of racisms" applied to colonial environments (Stoler, *Race*, 55–94; also see Greene, *Malthusian*, 34–38).

104. Foucault, "*Society*," 171–72.

105. Ibid., 216.

106. Ibid.

107. Ibid., 244.

108. Berlant, "Slow," 756.

109. Esposito, *Bios*, 46.

110. Ibid.

111. Hull and Hoffer, *Roe v. Wade*, 46.

112. Hale, *Systematic*, 236–37.

113. Luker, *Abortion*, 26. Meigs famously developed a treatment for the rectovaginal fistula and devised one of the most widely used specula of the nineteenth century, the duck-billed speculum. Bedford's lectures were serially published.

114. Dyer, *Champion*, 374–76.

Chapter 2

1. See Stormer, "Recursivity."

2. Augustine, *Confessions*, 179–220; Burke, *Religion*, 124–28. Also see Neisser, "Remembering."

3. Olick, *Politics*, 89.

4. Bratich, "Popular," 46–47. Also see duBois, *Torture*; E. Black, "Secrecy."

5. Assmann, *Religion*, 81–100; Halbwachs, *Collective*, 46–53; Olick, "Collective"; Olick and Robbins, "Social"; Zelizer, "Reading," 218–21.

6. Olick, *Politics*, 89, 91; original emphasis.

7. Connerton, *Societies*, 36.

8. Derrida, *Archive*, 12.

9. Irwin-Zarecka, *Frames*, 118. Also see Olick, *Politics*, 104–5.

10. Assmann, *Religion*, 81–100; Ricoeur, *Memory*, 21–44.

11. C. E. Scott, "Appearance"; de Certeau, *Practice*, 77–90.

12. De Certeau, *Capture*, 129.

13. Connerton, *Societies*, 72–104. Connerton discusses how bodily habitus produces memory, but not forgetfulness. Also see Bourdieu, *Logic*, 52–65.

14. De Certeau, *Capture*, 130.

15. Benjamin, *Illuminations*, 201–15.

16. Connerton, *Societies*, 13–21; Le Goff, *History*, 127–37; Olick and Robbins, "Social," 105–40; Casey, *Remembering*, 37–85, 146–215; Ricoeur, *Memory*, 24–30, 50–54.

17. Benjamin, *Illuminations*, 201–3.

18. Blair and Michel, "Reproducing," 41.

19. Connerton, *Societies*, 88–102; Bourdieu, *Logic*, 52–65.

20. Zerubavel, *Time*, 73–77.

21. On the present as a contraction of the past, see Deleuze, *Bergsonism*, 51–72.

22. I differ from Olick here. "The production and reception of memory occur through the textuality of memory, which is comprehensible only by attending to its intertextuality with other issues and earlier memories" (Olick, *Politics*, 104). By stressing genre, Olick reinforces the idea that studying mnesis is essentially about studying purposeful activations of recollection. Although very useful, it obscures the dynamism I want to highlight.

23. Browne, "Remembering," 169. For examples, see Biesecker, "Remembering"; Bruner, *Strategies*; Hasian, *Vectors*; Vivian, "Jefferson's"; Vivian, "Neoliberal," 1–26.

24. Todorov, *Memory*, 42–61; Todorov notes that forgiveness is etymologically and conceptually linked to forgetting.

25. Vivian, *Public*, 14; original emphasis. Also see Irwin-Zarecka, *Frames*, 133–60.

26. Olick, *Politics*, 104.

27. Campbell, *Philosophy*, bk. 1, chap. 1. Also see Foley, "Peri Ti?"

28. See Greene, "Rhetorical Materialism."

29. Connerton, *Societies*, 6. Also see de Certeau, *Capture*, 129–30.

30. Deleuze, *Fold*, 6.

31. Deleuze, *Bergsonism*, 74; original emphasis.

32. Deleuze, *Fold*, 22–26.

33. Burke, *Religion*, 124; also see 156–57. Also see Greene, "Rhetorical Pedagogy"; Chaput, "Rhetorical."

34. Casey, *Remembering*, 39.

35. Deleuze, *Fold*, 35.

36. Ibid., 79–80. Deleuze's discussion of Whitehead's "event" resonates with Scott's argument about "appearance" in public memory (C. E. Scott, "Appearance").

37. Deleuze, *Fold*, 37–38.

38. Hale, *Great*, 12–15.

39. Bourdieu, *Logic*, 52–65.

40. Foucault, "Nietzsche," 148–50; Massumi, "National," 177–78.

41. W. J. Robinson, *Law*, 5.

42. Benjamin, *Illuminations*, 202.

43. Deleuze, *Fold*, 23. I borrow liberally from and recombine Deleuze's *The Fold* with his *Bergsonism*. Also see Benjamin, *Illuminations*, 263.

44. *Proposition* is used broadly in a Whiteheadian sense. For discussion of propositions in Whitehead, see Stengers, *Thinking*, 406–22. I do not expand on the propositional quality of memory work in this book and so I will not elaborate at this time.

45. Burke, *Rhetoric of Motives*, 19–27, 37–39. Burke does not discuss identification in terms of remembering or forgetting per se, but the sense of place manifested within a discourse is resonant with creating a consubstantiality and thus supporting identification.

46. Simmel, *Sociology*, 330.

47. Kaplan, *Story*.

48. L. J. Reagan, *When*, 125. Thirteen doctors, nurses, and medical professionals were convicted in the Pacific Coast abortion ring case of 1936. For correspondence between the California state medical examiner's office and relevant agencies and organizations about the syndicate, see "Abortionists—Pacific Coast Abortion Ring 1834–56"; also see Solinger, *Abortionist*, 54–147. For a narrative of Ruth Barnett and Portland raids and news coverage, see Solinger, *Abortionist*, 169–93.

49. Sontheimer, "Abortion," 44–45, 96; L. J. Reagan, *When*, 125.

50. Fried, "Abortion."

51. Tillman, "Crossing"; Calhoun, "Rise"; Murtha, "Pennsylvania." Also see Grossman et al., "Self-Induction"; Jones and Jerman, "Abortion"; Mason Pieklo, "For Too Many."

52. Wiklund, *This*.

53. Foucault, *History*, 35; original emphasis.

54. Ibid., 33. Also see Esposito, *Bios*, 24–32; Dillon and Reid, *Liberal*, 24–30; Foucault, "Society," 171–81; Foucault, *Security*, 347–58; Foucault, *Biopolitics*, 35–37.

55. Messer and May, *Back*, 87–90.

56. Ibid., 7.

57. Joffe, *Doctors*, 55–142; Keemer, *Confessions*; Solinger, *Abortionist*.

58. Foucault, *History*, 22. The anonymous book is framed in almost Kinseyesque fashion as the sex life of not *the*, but *a*, human male; the author was, for Foucault, "the most direct and in a way the most naïve representative" of the injunction to expose sexual secrets.

59. Ibid., 32. Jouy was remanded to a hospital for the rest of his life. For Foucault, this case exemplified a "whole machinery for speechifying, analyzing, and investigating" to produce the truth of sexual (mis)conduct. That Foucault found Jouy's use of girls "bucolic" stakes out clearly both the accuracy of his argument—my judgment that his apparently tolerant

attitude toward Jouy's behavior is repulsive is no doubt conditioned by biopower—and the conflicted nature of biopower. The irony is that medicalized sexuality has demonstrated the great damage of pedophilia.

60. Nealon, *Foucault*, 91. A more elaborate and probably accurate phrasing would be "corporeal privacy as the horizon of secrecy, orientation toward which enables bodies to interiorize subjectivity."

61. Solinger, *Abortionist*, 87–116; Solinger, *Pregnancy*, 12–17, 66–79; Joffe, *Doctors*, 119–27; L. J. Reagan, *When*, 113–31.

62. Crimes against the family were housed together with sex crimes in earlier drafts of the model penal code (1956–59), but by the time the official draft was released, these were clearly separated (1962). "Press Release"; "Article 207—Vol. 1"; "Model Penal Code Tentative Draft No. 9"; "Model Penal Code Proposed Official Draft."

63. Deutscher, "Foucault's," 131.

64. Foucault, *History*, 25–26.

65. When studies of governmentality explore how different knowledge formations participate in the regulation of individual and communal conduct, they are indirectly elaborating on the horizons of secrecy associated with the private subject, the body, and the population that fuel the invention of biopolitical discourses. See Foucault, "Society," 190; Foucault, *Security*, 61–76.

66. Dean, *Publicity's*, 10.

67. Simmel, *Sociology*, 335.

68. E. Black, "Secrecy," 139. He is describing the way that representations of secrets function in arguments, which I have suspended as part of my analysis. Nevertheless, the basic relationship between disclosure-secrecy and remembering-forgetting holds.

69. Foucault, *History*, 57–70; Rose, *Governing*, 222–24, 244–49; Nadesan, *Governmentality*, 93–182.

70. Stafford, *Body*.

71. Deutscher, "Foucault's," 123–29.

72. A. N. Whitehead, *Process*, 25; Stengers, *Thinking*, 58–72. Whitehead uses the concept of the lure throughout *Process and Reality*, the reference for an initial orientation.

73. Deleuze and Guattari, *Thousand*, 217. Also see Thacker, "Shadows," 135.

74. Dean, *Publicity's*, 163; also see Hacking, *Taming*, 55–63.

75. Fox Keller, *Secrets*, 39–72. Fox Keller's discussion of secrecy and science takes on a different cast when scientific knowledge production is understood relative to biopower, bodies, and populations.

76. Hacking, *Taming*, 55–124.

77. Latour, *Politics*, 237; original emphasis. Also see Revel, "Identity," 52.

78. Van De Warker, "Detection," 357.

79. Hoitt, "Criminal," 541. Hoitt recalls eight cases, each notably different one from the other regarding motive and materials, then describes the nation as being in decline in the face of an "ever-growing evil" aided by the secrecy of the practice of abortion (542).

80. Potassium permanganate was used from the 1930s to the 1960s. See McDonough, "Vaginal"; Jetter and Hunter, "Death"; Carney, "Vaginal"; Marsh and Webster, "Vaginal"; St. Romain and Nix, "Chemical"; Wanamaker, "Lay"; Bobrow and Friedman, "Burns"; Vandergriff, "Intravaginal," 155–57.

81. See, for example, Rock, "Abortion." Rock's typology of causes is fairly standard.

82. Latour, *Politics*, 129. Also see Stormer, "Articulation."

83. See Lanham, *Handlist*. For a prime classical source, see Quintilian, *Institutes*, bk. 9.

84. J. Bennett, *Vibrant*, viii.

85. *Chiasmus* is a trope of reversal, and the basic figure of unveiling at the root of science is effectively chiastic. *Hysterologia* is a figure of interruption where material intercedes between the logic of a sentence and its object.

86. Latour, *Politics*, 67; original emphasis. Latour uses bench science in laboratories as his example, but the point applies equally well here. Although I am influenced by Latour's understanding of human-nonhuman relations, I do not use actor-network theory (ANT) for a number of reasons, but the prime one is that I am not intent on mapping a net. The scope of ANT is both too broad and too narrow for my purposes.

87. Burke wrote of rhetoric as the Wrangle, the Logomachy. A genealogy of rhetoric sees rhetoric not *as* the wrangle, but as various modes of wrangling produced from *and* for wrangling, the thing by which and for which there is struggle in Foucauldian terms. See Burke, *Rhetoric of Motives*, 23; Foucault, *Archaeology*, 216. Also see Greene, "Rhetorical Materialism," 60.

88. Canguilhem, *Normal*, 228.

Chapter 3

1. Nietzsche, "Truth," 250. Nietzsche described the worn metaphors as coins that had lost their embossing, seeming only as metal. A larger point can be derived. When modes of rhetoric are new, their freshness can distract one from the material that gives the rhetoric its value.

2. For example, see H. R. Storer, *Criminality*; H. R. Storer, *Why Not?*; Hale, *Great*.

3. Foucault, *Archaeology*, 21–77. This moment in the literature was strangely egalitarian with no primary texts through which others cycled.

4. Nebinger, *Criminal*; Thomas, *Abortion*. Major works prior to Nebinger include Hale, *Great*, 1867; Hodge, *Criminal*; H. R. Storer, *Criminal Abortion: Its Nature*; H. R. Storer, *Is It I?*; H. R. Storer, *Why Not?*

5. Taussig, "What to Teach," 514.

6. Berlant, "Slow," 754, 757–58, 779.

7. Fernald, "Sociological," 57–59.

8. Gordon, *Moral*, 55–71.

9. Fernald, "Sociological," 60. Also see Philbrick, "Social."

10. See Gordon, *Moral*, 86–91, 96–104; L. J. Reagan, *When*, 80–112; Solinger, *Pregnancy*, 63–129; Lovett, *Conceiving*, 2–16.

11. See Thiberge, "Criminal," 314; Crutcher, "Philosophic," 521.

12. Dixon-Jones, "Criminal," 14. Examples are legion—see Stockham, *Tokology*, 231; Lewis, "Clinical," 85; Gleason, *Talks*, 157–58; McCollom, "Criminal," 257; Oreman, "Medical"; Love, "Criminal," 57; Rogers, "Attitude," 149–50; Wetherill, "Remedies"; Crutcher, "Philosophic," 521–23; Hurley, "Prevention," 268; Ladova, "Discussion," 44; Somers, "Measures," 111; Grant, "Criminal," 517–18; Ghent, "Criminal," 3 (vol. 23, no. 5); Person, "Discussions," 11; Lyons, "Moral," 293–95; Thiberge, "Criminal," 316; Barbat, "Criminal," 70; Weiss, "Some," 77–78; Dakin, "Induced," 66.

13. Thomas, *Practical*, 43.

14. Burke, *Grammar*, xv–xviii, 3–20.

15. Ghent, "Criminal," 5–9 (vol. 23, no. 5).

16. Grant, "Criminal," 513–14.

17. Rudolph Weiner Holmes, "Criminal."

18. Crutcher, "Philosophic," 526.

19. The quote "great ignorance" is from McCollom, "Criminal," 257. The quote "utter ignorance" is from Johnson, "Abortion," 91. The "thoughtless" quote is from Dixon-Jones, "Criminal," 10.

20. Smith-Rosenberg, *Disorderly*, 167–296.

21. Fernald, "Sociological," 58.

22. Sturken, "Remembering," 120. Sturken discusses recovered memory but her observation is apropos. Also see Petchesky, *Abortion*, 74–75.

23. Pirkner, "Problem," 374; original emphasis.

24. L. J. Reagan, *When*, 19–45, 113–25; Bacon, "Duty," 22; Sheean, "Common," 38–39; Grant, "Criminal," 517.

25. Barbat, "Criminal," 70. Barbat reported abortionists to the Post Office for violation of the Comstock Laws' prohibition against sending abortion advertisements through the mail, thus prompting publishers to drop certain ads. Abortionists simply ran new ads under aliases. The idea originally was proposed by Rudolph Weiner Holmes, "Criminal," 31.

26. See Vivian, *Public*, 39–60.

27. Foucault, *Clinic*, 92.

28. Sturken, "Remembering," 115.

29. Foucault, *Clinic*, 94. Foucault explains further that "in its material reality, the sign is identified with the symptom itself; the symptom is the indispensible morphological support of the sign" (93). Foucault writes of medical perception of biological diseases, not social ones. Via Canguilhem, I have interpolated antiabortionists' idea of social disease into Foucault's work.

30. Rosenberg, "Pathologies," 729.

31. Johnson, "Abortion," 87–88, 88–89.

32. Foucault, *Security*, 17–22.

33. Pirkner, "Problem," 374.

34. J. F. Scott, "Criminal," 73.

35. Dixon-Jones, "Criminal," 10.

36. The range of turn-of-the century U.S. discourses connecting immigration to threats is overwhelming. For an excellent discussion, see Jacobson, *Barbarian*. For consideration of nativism of the era in relation to immigration, see Higham, *Strangers*, chaps. 3–5.

37. Dorsett, "Criminal," 958. Also see LeBeuf, "Attitude." LeBeuf is another perfect specimen of turn-of-the-century discourse, although he includes an elaborate table of fertility over time among different classes, locations, and ethnicities.

38. Crutcher, "Philosophic," 527; Fernald, "Sociological," 62; Reed, "Therapeutic," 27; Billings, "Diminishing"; Paterfamilias, "'Race'"; Thorndike, "Decrease."

39. Taussig, "Frequency," 46.

40. Suttner, "Plea," 307.

41. Dibrell, "Discussion," 273.

42. Zeisler, "Legal," 540.

43. Foucault, "*Society*," 79–83.

44. Esposito, *Immunitas*, 68.

45. Green, "Feticide," 590. Also see Nowlin, "Criminal," 179; Thomas, *Practical*, 43; Dixon-Jones, "Criminal," 9, 10; McCollom, "Criminal," 258; J. F. Scott, "Criminal," 73; Hawkins, "Abortion," 770, 772.

46. Fish, "Criminal," 107.

47. Rogers, "Attitude," 149. William Millar similarly noted that unborn rights were a slowly developing phenomenon. See Millar, "Human," 272.

48. Love, "Criminal," 55.

49. Ely, "Ethics," 98. Contrary views existed but were rare. See E. A. Ross, "Western"; Holmes et al., "'Why Race-Suicide'"; Schindler, "'Why Race-Suicide.'"

50. Esposito, *Bios*, 96.

51. Foucault, *Hermeneutics*, 129. Foucault discusses ancient philosophies of the care of self, here Socratic self-mastery through anamnesis.

52. Esposito, *Bios*, 92.

53. "If history is what hurts, nature is what heals" (Haraway, *Primate*, 156).

54. Foucault, *Hermeneutics*, 130–36. The "ignorant woman" exists in a space similar to that of the *stultus* as defined by Seneca in letter 52 to Lucilius, as read by Foucault. "The *stultus* is someone who remembers nothing, who lets life pass by, who does not try to restore unity to his [*sic*] life by recalling what is worth memorizing and [who does not] direct his attention and will to a precise and well-determined end" (131).

55. Esposito, *Immunitas*, 63–64; original emphasis.

56. Hull and Hoffer, *Roe v. Wade*, 34–35.

57. Cuthbert, "Discussion," 102.

58. Fish, "Criminal," 107.

59. Allen, *Population*, 12–15.

60. H. R. Storer, *Criminal Abortion in America*.

61. Thomas, *Practical*, 43; Winter, "Criminal," 91.

62. Philbrick, "Social," 102.

63. Taussig, *Prevention*, 78; Bacon, "Duty," 18.

64. It may be fairly objected that different places have different conditions, but New York's estimates rivaled the Michigan study's national estimate and Chicago had a thriving abortion underground.

65. Taussig, "Frequency," 46–47.

66. Sturken, "Remembering," 120; Foucault, *Hermeneutics*, 135. Foucault discusses how under guidance the *stultus* is transformed in the Stoical system to the *sapient* (sage), who masters will toward the self.

67. Thomas, *Practical*, 43.

68. Mapes, "Criminal," 677.

69. Dixon-Jones, "Criminal," 9. Also see McArdle, "Physical," 938; Saur, *Maternity*, 150; Fernald, "Sociological," 59.

70. A tampon-and-tent method uses a tent to dilate the cervix, usually followed by puncturing or tearing the amniotic sac, and then packing the vagina with a cotton tampon until the ovum has passed.

71. Foucault, *Clinic*, 163; original emphasis. Also see Stormer, *Articulating*, 41–88.

72. For more on Chicago's antiabortion campaigns, particularly the turn-of-the-century anti-midwife campaign and the Chicago Medical Society's Abortion Committee, see L. J. Reagan, *When*, 90–109.

73. Rudolph Weiner Holmes, "Criminal," 30.

74. Foucault, *Clinic*, 103; original emphasis.

75. Heiermann, "Ethical," 236.

76. Sontag, *Illness*, 43.

77. Russell, "Criminal," 304.

78. A. L. Smith, "Higher," 472.

79. Dubow, *Ourselves*, 22.

80. Ibid., 10–37.

81. Ibid., 25.

82. Lyons, "Moral."

83. Ibid., 292, 291.

84. Weiss, "Some," 74.

85. Green, "Feticide," 590, also 594.

86. Churchill, "Rise," 16–17.

87. Gould, *Ontogeny*, 198; also see 13–17, 197–202. The terms *preformationism* and *epigenesis* had been used in the seventeenth century and were revived at the turn of the twentieth, technically a kind neopreformationism and neoepigeneticism. The tension of an entelechial origin versus a contextual unfolding potential is evident in early Greek science and cosmology, notably in Aristotle's *Generation of Animals*. The debate mentioned here is one of several instances where principles of inherent design and potentiality clash in explanations of developmental biology. Also see Haraway, *Crystals*, 22–24, 33–42.

88. Gould, *Ontogeny*, 13–206.

89. Ibid., 167–206; Louis-Fischer, "Laurent Chabry"; Maienschein, "Origins"; Oppenheimer, "Curt Herbst's"; Haraway, *Crystals*, 1–32.

90. Morgan, *Icons*, 165–66.

91. Nick Hopwood demonstrates that nineteenth-century plating practices helped create a sense of staged progression through sequenced illustrations of multiple specimens. Green's reference to staged development stands out in that regard. See Hopwood, "Producing"; Hopwood, "Visual"; Hopwood, "History."

92. Morgan, *Icons*, 140–43.

93. Saur, *Maternity*, 150. For other examples, see Markham, "Fœticide"; Dixon-Jones, "Criminal," 16; Mapes, "Criminal," 684; Hurley, "Prevention," 266; Murphy, "Symposium," 189; Bacon, "Duty," 19; Reed, "Therapeutic," 26; Ghent, "Criminal," 16 (vol. 23, no. 5), 2 (vol. 23, no. 6); Pattison, "Abortion," 653; Suttner, "Plea," 305; Carroll, "Rights," 936; Parsons, "Written," 154; Green, "Feticide," 590, 594; Hood, *Girls*, 77.

94. Ashton, *Text-Book*, 145.

95. Latour, *Politics*, 237, also 65–70; Foucault, *Clinic*, 96.

96. Stafford, *Body*, 17.

97. Esposito, *Immunitas*, 8.

98. Ibid., 49.

99. Quintilian, *Institutes*, bk. 8, chap. 6, 37–39.

100. De Certeau, *Practice*, "Story Time," section titled "The Art of Memory and Circumstances"; original emphasis.

101. Ibid., "Spatial Stories," sections titled "Creating a Theater of Actions" and "Frontiers and Bridges"; original emphasis.

102. C. E. Scott, "Appearance." Scott argues that there is a "dimension of nondetermination in the occurrence of appearing" that makes memory mutable, transitory (153). Memory is irreducibly subjunctive, freighted with questions of "*might* rather than *is*" (155; original emphasis).

103. L. J. Reagan, *When*, 28–29. Many women were placed in maternity homes after failed attempts to abort. Maternity homes were not above suspicion, however. In Chicago, maternity homes came under investigation as a part of an antiabortion crackdown on midwives (ibid., 105–7). For more on turn-of-the-century maternity homes, see Kunzel, *Fallen*.

104. Foucault, *Hermeneutics*, 307–8. Foucault discusses the general ethical mandate of Marcus Aurelius's Stoic philosophy. With modification, the mandate broadly applies: the techniques of self were much less developed in gynecology, and the goal was to make women renounce their agency, not free them as responsible agents.

105. Ibid., 289, 305.

106. Ibid., 277. Here Foucault is discussing Seneca, not Marcus Aurelius, but the goal is the same. Where Seneca favored investigation of cosmic nature (self-in-universe at the macroscopic scale), Marcus Aurelius favored analysis of biotic nature (self-in-universe at the microscopic scale).

107. Ibid., 306.

108. Ibid., 257, 308–11.

109. Gordon, *Moral*, 114.

110. Suttner, "Plea," 305.

111. Foucault, *Security*, 172.

112. Unlike his peers, Suttner felt immigration replenished the national "stock." His species orientation was no less racially coded, only more pragmatic.

113. Foucault, *Security*, 207–12. Foucault discusses obedience and revolts of conduct in relation to pastoral power in Europe from the Middle Ages to the Enlightenment.

114. Suttner, "Plea," 307. McCollom had voiced this sentiment a decade earlier ("Criminal," 257).

115. E. A. Hall, "Discussion."

116. Foucault, *Security*, 196–97. This resonates with Seyla Benhabib's claim that disputes over the boundaries of culture and law are often centered around women's and children's bodies. See Benhabib, *Claims*, 82–104.

117. Foucault, *Security*, 129.

118. Rogers, "Attitude," 150.

119. The quotations are from different sources. As they appear: Lyons, "Moral," 294; Thiberge, "Criminal," 316. Also see Dixon-Jones, "Criminal"; Somers, "Measures," 112.

120. Suttner, "Plea," 306.

121. Lyons, "Moral," 294.

122. Fish, "Criminal," 107. Also see Rudolph Weiner Holmes, "Criminal," 30; Grant, "Criminal," 517.

123. Barbat, "Criminal," 70.

124. J. F. Scott, "Criminal," 79.

125. Gleason, *Talks*, 158.

126. Oreman, "Medical," 88.

127. Gleason, *Talks*, 158–61; Greenley, "Practice," 184–85; Hurley, "Prevention," 268; Rudolph Weiner Holmes, "Criminal," 30; Ghent, "Criminal," 7 (vol. 23, no. 6); Person, "Discussion," 11–12; Dabney, "Discussion"; Beckman, "Abortion," 450.

128. Greenley, "Practice," 184; Nelken, "Discussion," 320. Greenley's language of a good scolding is reflective of many physicians' tone, whereas grotesque flights of violent imagination were rare.

129. Rudolph Weiner Holmes, "Criminal," 30.

130. Thiberge, "Criminal," 317.

131. Ghent, "Criminal," 10 (vol. 23, no. 6).

132. Foucault argues that the clinical gaze became a mode of teaching as well as a diagnostic system of perception. As the clinical gaze "saw ever more clearly, it would be turned into speech which states and teaches; the truth, which events, in their repetitions and convergence, would outline under its gaze, would, by this same gaze and in the same order, be reserved, in the form of teaching, to those who do not know and have not yet seen" (*Clinic*, 114–15). The medical pastorate was roughly related to the educational mission embedded within the system of clinical perception that had developed over the nineteenth century.

133. Foucault, *Hermeneutics*, 282. Foucault is discussing the manner in which Stoicism, that of Seneca specifically, produces what I have termed a point of inclusion.

134. Mohanram, *Black*, 85. She is discussing racially regenerative discourses of colonialism, but her general observation is appropriate to U.S. discourse on abortion. Also see McClintock, *Imperial*, 24–61, 232–46, 352–60.

135. Foucault, *Hermeneutics*, 282. Foucault is discussing the general effect of Stoic self-inspection, but the language perfectly captures the ethical hopes of anti-Malthusian doctors.

136. De Certeau, *Practice*, "Spatial Stories," section titled "The Art of Memory and Circumstances"; original emphasis.

137. Casey, *Remembering*, 90–103, 122–40. Casey also touches on what de Certeau talks about as "founding" in terms of horizons and pathways constituted by place memory (203–5).

138. Foucault, *Clinic*, 164–71. This also explains why illness is more than metaphorically powerful within rhetoric. It is not only something to be diagnosed; it diagnoses us in return.

139. Casey, *Remembering*, 70, 75. I am tweaking Casey's discussions about the differences between remembering space and time here. I recognize that space is irretrievably confused with time in memory, but I foreground space because of the global positioning so common to medical discourse on abortion. I discuss the temporal entanglement below with Massey's description of modernist space-time.

140. Foucault, *Clinic*, 187, 189.

141. In general, the move from organic to molecular medicine is crucial to the arc of this visual expansion. For discussions of the expansiveness of biomedical inner space, see Duden, *Disembodying*, 34–42; Stafford, *Body*, 341–98; Rose, *Politics*, 9–15; Adams, *Reproducing*, 136–37.

142. Derrida, *Truth*, 138. Derrida discusses the inverted relation of the infinitesimal to size in relation to his concept of "cision" (119–47). Also see Duden, *Disembodying*, 34–42; and Nochlin, *Body*; Stafford, *Body*, 47–83, 131–58, 342–61. *Peristasis* is a specific form of the more general figure *enargia*, which includes figures of vivid description.

143. Foucault, *Clinic*, 191.

144. Deleuze, *Bergsonism*, 82–83.

145. Foucault, "Society," 43–111; also see Stoler, *Race*, 17–94. Foucault discusses how race as a justification for war between nations became an organizing principle of war within the nation, of war with itself. Stoler places this discussion more clearly within Foucault's framework for the history of sexuality. Also see Deutscher, "Foucault's," 131.

146. Deleuze, *Bergsonism*, 74.

147. Elias, *Civilizing*, 138–56, 294; Stoler, *Carnal*, 61–78. Also see Cott, afterword; Hodes, "Fractions"; Stoler, "Tense."

148. Stoler, *Race*, 95–101. Stoler notes how Foucault's argument that bourgeois subjectivity was anchored in a racialized sexuality does not strictly align with the colonial project. Rather, the racialized class distinctions that made an affluent white Anglo identity intelligible in contrast to working-class and antipode populations were a mobile set of elements that were deployed by the West generally. Also see Spivak, "Subaltern," 294. Spivak critiques Foucault's elision of imperialism and the manner in which his concept of power assumes a negligence of the colonial project (*Critique*, 277–79).

149. J. F. Scott, "Criminal," 76.

150. O'Callaghan, "Moral," 24.

151. Saur, *Maternity*, 149.

152. LeBeuf, "Attitude," 5; Russell, "Criminal," 299; J. F. Scott, "Criminal," 77.

153. Love, "Criminal," 56; Weiss, "Some," 74; Nowlin, "Criminal," 178. Hippocrates held that life began at thirty-two days for males, forty-two days for females; Aristotle held that life began at forty days for male fetuses, eighty days for females; Galen held that life began at forty days regardless of sex. For an excellent survey of early philosophy on humanity, animality, and vitality, see Simondon, *Two Lessons*.

154. Goodell, "Introductory," 19. Also see McNair, "Status"; Parish, "Criminal," 644; J. F. Scott, "Criminal," 77; Rudolph Weiner Holmes, "Criminal," 29; Love, "Criminal," 56; Ploss-Bartels, "Abortion," 272–73. Scott (77) cites Ovid's *Amores*, bk. 2, elegy 14, "Against Abortion" and Seneca's "Consolation to Helvia," xvi; and Ploss-Bartels (272) also notes Seneca's "Consolation to Helvia." References to early Greeks and Romans were not entirely consistent. Crutcher praised "pagan Rome" for rewarding families that bore children ("Philosophic," 524).

155. Ghent, "Criminal," 10 (vol. 23, no. 6); also see Reed, "Therapeutic," 27.

156. J. F. Scott, "Criminal," 73; Dixon-Jones, "Criminal," 9.

157. Grant, "Criminal," 517.

158. Massey, *Space*, 68.

159. Ibid., 68, 69. What Massey describes involves a specific variety of memory work where, as Casey describes it, "the spatiality and temporality of the mnemonic presentation [global emplacement] are often correlated to the point of becoming indissociable. The 'when' and 'where' are inextricably linked" (*Remembering*, 70).

160. Sturken, "Remembering," 119.

161. Esposito, *Immunitas*, 15.

Chapter 4

1. A. D. Black, "Social," 98. Abortion as "evil" continued from the turn of the century but with less frequency. See Dekker, "Is Abortion"; Findley, "Slaughter"; W. J. Robinson, *Law*, 6, 25; M. Davis, *Women's*, 59–61; Rongy, *Abortion*, 145–47; Lockridge, "Woman's."

2. See Poovey, *History*, 278–95; Gallagher, *Body*, 8–16; 36–50, 157–70; C. R. McCann, "Malthusian."

3. Dickinson called Sanger's activism "anathema." Dickinson, "Relation." Also see "National Committee on Maternal Health, Inc.: History"; Memo to Sub-committee on Social Studies, "Background of Conference on the Social Problems of Human Reproductions as They Relate to Medicine," n.d., National Committee on Maternal Health Collection (NCMHC), Countway Library of Medicine, Harvard University, BMS c78, box 10, folder 350; Committee on Maternal Health Biennial Report. Sexology, part of what Foucault called *scientia sexualis*, names the scientific study of sex. *Sexology* often refers to work of and influenced by Richard Freiherr von Krafft-Ebing and Havelock Ellis.

4. C. R. McCann, *Birth Control*, 80. Dickinson was influential in American sexology and to the NCMH research agenda, particularly in his empiricist approach. For Dickinson's influence on Kinsey, see J. H. Jones, *Kinsey*, 270, 291–93, 306; Gathorne-Hardy, *Sex*, 87–88, 156–57, 211–12, 235–37, 301, 345.

5. Gordon, *Moral*, 181–82, 189–90; C. R. McCann, *Birth Control*, 75–79. The bureau provided gynecological examinations and contraception services to married women and collected data for research on contraception.

6. C. R. McCann, *Birth Control*, 80–90. McCann describes complicated negotiations involving a petition for licensing to the New York State Board of Charities and courting the endorsement of the New York Academy of Medicine.

7. "National Committee on Maternal Health, Inc.: History." The NCMH was most productive prior to World War II, when funding was better, but it produced fourteen books and dozens of research papers.

8. Kopp, *Birth Control*; Whelpton, "Frequency"; Gebhard et al., *Pregnancy*.

9. Kinsey produced the third volume in his series on human sexuality partly because of conflicted assumptions on display at Arden House.

10. W. J. Robinson, *Law*; Rongy, *Abortion*.

11. C. R. McCann, *Birth Control*, 93–95; Solinger, *Pregnancy*, 107.

12. Beck, Newman, and Lewit, "Abortion," 2140.

13. Philbrick, "Social," 104–5; Ladova, "Discussion," 44; Hawkins, "Abortion," 770. Hawkins echoed Anna Galbraith, who in her 1899 valedictory address contested the idea of woman as a generative apparatus. Galbraith, "Dangers," 41.

14. See Gordon, *Moral*, 125–38; Bullough, "Development"; Bullough, *Science*, 92–119; Waters, "Sexology," 46–49; Robb, "Marriage," 95–100. U.S. medical literature appropriated European research questions through people like Margaret Sanger, Hannah Stone, William Robinson, Denslow Lewis, and Robert Latou Dickinson. In contrast to European psychology, in the United States, "more than elsewhere, concerns about public health, in addition to the strength of social purity movements, led to greater emphasis being placed on concrete empirical studies of urban vice and prostitution, along with developing programmes of sex education that would teach the importance of purity" (Waters, "Sexology," 46). For an excellent study of the rhetoric of sex education from the Progressive Era, see Jensen, *Dirty Words*.

15. Esposito, *Immunitas*, 163, 162. See Petchesky, *Abortion*, 123; for a summative view of underground abortion dangers in the mid-twentieth century, also see Gorney, *Articles*, 21–23.

16. L. Jacobi, "Infanticide," 455. Also see *Birth Control Movement*.

17. For examples, see Ploss-Bartels, "Abortion"; Dekker, "Is Abortion," 198; Becelaere, "Jurisprudence," 33; Taussig, *Abortion*, 44; Ayres, "Therapeutic"; Burgess, "Social," 115–17; V. Robinson, *Pioneers*, 94; W. J. Robinson, *Law*, 5, 69, 114; Rongy, *Abortion*, 24, 35; A. Stone, "Discussion," 172; Stopes, *Wise*, 11; Wile, "Birth Control," 147.

18. L. Jacobi, "Infanticide," 461. Also see W. J. Robinson, "Ethics." Robinson concludes his letter to the editor: "Freedom to teach the people the proper means of preventing conception would at once do away with seventy-five percent of all abortions. Wouldn't it be worth while?"

19. Rongy, "Abortion," 404.

20. Downie, "Interpretation," 30.

21. For discussions of the impact the Depression had on fertility control generally, see L. J. Reagan, *When*, 132–47; Gordon, *Moral*, 211–41; Solinger, *Pregnancy*, 103–29.

22. Florence Taussig, Frederick's wife, was active in the suffrage and peace movements, including in work with Alice Paul and the National Woman's Party. Linkage of overpopulation to war predated World War I in medical writing on abortion and continued into the 1960s. See L. Jacobi, "Infanticide," 452–53; Hubbard, "Abortion"; Rongy, "Abortion," 404; Taussig, *Abortion*, 6; Downie, "Interpretation," 28–30; Overstreet, foreword, 11.

23. Taussig, "Control of Criminal Abortion," 777. On Konikow, see Gordon, *Moral*, 142, 186–87.

24. Taussig, "Control of Criminal Abortion," 778.

25. Petchesky, *Abortion*, 72.

26. Taussig, "Abortion in Relation to Fetal and Maternal Welfare," in *Fetal*. Also see United States Department of Labor, Children's Bureau, *Maternal*. Taussig published his own findings in 1931, in advance of the 1933 release of the White House Conference report. Taussig, "Abortion in Relation to Fetal and Maternal Welfare," *American Journal*.

27. Taussig, *Abortion, Spontaneous*, 405; original emphasis.

28. Ibid., 5, 29.

29. Dickinson, "Discussion," 51. Dickinson convinced Taussig to significantly update the book, but Taussig passed away suddenly in 1943 on a vacation in Bar Harbor, Maine.

30. Taussig, *Abortion, Spontaneous*, 28.

31. Ibid., 29, 446. Comments on abortion's wastefulness are common to the literature, with authors seemingly vying for new ways to state conventional wisdom. See E. H. Stevenson,

"Tetanus," 258–59; Rongy, "Abortion," 404; Taussig, "Abortion in Relation to Fetal and Maternal Welfare," *American Journal*, 730; Watkins, "Five-Year," 161; Yarros, *Modern*, 128; Rongy, *Abortion*, 127; Stone and Stone, *Marriage*, 196; Bundesen, "Suggested," 156; Cosgrove and Carter, "Consideration," 299; Donnelly, "Are There," 118; Kummer and Leavy, "Criminal," 170.

32. Esposito, *Bios*, 58. Esposito elaborates on biopolitical reason in Hobbes: "If life is abandoned to its internal powers, to its natural dynamics, human life is destined to self-destruct because it carries with itself something that ineluctably places it in contradiction with itself." The negation of this negation was the antibody for moral restoration for anti-Malthusians and family planning for neo-Malthusians.

33. Taussig, *Prevention*. Sanger initially held abortion as a right but revised her stand before opening the Brownsville, New York, clinic. Havelock Ellis may have convinced Sanger to change her mind, although McCann notes that American Birth Control League records from at least 1926 to 1929 indicate that Sanger's clinics referred women to abortionists. Also see Hull and Hoffer, *Roe v. Wade*, 66.

34. Sanger, *Sanger*, 217. Sanger recounted the opening day of her first clinic: "We explained simply what contraception was; that abortion was the wrong way—no matter how early it was performed it was taking a life; that contraception was the better way, the safer way."

35. See Winslow, "Efficiency"; Bauer, "Half"; Imber, "First World War"; Dubos and Dubos, *White*, 131–84; Rothman, *Living*, 194–245; Patterson, "Germs."

36. Downie, "Interpretation," 29.

37. Bundesen, "Suggested," 157–58; for discussion of public health epidemiology, see 155; for discussions of women's ignorance, see 161.

38. Mary Steichen Calderone to Christopher Tietze, February 15, 1954, Mary Steichen Calderone Papers (MSCP), Schlesinger Library, Radcliffe Institute for Advanced Study, Harvard University, call no. 179, box 2, fol. 20. SIECUS was founded in 1964 and has become a leading sex education organization in the United States.

39. Calderone, *Abortion*, 181. Also see Gorney, *Articles*, 24–25.

40. Calderone's papers contain the draft of the unfavorable review by Charles Miller and her response to the editors of *Medical Economics* (Miller, Draft).

41. Newman, "Conference," 2.

42. M. E. Davis, "Review." The proceedings were also reviewed in *Eugenics Quarterly*, which used the language of a "disease in our society," while critiquing the conference for not giving enough weight to fetal life. See Buxton, review.

43. Rubin, "Illegal Abortion." The language of "communicable illness" persisted through the 1960s. See R. E. Hall, "Hospitals," 1933–34. Hall referred to abortion as a "pandemic."

44. Taussig, *Abortion, Spontaneous*, 44–45. Also see V. Robinson, *Pioneers*, 101; Rongy, *Abortion*, 36, 47–48; Greenhill, *Obstetrics*, 328; Kisch, *Sexual*, 8.

45. Burke, *Religion*, 20. Burke defined *scientism* as a way of distinguishing different orders of language: "First, I would set 'Dramatism' against 'Scientism.' In so doing, I do not necessarily imply a distrust of science as such. I mean simply that language in particular and human relations in general can be most directly approached in terms of *action* rather than in terms of *knowledge* (or terms of 'form' rather than in terms of 'perception'). The 'scientistic' approach is via such essentially epistemological question as 'What do I see when I look at this object?' or 'How do I see it?'" (38–39).

46. Many observers noted that the Church was antiquated and a source of primitivism through stringent moral codes and laws based on Christian morality, including Comstockery. See Stopes, *Wise*, 19–20; Sanger, *Woman*, 127–28; Schroeder, "Physiologic," 17; Dickinson, "Mailability"; Rongy, *Abortion*, 28, 30, 45–46, 53, 61; W. J. Robinson, *Law*, 20–21; Wile, "Birth Control," 144–45; Guttmacher, "Social," 301; Guttmacher, "United States," 456.

47. Taussig, "Effects," 39.

48. It is interesting that physicians made little use of graphical representations of data in the literature examined, preferring tabular representation, despite an enthusiasm for graphical displays of data after the ninth census. See Funkhouser, "Historical," 337–42.

49. Curtis, *Politics*, 8, 40. Also see C. R. McCann, "Malthusian," 144–46.

50. Early probabilistic understandings of public heath risks began in the nineteenth-century insurance industry. Key moments in the rise of public health include antidiphtheria and antituberculosis campaigns, as well as efforts to curb infant mortality at the end of the nineteenth and beginning of the twentieth century. See Rothstein, *Public*, 1–175.

51. Kross, "Abortion," 107–8.

52. Esposito, *Immunitas*, 16, 162–65.

53. Kross, "Discussion," 146–47.

54. Clair E. Fulsome to Fred J. Taussig, March 5, 1942, 4–5, Florence Taussig Papers (FTP), Western Historical Manuscript Collection, University of Missouri–St. Louis, sl 590, box 1, folder 1. Taussig was formally invited the next month. Fulsome to Taussig, April 28, 1942, FTP, sl 590, box 1, folder 1.

55. Fulsome to Taussig, March 5, 1942, 6–7; original emphasis. See Dickinson, foreword to *Abortion*, 8; Dickinson, "Discussion," 50; Bundesen, "Suggested"; Whelpton, "Frequency," 29; Taussig, "Discussion," 52; Beck, Newman, and Lewit, "Abortion," 2135.

56. The NCMH call to adopt a public health footing toward abortion parallels a general move to broaden public health initiatives to include the general well-being of all citizens. Edgar Sydenstricker wrote in 1935, "It is restricted to a few activities such as community sanitation, water supplies and food inspection, control of infectious diseases, education in hygiene, the medical care of the tuberculous and mentally diseased, and the medical care of the indigent. A newer concept which many sanitarians are coming to accept is much broader and far more sound. It may be stated in terms somewhat as follows: Society has a basic responsibility for assuring, to all of its members, healthful conditions of housing and living, a reasonable degree of economic security, proper facilities for curative and preventive medicine and adequate medical care—in fact the control, so far as means are known to science, of all of the environmental factors that affect physical and mental well-being" ("Changing," 305).

57. Without doubt, *economics* was the favored material explanation. See Dekker, "Is Abortion," 197; Yarros, "Obstetrics"; Taussig, "Abortion in Relation to Fetal and Maternal Welfare," *American Journal*, 735; Frackman, "Present," 163; Taussig, "Control of Abortion," 113; Welsh, "Problem," 13; Stix and Wiehl, "Abortion," 624; Sangmeister, "Survey," 758.

58. Goss, Slate, and Paul, "Induced," 325; Rapaport, "American," 25–26.

59. *Vanity* was not often brought up. See Rongy, *Abortion*, 100. *Urbanism* featured as well, but it was more of a catchall reason that could easily mean something else. See Dekker, "Is Abortion," 197; Wynne, "Abortion," 21; Burgess, "Social," 124. A physician might mention the *physical burden* of too many children. See Berenson, "'Contraception,'" 19.

60. Each of the following writers offered a nest of material causes, plucking one or another out for emphasis, although economic reasons were typically paramount: Ploss-Bartels, "Abortion," 264–65; Rongy, *Abortion*, 100, 111, 116; Taussig, *Abortion, Spontaneous*, 44–45, 372, 389; Taussig, "Abortion: Cause," 859; Burgess, "Social," 115–16, 123–26; Olson, "Problem"; Shipps, "Some."

61. Prior to 1920, the occasional writer asserted an unqualified right to choose, the very thing that Taussig had marked as a radical socialist position. See Dakin, "Induced," 65–66; Dekker, "Is Abortion," 198.

62. V. Robinson, *Pioneers*, 101–2; W. J. Robinson, "Abortion," 117; W. J. Robinson, *Law*, 24; Stopes, *Wise*, 15; Frackman, "Present," 162; Mayer, Harris, and Wimpfheimer, "Therapeutic,"

945; Taussig, "Abortion and Its Relation to Fetal and Maternal Mortality," 713; Yarros, "Obstetrics," 308; Welsh, "Problem," 18; Bundesen, "Suggested," 155; Rout, "Contraception"; Nobel, "Abortion," 14.

63. Hacking, *Taming*, 64–86; Foucault, *Biopolitics*, 273–78, 349–57.

64. Rudolph W. Holmes, "Discussion," 848. Also see Meyer, "Frequency," 138, 140; Millar, "Human," 282; Simons, "Statistical," 840; M. Davis, *Women's*, 53; Jesse and Spencer, "Abortion," 447; Beck, Newman, and Lewit, "Abortion," 2132, 2134.

65. For a discussion of determinism and chance in statistical theory, see Gigerenzer et al., *Empire*, 59–68, 132–35.

66. See Rose, *Inventing*, 37–38; Curtis, *Politics*, 40–41. Rose argues that "regimes of bureaucracy" are part of the arts of memory used to constitute subjects, or create "folds in the soul," in Deleuzian terms. Curtis also describes the memory work of governmentality as it mediates between individualization and totalization of bodies.

67. Igo, *Averaged*, 282. Igo is speaking of the kind of subjectivity generated in relation to social data derived from surveys.

68. Casey, *Remembering*, 99; original emphasis.

69. For a critique of Foucault's naturalization of population as an entity, see Curtis, *Politics*, 41–42.

70. For a quick overview of statistical research from the 1930s, see Rock, "Abortion," 1020–21.

71. Kopp, *Birth Control*. Clinical series at the hospital, city, or state level rapidly became one of the most common studies on abortion, with Hillis's study being the earliest large clinical series on abortion I have come across and Pearl's study the largest overall, with nearly thirty-one thousand clinical histories compared. See Hillis, "Experience"; Watkins, "Five-Year"; Witherspoon, "Analysis"; Millar, "Human"; Stewart, "Analysis"; Simons, "Statistical"; Pearl, "Fertility"; Brunner and Nelson, "Abortions"; Brunner, "Outcome"; McIver and Rucker, "Survey"; Sangmeister, "Survey"; L. B. Stevenson, "Maternal"; OSMA Committee on Maternal Health, "Maternal Deaths with Septic Shock."

72. Taussig, "Abortion in Relation to Fetal and Maternal Welfare," *American Journal*. Also see Tietze, "Therapeutic."

73. For examples of the range of survey methods, see Whelpton, "Frequency"; Stix, "Study"; Stix and Wiehl, "Abortion"; Hamilton, "Some"; Hefferman and Lynch, "What Is"; Rapaport, "American"; Harter and Beasley, "Survey."

74. Foucault, *Security*, 29–79. Foucault discusses the spatialization of risk in regard to the emergence of the concept of population, which involved treating threats as events. For a discussion of the administrative gaze relative to state formation and census making, see Curtis, *Politics*, 38–44.

75. Deem, "Stranger"; M. Warner, "Mass"; M. Warner, *Publics*, 159–86. Deem might refer to the statistical production of the average abortion as a "rhetoric of disincorporation" (449–51), involving abstracting embodied differences into an anonymous, private public.

76. Gigerenzer et al., *Empire*, 37–45; T. M. Porter, *Rise*, 52–54, 103, 151–92. Adolphe Quetelet had made a statistical *l'homme moyen* (the average man) his ideal in the nineteenth century. The average abortion I describe was not an ideal but an abnormal mode, which pointed to an unrealized, normative ideal. See Canguilhem, *Normal*.

77. Burke, *Grammar*, 59–61. The quotation is from Casey, *Remembering*, 97; original emphasis. Burke describes the "representative anecdote" as containing the germ of the "terminological structure" that evolves from it. "Thus," he writes, "the anecdote is in a sense a *summation* containing implicitly what the system that developed from it contains explicitly" (60; original emphasis). In terms of memory, the representative anecdote is a recursive structuration of rhetorical development.

78. Dunn, "Frequency," 2.

79. World Health Organization. At the time of Dunn's remarks, the ICD had been through four revisions and currently is in its tenth. Revision of the ICD was taken over by the World Health Organization in 1948. The ICD was itself a revision of the 1893 classification system by Jacques Bertillon (the Chief of Statistical Services for Paris) that had been commissioned by the International Statistical Congress, predecessor to the International Statistical Institute. Bertillon's list superseded William Farr's 1855 classification, also commissioned by the International Statistical Congress, which was revised in 1864, 1874, 1880, and 1886. Farr's principle of categorizing disease by anatomical site was retained through Bertillon to the ICD. François Bossier de Lacroix is credited as the first to attempt, in the eighteenth century, a systematic delineation of diseases. For a history of statistical societies, see T. M. Porter, *Rise*, 26–39.

80. Dunn, "Frequency," 11. The 1929 revision listed nonseptic abortion as a factor of multiple problems stemming from hemorrhages and criminal abortion as a homicide, not maternal death.

81. Ibid., 11. The first edition of the *Manual of Joint Causes of Death* was produced in 1914.

82. Whelpton, "Frequency," 31; original emphasis. Also see Taussig, *Abortion, Spontaneous*, 24; Nobel, "Abortion," 15; Hamilton, "Some," 920.

83. Tietze, "Introduction." For a history of inferential methods in statistics, see Gigerenzer et al., *Empire*, 74–109. Biostatisticians like Tietze did not report the methods they used to correct for deficiencies in descriptive data.

84. Casey, *Remembering*, 98. From M. Warner's perspective, the adumbration inherent to recollection would mean that the abstraction of a mass subject, whether statistically or otherwise, is part of addressivity; hence, mnestic relations are incumbent on forming a point of address (*Publics*).

85. Taussig, *Abortion, Spontaneous*, 24–28, 361–68. Taussig's estimate of total births was similar to census data. He derived his ratio of urban abortions to confinements (one termination per 2.5) from Marie Kopp's study of ten thousand birth control clients and his ratio of rural abortions (one termination per 5) on E. D. Plass's questionnaire of Iowa physicians. Further, he relied on K. Freudenberg's mortality estimate because he felt that a 1.2 percent mortality rate reflected the gradually improving safety of abortion, as compared with most U.S. estimates of 2 to 4 percent mortality. A mortality figure closer to one percent was replicated many times by analysis of data from various hospitals over the subsequent years. Kopp, *Birth Control*; Plass, "Personal," as quoted by Taussig, *Abortion, Spontaneous*, 25, 364, 366, 502; Freudenberg, "Frequency," 758, as quoted by Taussig, *Abortion, Spontaneous*, 26, 493.

86. For figures from the Michigan study, see Philbrick, "Social," 102; Gordon, *Moral*, 25.

87. W. J. Robinson, "Abortion," 117; Rongy, "Abortion," 402. Meyer provided one of the earliest comparative assessments of available data and their limitations ("Frequency").

88. Initially, an estimate of 750,000 was written into a draft of the final statement, only to be beaten back by Tietze and Whelpton, who were concerned that statement would contradict the Statistics Committee report in the proceedings. See "Summarizing Statement by the Abortion Conference"; Winfield Best to Alan Guttmacher, December 13, 1955, MSCP, call no. 179, box 2, folder 20; Mary Steichen Calderone to Christopher Tietze, April 26, 1957, MSCP, call no. 179, box 2, folder 20; Christopher Tietze to Mary Steichen Calderone, April 22, 1957, MSCP, call no. 179, box 2, folder 20; P. K. Whelpton to Mary Steichen Calderone, May 6, 1957, MSCP, call no. 179, box 2, folder 20.

89. Tietze and Lewit, "Abortion," 23. For examples of citations of the Arden House estimate, see Goodno, Cushner, and Molumphy, "Management," 16; Harter and Beasley, "Survey"; Hershey, "Society's," 2312; E. A. Bennett, "Abortion," 248; R. A. Schwartz, "Psychiatry," 100.

90. One is reminded of Benjamin's sixth aphoristic thesis on the philosophy of history: "To articulate the past historically does not mean to recognize it 'the way it really was' (Ranke). It means to seize hold of a memory as it flashes up at a moment of danger." The distribution of danger into a table of probabilities converts flashes of memory into a highly plastic, recursive resource that allows the past to be seized indefinitely (Benjamin, *Illuminations*, 255).

91. Hamilton, "Some," 920.

92. Dunn, "Frequency," 11. Similar to Taussig's 1936 calculations, Dunn's work averaged ratios of abortions to confinements sampled from urban and rural areas in order to approximate the total number of abortions and then applied a rationalized fatality rate of 1 percent, whereas Taussig had assumed a 1.2 fatality rate. The great difference came from Dunn's assuming a lower overall number of abortions.

93. Taussig, "Discussion," 28. Taussig had reviewed available data from 1936 onward and had arrived at a similar conclusion to Dunn's, although Taussig felt Dunn's corrections were too conservative.

94. Tietze, "Abortion as a Cause," 1435–36. The 1944 Special Study classified deaths for 1940 according to both the fourth and fifth iterations of the ICD. By comparing the discrepancy, Tietze was able to apply a percentage correction to mortality rates from data for 1927–38. Despite census modifications, the rough figure of about a quarter of maternal deaths from abortion was a mainstay. For an earlier estimate of the proportion of maternal deaths from abortion, see F. J. McCann, "Criminal," 111; Hillis, "Experience," 84. The most sophisticated discussion of mortality pre-*Roe* is Tietze, "Mortality."

95. Kummer and Leavy, "Criminal"; Barno, "Criminal," 11. It is possible that Russell S. Fisher's estimation was an additional source for the lower limit of five thousand annual deaths (Fisher, "Criminal," 248). For one of the rare instances where Dunn's revision was used (and then only in a review of the conference), see Popenoe, "Abortion," 1.

96. Gebhard et al., *Pregnancy*, 204. The discussion of maternal mortality rates is extensive, in all cases working from Taussig's research and revisions thereof. For examples, see Yarros, *Modern*, 135–36; OSMA Committee on Maternal Health, "Maternal Deaths Involving Criminal Abortion"; Fox, "Abortion"; Sangmeister, "Survey," 756; Committee on Maternal and Child Welfare, "Maternal," 72; M. Davis, *Women's*, 54; Harter and Beasley, "Survey," 1937.

97. It is common for today's antiabortion advocates to argue that because the numbers were hard to pin down and often exaggerated, the danger of illegal abortion was cynically overblown in an attempt to legalize it. Setting aside the contradiction of considering abortion to be murder yet not as dangerous as claimed, there are counterfactual problems with seeing a left-wing plot to defraud the public about induced abortion's risk on the way to *Roe v. Wade*. One is that most physicians in question did not want abortion deregulated. Alan Guttmacher himself only favored a full repeal after studying the effect of partial liberalization post-1967. He explained the evolution of his thinking in testimony before the Subcommittee on Criminal Laws and Procedures of the U.S. Senate Committee on the Judiciary in 1973 (Guttmacher, Testimony).

98. Galdston in Calderone, *Abortion*, 163. Galdston spoke in regard to what should be in the concluding statement of the conference. He was executive secretary of the Medical Information Bureau of the New York Academy of Medicine at the time.

99. Taussig, *Abortion, Spontaneous*, 400–401. Also see Taussig, "Abortion and Its Relation to Fetal and Maternal Mortality," 713; Taussig, "Control of Criminal Abortion."

100. See Gampell, "Legal," 22–23. Also see Greeley, "Abortion," 26.

101. Donnelly, "Are There," 113; also see Joseph P. Donnelly to Mary Steichen Calderone, May 16, 1956, MSCP, call no. 179, box 2, folder 15. For other instances of life-at-conception advocacy during and after World War II, see Taylor, "Summary," 174; Cosgrove and Carter,

"Consideration," 300, 303; Friedman, "Abortion," 659; Rubin and Novak, *Integrated*, 391. For discussions of abortion as justifiable homicide, see Taussig, "Abortion and Its Relation to Fetal and Maternal Mortality," 713; Taussig, *Abortion, Spontaneous*, 400, 401; Nobel, "Abortion," 7; A. D. Black, "Social," 100, 101.

102. W. J. Robinson, *Law*, 34. Also see R. E. Hall, "Non-Catholic," 83.

103. Dubow, *Ourselves*, 42–51.

104. Casper, *Making*, 30–72.

105. The conversation on the harm to women is extensive, as one might expect. For a sampling of opinion from clinical, to experimental, to statistical, see L. S. Schwartz, "Treatment"; W. J. Robinson, *Law*, 27, 55, 73, 75; D'Amour and Kiven, "Harmful," 506; Taussig, "Effects," 46–47; Dickinson, "Discussion," 51.

106. Although the 22 percent figure is taken from Kinsey's report at the PPFA conference, the one-in-five ratio was generally confirmed by other statistical analyses. See Bates and Zawadzki, *Criminal*, 3.

107. Casey, *Remembering*, 99. Rather than focus on interpellation in relation to such categories, as M. Warner (*Publics*) might be concerned with, I am interested in how the measurement of such dangers is interwoven with collective memory.

108. Casey, *Remembering*, 123–24. Casey marks availability and consolidation as two attributes of recognition in regard to establishing "presentness" in recollection.

109. Mary Steichen Calderone to William C. Menninger, June 4, 1957, MSCP, call no. 179, box 2, fol. 20.

110. Ibid. An earlier volume, *Therapeutic Abortion*, edited by psychiatrist Harold Rosen, was an important moment in professional discourse about psychiatric indicators of abortion. The book developed from two psychiatric conference panels, the first at the Maryland Society of Private Practicing Psychiatrists in 1951 and the second at the American Psychiatric Association in 1952. See Rosen, *Therapeutic*.

111. Bellhouse et al. in Calderone, *Abortion*, 181–82.

112. Guttmacher in Calderone, *Abortion*, 167.

113. Finn, "Risky," 10; original emphasis.

114. Well before the upsurge in descriptive data on abortion, that "all roads lead to abortion" was apparent to some. See Meyer, "Frequency," 144.

115. Gordon, "Teenage," 253–60; L. J. Reagan, *When*, 28–29; Solinger, *Pregnancy*, 67–69.

116. Gilman Srebnick, *Mysterious*, 3–12.

117. W. J. Robinson, *Law*, 83–104.

118. Kinsey in Calderone, *Abortion*, 54, 56.

119. See Greenley, "Practice"; Bates and Zawadzki, *Criminal*, 4. Greenley wrote, "It would seem to the ordinary mind, that if a married woman wishes an act of that kind, she must be to some extent, at least, demented" (184), which is reminiscent of H. R. Storer and Edwin Hale, among others, from thirty years prior. The "ignorant" woman encompasses a broad explanation for abortion, but there is a specific, if loose, subdiscourse that produces the unthinkable subject of a mother who chooses abortion over more children.

120. Kinsey in Calderone, *Abortion*, 54–55. Also see Downie, "Interpretation," 27; Dekker, "Is Abortion," 200; Watkins, "Five-Year," 162; Stewart, "Analysis," 873; Palmer and Greenberg, *Facts*, 159; Moses, *Contraception*, 22–23; Simons, "Statistical," 846; Willson et al., *Obstetrics*, 162, 183; Kummer, "Therapeutic," 140; Harter and Beasely, "Survey"; Bates and Zawadzki, *Criminal*, 4; Lyon, "Abortion," 21.

121. Kinsey in Calderone, *Abortion*, 55. Also see Gebhard et al., *Pregnancy*, 165; R. A. Schwartz, "Psychiatry," 100. Schwartz summarizes Gebhard et al.

122. The earliest and most forceful statement on mothers aborting came from the anonymous "Wife of a Christian Physician" in an 1866 letter published by the *Boston Medical and*

Surgical Journal (the forerunner of the *New England Journal of Medicine*). (Wife of a Christian Physician, "'Why Not?'"; the letter is reprinted in an appendix to Stormer, "*Why Not?*")

123. Calderone in Calderone, *Abortion*, 160. Also see Korentzwitt, "Modern," 14.

124. See conversations in Calderone, *Abortion*, 77, 80, 93, 101.

125. Kleegman in Calderone, *Abortion*, 111–12, 183. Kleegman attended the 1942 NCMH conference and, an interesting side note, was also R. L. Dickinson's niece. For discussions of class difference in rates and in relation to law, see Millar, "Human," 272; Palmer and Greenberg, *Facts*, 161; Pavey, "Conservative," 164; Guttmacher, "Social," 303; Guttmacher, "United States," 456; Roemer, "Abortion," 1907; R. E. Hall, "Hospitals," 1934; Lyon, "Abortion," 21.

126. Taussig, *Abortion, Spontaneous*, 45; Wile, "Birth Control," 144; Rongy, *Abortion*, 126. Wile and Rongy both argued along different lines from Taussig. Where Taussig wrote, "Such views are often the result of wishful thinking; they are too frequently an attempt to bolster up preconceived theological opinions by the use of limited and false interpretations of history," they contended that racial improvement (ostensibly race as species) was the antithesis of race suicide.

127. Solinger, *Wake Up*, 20–40; Solinger, *Beggars*, 65–71. For a discussion of the largely unwritten African American history of abortion, see L. J. Ross, "African-American."

128. Tietze in Calderone, *Abortion*, 211–17. The exclusion of data on African American women was all the more curious given that Tietze himself had previously noted with horror that, although the incidence rate was lower, the mortality rate was several times higher among African American women. See Tietze, "Abortion as a Cause," 1438.

129. There was concern with the separate publication of Kinsey's data by the ISR—that if its volume was published at the same time as PPFA's proceedings, the ISR volume would dominate reception, and that if the two were not coordinated, ISR's book could contradict PPFA's findings. For background on the editorial process relative to Kinsey's data being published by the ISR, see Mary Steichen Calderone to Christopher Tietze, October 16, 1956, MSCP, call no. 179, box 9, fol. 157; Winfield Best to Mary Steichen Calderone, March 28, 1957, MSCP, call no. 179, box 2, fol. 21; Whelpton to Calderone, May 6, 1957; Mary Steichen Calderone to members of Editorial Committee, memorandum, May 21, 1957, MSCP, call no. 179, box 2, fol. 20.

130. Witherspoon, "Analysis," 368; Moses, *Contraception*, 24–25; Tietze, "Therapeutic," 147; Spengler, "Notes"; Stormer, *Articulating*, 21–39.

131. Finn, "Risky," 6.

132. Esposito, *Immunitas*, 170. Esposito is discussing the pregnant body's immune system that blocks ordinary immunological reactions that would attack the embryo as an invader. Physicians' effort to make women immune to abortion as a social disease has an unexpected similarity.

133. L. J. Reagan, *When*, 195.

134. Stormer, *Articulating*, 21–39. Also see Lovett, *Conceiving*, 93–102.

135. Deleuze and Guattari, *Thousand*, 486.

136. De Certeau, *Practice*, "Spatial Stories," sections titled "Creating a Theater of Actions" and "Frontiers and Bridges"; original emphasis.

137. Fulsome to Taussig, March 5, 1942, 5; emphasis added.

138. Canguilhem, *Normal*, 247.

139. Collier and Lakoff, "Regimes," 23.

140. Berlant, "Slow," 767–76.

141. Taussig, *Abortion, Spontaneous*, 446–52.

142. The more radical and sweeping elements of Taussig's program such as forced sterilization, positive improvements in abortion provision, and remedying economic opportunity nationally fell away soon after the Depression, however.

143. Gordon, *Moral*, 125–68.

144. Collier and Lakoff, "Regimes," 23.

145. Welsh, "Problem," 19.

146. A. D. Black, "Social," 98. One conferee grasped the nettle of moving from a failed disciplinary model as desired by a medical pastorate to a more indirect biopolitical model: "We cannot reform or discipline women to welcome and continue every pregnancy. We must realistically adapt our legal structure and medical philosophy to fit our patients, just as in any field of legal and medical practice." See Squier, "Discussion," 171.

147. Amen, "Some"; Pink, "Motherhood"; Bundesen, "Suggested," 155–62; Cooper, "Possibilities."

148. Lidz in Calderone, *Abortion*, 166.

149. Kosmak, "Introductory." For background on Kosmak's reproductive politics, see Gordon, *Moral*, 179–84.

150. Taylor, "Summary," 175.

151. For background on Taylor's refusal to sign, see Howard C. Taylor to Mary S. Calderone, May 2, 1957, MSCP, call no. 179, box 2, folder 15; Mary Steichen Calderone to Howard C. Taylor, May 6, 1957, MSCP, call no. 179, box 2, folder 15; Mary Steichen Calderone to Alan Guttmacher, July 1, 1957, MSCP, call no. 179, box 2, folder 15.

152. Collier and Lakoff, "Regimes," 31.

153. Merismus is related to synecdoche, but *synecdoche* refers to the identification of the part by its whole or the other way around. So synecdoche is a naming figure that operates between the composition and its constituent elements—a song is known by its hook, for instance. *Merismus* refers to the elaboration of divisible parts, not the shorthand by which whole-to-part relations are signified.

154. De Certeau, *Practice*, "Spatial Stories," section titled "The Art of Memory and Circumstances"; original emphasis.

155. Hodann, "New," 180. As with most subjects on abortion, the 1955 PPFA conference provides the most extensive discussion of Scandinavian law and policy. One entire session of the conference was devoted to it. For greater detail, see discussion in Calderone, *Abortion*, 14–32.

156. Brekke in Calderone, *Abortion*, 15.

157. Hodann, "New."

158. Geijerstam in Calderone, *Abortion*, 25–27. Humanitarian indicators included girls under fifteen, rape, incest, criminal coercion, insanity, or imbecility. Eugenic indicators included hereditary mental and physical disease. Normal approval was available before the twentieth week. The special committee heard cases occurring up to the twenty-fourth week. Also see Rapaport, "American," 24–33.

159. Clemmesen in Calderone, *Abortion*, 21–22. The 1956 revision specified existing or threatened illness (mental or physical) and social circumstances that would affect the woman's future well-being.

160. Brekke in Calderone, *Abortion*, 15–16. Norway had a 1902 statute that allowed for abortions by physicians for medical reasons alone. "Humanitarian" was actually quite narrow, referring to cases of rape, incest, or pregnancy before sixteen years, the age of consent. Eugenic indicators required compulsory abortion in the proposed law. Norway also established maternal health centers beginning in 1951 modeled on the Danish Mother's Aid model (ibid., 19).

161. "Norway."

162. Stone in Calderone, *Abortion*, 209.

163. Simon, "Psychiatric," 79. Also see "Therapeutic Abortion"; Tietze, "Abortion in Europe," 1931; Tietze and Lewit, "Abortion," 27.

164. Guttmacher, "Therapeutic," 118; Guttmacher, "Psychiatric"; Guttmacher, "Abortion," 6; Savel, "Adjudication," 17. Also see Solinger, "'Complete.'" Hull and Hoffer argue that the first review committees began in Detroit in the late 1930s, although Guttmacher claimed to have inaugurated the practice (*Roe v. Wade*, 72).

165. See discussion in Calderone, *Abortion*, 166, 176, 182–83.

166. The 1905 Women's Congress did have some influence in the United States at the time, as socialist physicians in the United States such as Ladova pointed to it as a modern model for reproductive rights. Debates about legalizing abortion began to emerge in Italy and Germany as well. See Ladova, "Discussion," 44; L. Jacobi, "Infanticide," 456–57.

167. "Abortion: Translation of the Russian Law." This law repealed the existing law on abortion and replaced it with requirements for maternity homes and state support for large families as well as divorce reform and increased penalties for failure to pay alimony.

168. Taussig, "Abortion Problem in Russia"; Taussig, *Abortion, Spontaneous*, 405–20; Ferguson, "Abortion," 892. For examples of U.S. medical reception of the Soviet abortion experiment, see Yarros, *Modern*, 135, 142; W. J. Robinson, *Law*, 41; Rongy, *Abortion*, 79; Palmer and Greenberg, *Facts*, 163; Nobel, "Abortion," 1; Eliasberg, "Psychiatry," 27; Guttmacher, "Therapeutic," 113; Taussig, "Abortion and Its Relation to Fetal and Maternal Mortality," 713; Field, "Re-legalization," 422–26. Field's discussion is the only one that discusses Soviet relegalization in 1955.

169. Taussig, *Abortion, Spontaneous*, 413–14.

170. Ibid., 414–15. Gradually, Soviets restricted availability to abortion and increased support for contraception as the negative consequences became apparent of "wholesale" manual abortions (Taussig's adjective).

171. See discussion in Calderone, *Abortion*, 149–50, 200–202, 203–6. Guttmacher had previously noted at the conference the impact of Japan's policy as creating a rapid rise in numbers of abortions (ibid., 114).

172. Massey, *Space*, 69.

173. Casey, *Remembering*, 68–69. Casey refers to "worldhood" as an aspect of memory-frames that involves situating the object of memory within a scene and its surroundings.

Chapter 5

1. Gorney, *Articles*, 43–44; Hull and Hoffer, *Roe v. Wade*, 21. New York was the first state to pass an antiabortion law with a "therapeutic" exception to preserve the woman's life.

2. Packer and Gampell, "Therapeutic," 418. Also see Hull and Hoffer, *Roe v. Wade*, 69–72.

3. Deutscher, "Inversion," 62–63. Also see Solinger, "'Complete,'" 245.

4. Derrida, *Dissemination*, 95–117; Esposito, *Immunitas*, 121–27.

5. Fulsome to Taussig, March 5, 1942, 4–5.

6. Studdiford, "Common," 721.

7. Deutscher, "Inversion," 65. Deutscher modifies Agamben's analysis of Schmitt. Also see Wolfe, *Before*, 41–54.

8. Guttmacher, "Shrinking," 14.

9. Hannah Arendt and the recent literature on compassion inform my use of the concepts "pity" and "compassion." As Spelman notes, Arendt uses *compassion* more like *empathy* and sets it against *pity*, whereas *compassion* and *pity* are used "interchangeably" in ordinary English usage. As I am not discussing empathy, I use *compassion* and *pity* as rough synonyms (Spelman, *Fruits*, 67–68).

10. Packer and Gampell, "Therapeutic," 419.

11. Vivian, *Public*, 48–50, 55–60.

12. Arendt, *Human*, 237. Arendt considers forgiveness in regard to the consequences of action when one is "unable to undo what one has done though one did not, and could not, have known what he [*sic*] was doing" (237).

13. Vivian, *Public*, 37.

14. Govier, "Forgiveness," 61–62. Also see Holmgren, *Forgiveness*, 84–103, 193–210, 228–56, 257–78.

15. Brown, *Regulating*, 9.

16. Esposito, *Immunitas*, 167. Esposito is discussing immunological theory but the lesson applies here.

17. Vivian, *Public*, 47.

18. Govier, "Forgiveness," 70.

19. Foucault, *Archaeology*, 216–17. Regulation of the conditions under which what is sayable about abortion can be true would qualify as a principle of exclusion. Women's voices on the rationality of abortion were excluded except as translated and interpreted through the episteme of reproductive medicine as determined by a duly recognized authority. Also see Spelman, *Fruits*, 70.

20. Brown, *Regulating*, 93. Also see Berlant, *Female*, 34–35.

21. Garber, "Compassion," 26; Boltanski, *Distant*, 3–5.

22. Peritonitis is inflammation of the peritoneum, the lining that covers many of the abdominal organs and lines the abdomen.

23. Berlant, "Slow," 779; Brown, *Regulating*, 25–45.

24. Esposito, *Immunitas*, 167.

25. Solinger, *Beggars*, 37–64.

26. L. J. Reagan, *When*, 148–59. Also see discussion in Calderone, *Abortion*, 59–65; Keemer, *Confessions*; Joffe, *Doctors*, 108–27.

27. Guttmacher, "Shrinking," 12.

28. N. J. Davis, *From*, 89–107.

29. Arendt, *Human*, 241.

30. Govier, "Forgiveness," 62–71; Holmgren, *Forgiveness*, 84–103.

31. Deutscher, "Inversion," 65.

32. Esposito, *Immunitas*, 15.

33. Thomas, *Abortion*, 44.

34. Welsh, "Problem," 1. Welsh's estimate is very high compared with other statistics of the time.

35. Foucault, "On the Genealogy," 231.

36. Wolfe, *Before*, 36–39; Esposito, *Immunitas*, 29–34; Esposito, *Bios*, 46–47; Foucault, *Clinic*, 158–59; Foucault, *History*, 136–39.

37. Foucault, "Society," 248.

38. Esposito, *Immunitas*, 105; original emphasis. Esposito is discussing the work of Arnold Gehlen and speaking of Man in the generic.

39. Derrida, *Dissemination*, 153; original emphasis. Derrida deconstructs Plato's use of *pharmakon* as a metaphor for writing so as to oppose writing to speech. Plato only describes writing as a bad drug (by his account, it thoughtlessly repeats itself and so induces amnesia of the living truth) by availing himself of writing that is a good drug. The opposition of writing to speech is made possible through a certain practice of writing, hence displacing the opposition. Derrida stops short of life-death as *pharmakon* itself and instead uses life and death as settled values to establish the critical poles by which writing is conceived as *pharmakon*.

40. Esposito, *Immunitas*, 121–27.

41. For example, see M. Davis, *Women's*, 59.

42. W. J. Robinson, *Law*, 28.

43. Derrida, *Dissemination*, 162; Esposito, *Immunitas*, 127.

44. For differing analyses of the convertability of life into death, see Agamben, *Homo Sacer*, 71–86, 160–65; Dillon and Reid, *Liberal*, 15–33; Mbembe, "Necropolitics," 12–16; Esposito, *Bios*, 110–45; Mason, *Killing*, 9–71.

45. Studdiford, "Common," 721.

46. Colpitts, "Trends," 988; also see Guttmacher, "Shrinking," 13. Colpitts considers only European history. Experts contemporaneous with Colpitts were well aware of therapeutic applications of abortion in other cultural traditions. See Devereux, "Typological." Further, J. C. Ayres argued that a "German midwife, Justin Siegmundin, used it in placent praevia [the placenta blocks the cervix]" in the early 1700s ("Therapeutic," 41).

47. Graham, *Eternal*, 274–90. William Smellie in England and André Levret in France were central to innovations in the use of forceps in delivery, Smellie especially in that he developed a simple practice for determining contracted pelvis (278). Peter Chamberlen developed the forceps initially in the late 1600s (191).

48. W. H. Jones, *Management*, 33.

49. As quoted in Colpitts, "Trends," 988.

50. Colpitts, "Trends," 988. Also see Taussig, *Abortion, Spontaneous*, 277–78.

51. Dekker, "Is Abortion," 194.

52. Findley, "Slaughter," 35.

53. Hefferman and Lynch, "What Is"; Beck, Newman, and Lewit, "Abortion." Hefferman and Lynch sent a questionnaire to 367 U.S. hospitals, receiving 171 respondents, 152 providing detailed information on therapeutic abortions from 1941 to 1950. The average was 2.3 percent with a range of 0.2 to 7.3 per 1,000 pregnancies. Estimates prior to the 1940s and 1950s on therapeutic abortion were largely conjectural or based on very limited pools of data. Beck, Newman, and Lewit wrote, "Adequate data do not exist on legal or therapeutic abortions performed to save the life of the pregnant woman and, in a few states, to safeguard her physical or mental health as well" (2132).

54. Solinger, "'Complete,'" 245; Packer and Gampell, "Therapeutic," 420.

55. Taussig, "Effects," 46–47. Taussig died not long after the 1942 National Committee on Maternal Health conference was held, so it is unclear what he might have felt on consideration of findings from the 1950s, which undid much of the premise of inherent danger.

56. Solinger, *Wake Up*; Donnelly, "Are There," 118.

57. Tietze and Lewit, "Abortion," 22.

58. Calderone, "Illegal," 949.

59. Tietze, "Abortion as a Cause," 1437.

60. Timanus in Calderone, *Abortion*, 59–62, 66. Timanus also mentioned his familiarity with another practitioner, who had conducted approximately forty thousand abortions with only two deaths.

61. Joffe, *Doctors*, 42. See G. L. Timanus to Mary Steichen Calderone, February 11, 1956, MSCP, call no. 179, box 2, folder 19.

62. Kummer and Leavy, "Criminal," 170–71. Also see Kummer, "Post-abortion," 980. Kummer noted this was endemic to American literature while speaking before the International Congress of Psychosomatic Medicine and Maternity, Paris, July 11, 1962.

63. Guttmacher, "Abortion," 5. Guttmacher does not name G. Lotrell Timanus, but he is referring to him.

64. Zakin, Godsick, and Segal, "Foreign," 233.

65. Tietze, "Abortion as a Cause," 1437; Nobel, "Abortion," 3.

66. Thomas, *Abortion*, 79–89. Prior to Taussig's extensive discussion in *Abortion*, Thomas provided one of the more detailed explanations of antiseptic practices regarding abortion in his book *Abortion and Its Treatment*.

67. Latour, *Pasteurization*, 111–45; R. Porter, *Greatest*, 428–61.

68. Petchesky, *Abortion*, 80.

69. R. Porter, *Greatest*, 370–74.

70. Ibid., 453–58.

71. Esposito, *Immunitas*, 141.

72. Monica Casper notes the emergence of the fetal patient in the 1960s with the advent of amniocentesis and Rh treatments, which eventually led to fetal surgery. I suggest that the fetal patient becomes possible when abortion becomes a last resort. Casper, *Making*, 30–72; Rapp, *Testing*, 23–35.

73. Hodge, *Principles*, 301. Also see Taussig, *Abortion, Spontaneous*, 277.

74. Velpeau, *Elementary*, 489. His reference to a plant reflects an Aristotelian biology in which there are vegetative souls that are more primitive than animals or humans.

75. H. R. Storer, *Criminal Abortion in America*, 59–73, 99.

76. Hale, *Systematic*, 263–89. Hale based his argument only on the indication of contracted pelvis, but he fully supported Cooper's argument that if it is clearly unlikely that the fetus can be born without harm, abortion is necessary as soon as feasible.

77. W. J. Robinson, *Law*, 17.

78. Thomas, *Abortion*, 99.

79. Laqueur, "Mourning," 48; Boltanski, *Distant*, 6–7.

80. Rongy, *Abortion*, 90; original emphasis.

81. Taussig, *Abortion, Spontaneous*, 278. Taussig is quoting Dr. Winter without citation.

82. Ibid., 279. Taussig noted only the Soviet example, but physicians had charged abortionists and their clients with wrongly responding to socioeconomic and eugenic reasons. See L. J. Reagan, *Dangerous*, 76–104.

83. Packer and Gampell, "Therapeutic," 418–19.

84. Ibid., 447; Solinger, "'Complete,'" 242; Calderone, "Illegal," 949. Rh incompatibility occurs when the fetus and mother have different Rh blood types, which can, particularly in pregnancies after the first, produce "a jaundiced, anemic infant whose life may often only be saved by prompt blood transfusions. A subsequent pregnancy may give rise to even greater fetal damage resulting in stillbirth" (Packer and Gampell, "Therapeutic," 440). Also see Casper, *Making*, 31–34; Rapp, *Testing*, 24–31.

85. Guttmacher, "Shrinking," 14.

86. Ibid., 16–19; also see Taussig, *Abortion, Spontaneous*, 283–317. Taussig provides the most extensive discussion of indicators. According to Guttmacher, conditions such as preeclampsia that develop later in pregnancy did not meet criteria for therapeutic abortion, which usually referred to previable termination. As with all things abortion related, the generality comes with great variety. For example, Sophia Kleegman stated in 1955 that tuberculosis was the leading indicator for therapeutic abortion at Bellevue Hospital in New York because of its extensive "chest service" (Kleegman in Calderone, *Abortion*, 110).

87. Guttmacher, "Shrinking," 19–20.

88. Taussig, *Abortion, Spontaneous*, 279.

89. Calderone to Guttmacher, July 1, 1957. See Taylor to Calderone, May 2, 1957.

90. Bellhouse et al. in Calderone, *Abortion*, 181, 183.

91. Donnelly, "Are There," 113.

92. Ibid., 112–13. Also see Cosgrove and Carter, "Consideration," 304.

93. Indeed, Donnelly was referencing a 1931 article by Charles Gardner Child. The language of justifiable homicide was not present, but Storer articulated the legal rationale of intervening to prevent her death (H. R. Storer, *Criminal Abortion: Its Nature*, 114). Everett W. Burdett moved closer with a description of "justifiable abortion." See Burdett, "Medical," 201–5.

94. Donnelly, "Are There." Hague Clinic's remarkably low incidence of therapeutic practice had no corresponding increase in maternal mortality (fewer abortions did not mean more maternal death).

95. Ayres, "Therapeutic," 43.

96. Galdston and Guttmacher in Calderone, *Abortion*, 163.

97. W. J. Robinson, *Law*, 6; H. R. Storer, *Criminal Abortion in America*, 59.

98. Erhardt in Calderone, *Abortion*, 78–80.

99. Tietze in ibid., 83–85. Also see Laidlaw in ibid., 107; Gold et al., "Therapeutic."

100. Lyon, "Abortion," 21.

101. Lidz, "Reflections," 278.

102. Jenkins, "Significance."

103. For discussion of adoption practices in postwar America relative to abortion, see Solinger, *Wake Up*, 148–86.

104. Lidz, "Reflections," 279.

105. Romm, "Psychoanalytic," 210.

106. Eliasberg, "Psychiatry"; Lidz, "Reflections," 281; Murdock, "Experiences," 204.

107. Rosen, "Emotionally," 221.

108. Galdston in Calderone, *Abortion*, 119; first emphasis added.

109. Rosen, "Emotionally," 243. Rosen remarked that it is obvious that rape should be a legal exception, noting that the *illegality*, not the experience, "introduces complications with emotional overtones." However, rape and incest were added to the American Law Institute model penal code only in 1958, when the drafting was nearing completion. See "Model Penal Code Preliminary Draft."

110. Galdston in Calderone, *Abortion*, 118.

111. H. R. Storer, *Criminal Abortion: Its Nature*, 78. Also see Hull and Hoffer, *Roe v. Wade*, 41–42.

112. Galdston in Calderone, *Abortion*, 120.

113. See Lidz in ibid., 125; Rosen in ibid., 124; Kleegman in ibid., 112.

114. Kinsey in ibid., 143.

115. Eliasberg, "Prenatal."

116. Kolb in Calderone, *Abortion*, 140.

117. Eliasberg, "Prenatal," 214.

118. See discussion in Calderone, *Abortion*, 108, 128–32, 138–40. Corresponding to the medical dialogue, the American Law Institute model code committee struck suicide as a reason from early drafts (confidential memorandum—Louis B. Schwarz Reporter, n.d., American Law Institute Model Penal Code Collection [ALIMPCC], Biddle Law Library, University of Pennsylvania, box 7, folder 28).

119. Philbrick, "Social," 104–5; Ladova, "Discussion," 44; Hawkins, "Abortion," 769–72.

120. Hawkins, "Abortion," 769.

121. Fernald, "Sociological," 57–60.

122. Hawkins, "Abortion," 770, 772.

123. Brown, *Regulating*.

124. Stormer, "*Why Not?*"

125. Wife of a Christian Physician, "'Why Not?,'" 273.

126. Ibid., 274; original emphasis.

127. Ibid. On free love, see Battan, "'Marriage,'" 209–10.

128. H. R. Storer, *Is It I?* In the literature this is the only extended, direct address by a physician to men about their culpability for unwanted pregnancy.

129. *Stigma* normally referred to pregnancy outside marriage, but it broadly referred to social ostracisms connected with pregnancy under deplorable circumstances. Physicians faced

requests for abortion to avoid unwed motherhood more frequently. Ploss-Bartels, "Abortion," 264–65; Rongy, *Abortion*, 100; Taussig, *Abortion, Spontaneous*, 389; Taussig, "Abortion: Cause," 859; Hamilton, "Some," 919; Olson, "Problem," 672; Burgess, "Social," 115–16; Shipps, "Some," 311; Goss, Slate, and Paul, "Induced," 325; Rapaport, "American," 26.

130. See Brownmiller, *Against*; Bevacqua, *Rape*, 19–26; Battan, "'Marriage'"; Goldman, "'Most'"; Lindquist Dorr, "'Another.'" Susan Brownmiller is credited with initiating the rhetoric of rape-as-violence, but Bevacqua notes that Ruth Herschberger made that case in 1948, so it is unsurprising that medical literature is nearly silent on rape and abortion. Into the twentieth century, rape was frequently understood as a racial crime of African American men assaulting white women; marital rape was a nebulous, highly contested idea; coercion was hard to establish; and men were assumed to have the right to sex, coerced or not.

131. Hammett, letter, 773.

132. Rongy, *Abortion*, 201.

133. R. E. Hall, "Hospitals," 1934; Pavey, "Conservative," 164; Janovski, Wiener, and Ober, "Soap."

134. Konikow, *Physician's*, 9.

135. W. J. Robinson, *Abortion*, 89; see 83–104.

136. Downie, "Interpretation," 30.

137. Kleegman, "Planned Parenthood." Brown discusses tolerance discourse principally as the state deployed in "response to a legitimacy deficit and, in particular, to its historically diminished capacity to embody universal representation" (*Regulating*, 83–84).

138. Kleegman, "Planned Parenthood," 254–57; Kleegman in Calderone, *Abortion*, 115.

139. Dekker, "Is Abortion," 197, 198.

140. The reasoning for humanitarian exceptions resonates with the charity ethic that informed the development of Aid for Dependent Children, as Gordon discusses in *Pitied but Not Entitled*.

141. Brown, *Regulating*, 84. The quote concludes with "when those who have been historically excluded by norms of sex, race, ethnicity, and religion are vocal about such exclusion" (84). She is most concerned with the moment of vocal contestation of dominance, which is not apropos of therapeutic abortion until the 1960s, when women began to organize around rubella and thalidomide, as discussed below.

142. W. J. Robinson, *Law*, 281; Taussig, "Control of Abortion," 113; Kleegman in Calderone, *Abortion*, 109–16.

143. This counterrecollection became routine after World War I. For examples, see Dekker, "Is Abortion," 198; Taussig, "Abortion in Relation to Fetal and Maternal Welfare," *American Journal*, 735; Taussig, "Abortion: Cause," 859; Rongy, *Abortion*, 111; Guttmacher, "Social," 303; Guttmacher, "United States," 456; Palmer and Greenberg, *Facts*, 161; Welsh, "Problem," 13; Hamilton, "Some," 919; Fulsome to Taussig, March 5, 1942, 6–7; Burgess, "Social," 115–16; Roemer, "Abortion," 1907.

144. Petchesky, *Abortion*, 123.

145. C. R. McCann, *Birth Control*, 101–27; Kevles, *Name*, 85–95. Also see Happe, *Material*, 24–33; Hasian, *Eugenics*, 1–50, 80–88; Hodgson, "Ideological," 4–16; Rapp, *Testing*, 35–39; Gordon, *Moral*, 72–85; Petchesky, *Abortion*, 84–89, 92–94; Stern, *Eugenic*, 82–114.

146. Hodgson, "Ideological," 4–16; Hasian, *Eugenics*, 14–24.

147. Taussig, *Abortion, Spontaneous*, 317.

148. Kevles, *Name*, 3–19; Esposito, *Bios*, 127–35. For a discussion of biopower and eugenics illuminated by factory farming, see Wolfe, *Before*, 39–48. For more on Galton's use of statistics, see T. M. Porter, *Rise*, 128–46.

149. Kevles, *Name*, 57–69. Also see Hull and Hoffer, *Roe v. Wade*, 61–65.

150. Hodgson, "Ideological," 4–6; Hasian, *Eugenics*, 14–21.

151. Taussig, *Abortion, Spontaneous*, 45. He continued, "Such views are often the result of wishful thinking; they are too frequently an attempt to bolster up preconceived theological opinions by the use of limited and false interpretations of history."

152. Wile, "Birth Control," 144. Also see Rongy, *Abortion*, 126. Wile and Rongy both argued along different lines from Taussig. They contended that racial improvement (ostensibly race as species) was the antithesis of race suicide.

153. Kevles, *Name*, 118–22.

154. Hodgson, "Ideological," 9–13; C. R. McCann, *Birth Control*, 109–13; Kevles, *Name*, 70–84; Hasian, *Eugenics*, 25–138; Gordon, *Moral*, 80–85.

155. A. Jacobi, "Best," 1736.

156. See discussion in Calderone, *Abortion*, 117–53.

157. Taussig, *Abortion, Spontaneous*, 317–20.

158. Rongy, *Abortion*, 145–50, 120–29, 186.

159. Ibid., 186.

160. Ibid., 124, 126. Also see Hull and Hoffer, *Roe v. Wade*, 68–69.

161. Rongy, *Abortion*, 98.

162. W. J. Robinson, *Law*, 12 (all capitalized in the original; I have decapitalized the quotation for readability). Robinson also held biologically Malthusian views, contending that "*morons and imbeciles should not be allowed to get pregnant at all; they should be sterilized*" (69; original emphasis).

163. L. J. Reagan, *Dangerous*, 105–79. Also see Gorney, *Articles*, 49–55; Hull and Hoffer, *Roe v. Wade*, 100.

164. L. J. Reagan, *Dangerous*, 4.

165. Ibid., 103.

166. Ibid., 58.

167. Ibid., 58–59; Condit, *Decoding*, 28–31.

168. L. J. Reagan, *Dangerous*, 7–16.

169. Ibid., 105–38. Also see Rapp, *Testing*, 23–35.

170. W. J. Robinson, *Law*, 18.

171. Taussig, *Abortion, Spontaneous*, 319; emphasis added.

172. Rongy, *Abortion*, 24.

173. Greene's thesis is that the United States is both "subject and object" of the population apparatus, that is, both governs and is governed by the population crisis (*Malthusian*, 2).

174. Calderone to Tietze, February 15, 1954.

175. Whelpton, "Discussion," 36.

176. Douglas in Calderone, *Abortion*, 109.

177. Guttmacher, "Shrinking," 20.

178. Overstreet, foreword, 11. Also see Downie, "Interpretation," 30.

179. Yarros, *Modern*, 171–72.

180. Kleegman in Calderone, *Abortion*, 115. Also see Kleegman, "Planned Parenthood."

181. A doctor might acknowledge its inevitability, as Guttmacher did at the PPFA conference, but that was not why exceptions were made. See Guttmacher in Calderone, *Abortion*, 167.

182. Schermer, "Abortion," 223; Packer and Gampell, "Therapeutic," 449.

183. Bellhouse et al. in Calderone, *Abortion*, 181–82.

184. For example, see Scherman, "Therapeutic," 333. Also see Solinger, "'Complete,'" 248–54.

185. R. E. Hall, "Non-Catholic," 80; Saxon, "Robert E. Hall."

186. Solinger, "'Complete,'" 248, 257–58.

187. Guttmacher, "Therapeutic."

188. Solinger, "'Complete,'" 242.

189. Esposito, *Immunitas*, 171.

190. Arendt, *Revolution*, 79–80.

191. Scherman, "Therapeutic," 333.

192. R. E. Hall, "Non-Catholic," 77.

193. Ibid., 80.

194. Ibid., 84.

195. "Model Penal Code Proposed Official Draft." See Gorney, *Articles*, 45–48, 56–59; Hull and Hoffer, *Roe v. Wade*, 97–99.

196. Guttmacher, "Abortion," 6.

197. Confidential memoranda on the code's development are replete with support from medical authorities, demonstrating that Taussig's research in particular was critical to the development of the code ("Article 207—Vol. 1"). The law mimicked medical reasoning and was conceived strictly as related to harm, not morality, in the case of medically authorized necessity ("Model Penal Code Council Draft No. 16"). Further, ALI committee members were influenced by fetal deformation from thalidomide (Louis B. Schwartz to Max Ascoli, December 17, 1962, ALIMPCC, box 2, folder 16).

198. Guttmacher, "Abortion," 6. Guttmacher was at the public unveiling in December, not at the final vote on the code in May.

199. Ibid., 7.

200. N. J. Davis, *From*, 65–87.

201. Ibid.

Conclusion

1. Esposito, *Immunitas*, 174.

2. Foucault, *History*, 95. For a discussion of the pregnant body as permeable and vulnerable, see Kukla, *Mass*, 10–19, 65–143.

3. Nietzsche, *Genealogy*, Second Essay, I.

4. It is possible to extend this approach to mnestic dynamism beyond abortion, certainly, and biopolitics as well, but I have discussed that elsewhere.

5. Allen, "Law," 210–11.

6. Carol Mason explores how protection for and from the unborn are paired in militant pro-life rhetoric (*Killing*, 72–98).

7. Cooke et al., *Terrible*, 35.

8. N. J. Davis argues, and I agree, that the abortion rights movement marked an ideological rupture from the previous centuries' abortion control models (*From*, 109–28). However, an ideological rupture, even one as stark as abortion rights, does not always accompany a fundamental rupture in the rhetoric.

9. I realized this reviewing Kelly E. Happe's book, *The Material Gene*. Her excellent book concludes with an argument for biosociality without genetics, but it strikes me that the larger problem is disease as a means of struggle within biopower, not specific knowledges that mobilize disease in the name of cultural conflict.

10. For an excellent discussion of different control models in relation to social problems, see N. J. Davis, *From*, 210–36.

11. Foucault, *Order*, xv. Foucault's use of Orientalist figures to talk about exoticism is well noted.

12. Foucault, "What Is," 42, 65, 45.

Bibliography

Abdullaeva, Mehribon. "Abortion Around the World—Overview." NOW Foundation, n.d. http://www.nowfoundation.org/issues/reproductive/050808_abortion_worldwide.html.

"Abortion: Translation of the Russian Law." Draft manuscript. 1936. Margaret Sanger Papers, Sophia Smith Collection, Smith College, MS 138, box 73, folder 1.

"Abortionists—Pacific Coast Abortion Ring 1834–56." Correspondence between Charles B. Pinkham, investigators, and prosecutors. American Medical Association Archives, Chicago, HHF, 0003–15.

Adams, Alice. *Reproducing the Womb: Images of Childbirth in Science, Feminist Theory, and Literature*. Ithaca: Cornell University Press, 1994.

Agamben, Giorgio. *Homo Sacer: Sovereign Power and Bare Life*. Translated by Daniel Heller-Roazen. Stanford: Stanford University Press, 1998.

———. *The Kingdom and the Glory: For a Theological Genealogy of Economy and Government ("Homo Sacer" II, 2.)* Translated by Lorenzo Chiesa. Stanford: Stanford University Press, 2011. Kindle edition.

———. *The Sacrament of Language: An Archaeology of the Oath*. Translated by Adam Kotsko. Stanford: Stanford University Press, 2011.

———. *State of Exception*. Translated by Kevin Attell. Chicago: University of Chicago Press, 2005.

Allen, Nathan. "Changes in New England Population." *Popular Science Monthly* 23 (1883): 433–44.

———. "Changes in the Population." *Harper's Magazine* 38 (1868–69): 386–92.

———. "The Law of Human Increase." *Quarterly Journal of Psychological Medicine and Medical Jurisprudence* 2, no. 2 (1868): 209–66.

———. *Population: Its Law of Increase*. Lowell, Mass.: Stone and Huse, 1870.

———. "Vital Statistics." *Congressional Quarterly* 5 (1877): 241–52.

Amen, John Harlan. "Some Obstacles to Effective Legal Control of Criminal Abortions." In National Committee, *Abortion*, 134–47.

Anonymous. "Criminal Abortion." *Boston Medical and Surgical Journal* 63 (1860): 66.

Arendt, Hannah. *The Human Condition*. With an introduction by Margaret Canovan. 2nd ed. Chicago: University of Chicago Press, 2008.

———. *On Revolution*. With an introduction by Jonathan Schell. New York: Penguin Books, 2006.

"Article 207—Vol. 1." Draft article with comments. January 16, 1956. American Law Institute Model Penal Code Collection, Biddle Law Library, University of Pennsylvania, box 8, folder 9.

Ashton, William Easterly. *A Text-Book on the Practice of Gynecology: For Practitioners and Students*. Philadelphia: W. B. Saunders, 1907.

Assmann, Jan. *Religion and Cultural Memory: Ten Studies*. Translated by Rodney Livingstone. Stanford: Stanford University Press, 2006.

Augustine. *Confessions*. Translated with an introduction by Henry Chadwick. New York: Oxford University Press, 1998. Kindle edition.

Ayres, J. C. "Therapeutic Abortion: Indication and Technique." *Journal of the Tennessee State Medical Association* 31, no. 2 (1938): 41–45.

Bacon, C. S. "The Duty of the Medical Profession in Relation to Criminal Abortion." *Illinois Medical Journal* 7 (1905): 18–24.

Barbat, J. Henry. "Criminal Abortion." *California State Journal of Medicine* 9, no. 2 (1911): 69–71.

Barno, Alex. "Criminal Abortion: Death and Suicides in Pregnancy in Minnesota, 1950–1964." *Minnesota Medicine* 50 (1967): 11–16.

Barthes, Roland. *Mythologies.* Translated by Annette Lavers. New York: Hill and Wang, 1972.

Bates, Jerome E., and Edward Z. Zawadzki. *Criminal Abortion: A Study in Medical Sociology.* Springfield, Ill.: Charles C. Thomas, 1964.

Battan, Jesse F. "'In the Marriage Bed Women's Sex Has Been Enslaved and Abused': Defining and Exposing Marital Rape in Late Nineteenth-Century America." In Smith, *Sex Without Consent,* 204–29.

Bauer, Theodore J. "Half a Century of International Control of the Venereal Diseases." *Public Health Reports* 68, no. 8 (1953): 779–87.

Becelaere, J. Van. "The Jurisprudence of Provoked Abortion." *Western Medical Times* 48, no. 2 (1928): 33–34.

Beck, Mildred B., Sidney H. Newman, and Sarah Lewit. "Abortion: A National Public and Mental Health Problem—Past, Present, and Proposed Research." *American Journal of Public Health* 59, no. 12 (1969): 2131–43.

Beckman, Oswald H. "Abortion, and Some Suggestions How to Lesson Criminal Abortion." *California State Journal of Medicine* 14, no. 11 (1916): 447–50.

Benhabib, Seyla. *Claims of Culture: Equality and Diversity in the Global Era.* Princeton: Princeton University Press, 2002.

Benjamin, Walter. *Illuminations: Essays and Reflections.* Edited with an introduction by Hannah Arendt. New York: Schocken Books, 1968.

Bennett, Elizabeth A. "Abortion." *Nursing Clinics of North America* 3, no. 2 (1968): 243–51.

Bennett, Jane. *Vibrant Matter: A Political Ecology of Things.* Durham: Duke University Press, 2010.

Berenson, Freida. "'Contraception': Its Present Status in Relation to Public Health." Unpublished manuscript. 1936. Women's Medical College, Allegheny University, Allegheny Special Collection on Women Physicians.

Berlant, Lauren. *The Female Complaint: The Unfinished Business of Sentimentality in American Culture.* Durham: Duke University Press, 2008.

———. "Slow Death (Sovereignty, Obesity, Lateral Agency)." *Critical Inquiry* 33 (2007): 754–80.

Bevacqua, Maria. *Rape on the Agenda: Feminism and the Politics of Sexual Assault.* Boston: Northeastern University Press, 2000.

Biesecker, Barbara. "Remembering World War II: The Rhetoric and Politics of National Commemoration at the Turn of the 21st Century." *Quarterly Journal of Speech* 88 (2002): 393–409.

———. "Rethinking the Rhetorical Situation from Within the Thematic of *Différance.*" *Philosophy and Rhetoric* 22, no. 2 (1989): 110–30.

Biesecker, Barbara A., and John Louis Lucaites, eds. *Rhetoric, Materiality, and Politics.* New York: Peter Lang, 2009.

Billings, John S. "The Diminishing Birth-Rate in the United States." *Forum* 15 (1893): 467–77.

Binion, Rudolph. "'More Men Than Corn': Malthus Versus the Enlightenment." *Eighteenth-Century Studies* 32 (1999): 564–69.

The Birth Control Movement. Pamphlet. 1917. Margaret Sanger Papers, Sophia Smith Collection, Smith College, MS 138, box 48, folder 12.

Bitzer, Lloyd F. "Rhetorical Situation." *Philosophy and Rhetoric* 1 (1968): 1–14.

Black, Algernon D. "Social, Moral, and Economic Causes and Control of Abortion." In National Committee, *Abortion,* 98–106.

Black, Edwin. "Secrecy and Disclosure as Rhetorical Forms." *Quarterly Journal of Speech* 74 (1988): 133–50.

Blair, Carole, and Neil Michel. "Reproducing Civil Rights Tactics: The Rhetorical Performances of the Civil Rights Memorial." *Rhetoric Society Quarterly* 30 (2000): 31–55.

Bobrow, M. Leo, and Stanley Friedman. "Burns of the Vagina and Cervix Following the Use of Potassium Permanganate." *New York State Journal of Medicine* 58 (1958): 527–29.

Boltanski, Luc. *Distant Suffering: Morality, Media, and Politics.* Translated by Graham Burchell. Cambridge, U.K.: Cambridge University Press, 1999.

Bordo, Susan. *Unbearable Weight: Feminism, Western Culture, and the Body.* Berkeley: University of California Press, 1993.

Bourdieu, Pierre. *Logic of Practice.* Translated by Richard Nice. Stanford: Stanford University Press, 1990.

Bratich, Jack. "Popular Secrecy and Occultural Studies." *Cultural Studies* 21 (2007): 42–58.

Brown, Wendy. *Regulating Aversion: Tolerance in the Age of Identity and Empire.* Princeton: Princeton University Press, 2006.

Browne, Stephen H. "Remembering Crispus Attucks: Race, Rhetoric, and the Politics of Commemoration." *Quarterly Journal of Speech* 85 (1999): 169–87.

Brownmiller, Susan. *Against Our Will: Men, Women, and Rape.* New York: Simon and Schuster, 1975.

Bruner, M. Lane. *Strategies of Remembrance: The Rhetorical Dimensions of National Identity Construction.* Columbia: University of South Carolina Press, 2002.

Brunner, Endre K. "The Outcome of 1556 Conceptions: A Medical and Sociology Study." *Human Biology* 13 (1941): 159–76.

Brunner, Endre K., and Louis Nelson. "Abortions in Relation to Viable Births in 10,069 Pregnancies: A Study Based on 4,500 Clinical Histories." *American Journal of Obstetrics and Gynecology* 38 (1939): 82–90.

Bullough, Vern L. "The Development of Sexology in the USA in the Early Twentieth Century." In *Sexual Knowledge, Sexual Science,* edited by Roy Porter and Mikuláš Teich, 303–22. Cambridge, U.K.: Cambridge University Press, 1994.

———. *Science in the Bedroom: A History of Sex Research.* New York: Basic Books, 1994.

Bundesen, Herman N. "Suggested Public Health Procedure for the Control of Abortions." In National Committee, *Abortion,* 155–62.

Burdett, Everett W. "The Medical Jurisprudence of Criminal Abortion." *New England Medical Gazette* 18 (1883): 200–214.

Burgess, Ernest. "Social and Economic Aspects of Abortion." In National Committee, *Abortion,* 115–32.

Burke, Kenneth. *Grammar of Motives.* Berkeley: University of California Press, 1969.

———. *Rhetoric of Motives.* Berkeley: University of California Press, 1969.

———. *The Rhetoric of Religion: Studies in Logology.* Berkeley: University of California Press, 1970.

Buxton, C. Lee. Review of *Abortion in the United States.* Mary Steichen Calderone Papers, Schlesinger Library, Radcliffe Institute for Advanced Study, Harvard University, call no. 179, box 3, folder 24.

Calderone, Mary Steichen, ed. *Abortion in the United States: A Conference Sponsored by the Planned Parenthood Foundation of America, Inc. at Arden House and the New York Academy of Medicine.* New York: Hoeber-Harper Book, 1958.

———. "Illegal Abortion as a Public Health Threat." *American Journal of Public Health* 50, no. 7 (1960): 948–54.

Calhoun, Ada. "The Rise of DIY Abortions: An Idaho Woman Could Change the Course of American Abortion Law." *New Republic,* December 21, 2012. http://www.newrepublic .com/article/politics/magazine/111368/the-rise-diy-abortions.

Campbell, George. *Philosophy of Rhetoric.* N.p.: FQ Legacy Books, 2010. Kindle edition.

Canguilhem, Georges. *The Normal and the Pathological.* Translated by Carolyn R. Fawcett in collaboration with Robert S. Cohen. Introduction by Michel Foucault. New York: Zone Books, 1991.

Carlyle, Thomas. *Chartism.* 1840. Reprint. N.p.: Evergreen Books, 2011. Kindle edition.

Carney, Bruce H. "Vaginal Burns from Potassium Permanganate." *American Journal of Obstetrics and Gynecology* 63 (1953): 127–30.

Carroll, W. S. "The Rights of the Unborn Child." *Pennsylvania Medical Journal* 13 (1909–10): 936–41.

Casey, Edward S. "Public Memory in Place and Time." In *Framing Public Memory,* edited by Kendall R. Phillips, 17–44. Tuscaloosa: University of Alabama Press, 2004.

———. *Remembering: A Phenomenological Study.* 2nd ed. Bloomington: Indiana University Press, 2000.

Casper, Monica J. *Making of the Unborn Patient: A Social Anatomy of Fetal Surgery.* New Brunswick: Rutgers University Press, 1998.

Chaput, Catherine. "Rhetorical Circulation in Late Capitalism: Neoliberalism and the Overdetermination of Affective Energy." *Philosophy and Rhetoric* 43, no. 1 (2010): 1–25.

Churchill, Frederick B. "The Rise of Classical Descriptive Embryology." In Gilbert, *Conceptual,* 1–29.

Collier, Stephen J., and Andrew Lakoff. "On Regimes of Living." In *Global Assemblages: Technology, Politics, and Ethics as Anthropological Problems,* edited by Aihwa Ong and Stephen J. Collier, 22–39. Malden, Mass.: Blackwell, 2005.

Collins, Clarkson T. "Diseases of Females." *Boston Medical and Surgical Journal* 47, no. 23 (1853): 475–80.

Colpitts, R. Vernon. "Trends in Therapeutic Abortion." *American Journal of Obstetrics and Gynecology* 68, no. 4 (1954): 988–97.

Committee on Maternal and Child Welfare. "Maternal and Child Welfare: Abortion." *Journal of the Maine Medical Association* 34 (1943): 72–74.

Committee on Maternal Health Biennial Report. 1928. Margaret Sanger Papers, Sophia Smith Collection, Smith College, MS 138, box 49, folder 5.

Condit, Celeste. *Decoding Abortion Rhetoric: Communicating Social Change.* Urbana: University of Illinois Press, 1990.

Connerton, Paul. *How Societies Remember.* Cambridge, U.K.: Cambridge University Press, 1989.

Cooke, Robert E., André E. Hellegers, Robert G. Hoyt, and Herbert W. Richardson, eds. *The Terrible Choice: The Abortion Dilemma.* Foreword by Pearl S. Buck. New York: Bantam, 1968.

Cooper, George M. "The Possibilities of a Statewide Program of Abortion Control." In National Committee, *Abortion,* 163–73.

Cornell, Drucilla. *The Imaginary Domain: Abortion, Pornography, and Sexual Harassment.* New York: Routledge, 1995.

Cosgrove, S. A., and Patricia A. Carter. "A Consideration of Therapeutic Abortion." *American Journal of Obstetrics and Gynecology* 48, no. 3 (1944): 299–314.

Cott, Nancy F. Afterword to Stoler, *Haunted*, 469–72.

Crutcher, Ernest. "A Philosophic Review of the Crowning Sin of Civilization." *Northwest Medicine* 1 (1903): 521–28.

Curtis, Bruce. *The Politics of Population: State Formation, Statistics, and the Census of Canada, 1840–1875*. Toronto: University of Toronto Press, 2002.

Cuthbert, M. F. "Discussion." *American Journal of Obstetrics* 38 (1898): 101–2.

Dabney. "Discussion." *New Orleans Medical and Surgical Journal* 57 (1907): 320.

Dakin, C. E. "Induced Abortion." *Journal of the Iowa State Medical Society* 6, no. 2 (1916): 65–68.

D'Amour, Fred E., and Nathan Kiven. "Harmful Effects of Certain Chemical Substances upon the Uterus of a Rat." *American Journal of Obstetrics and Gynecology* 29 (1935): 503–9.

Davis, M. Edward. "Review." *Science* 129, no. 3339 (1959): 36. Mary Steichen Calderone Papers, Schlesinger Library, Radcliffe Institute for Advanced Study, Harvard University, call no. 179, box 3, folder 24.

Davis, Maxine. *Women's Medical Problems*. New York: McGraw-Hill, 1945.

Davis, Nanette J. *From Crime to Choice: The Transformation of Abortion in America*. Westport, Conn.: Greenwood Press, 1985.

Dean, Jodi. *Publicity's Secret: How Technoculture Capitalizes on Democracy*. Ithaca: Cornell University Press, 2002.

de Certeau, Michel. *The Capture of Speech and Other Political Writings*. Translated by Tom Conley. With an introduction by Luce Giard. Minneapolis: University of Minnesota Press, 1997.

———. *The Practice of Everyday Life*. Translated by Steven Randall. Berkeley: University of California Press, 1984. Kindle edition.

Deem, Melissa. "Stranger Sociability, Public Hope, and the Limits of Political Transformation." *Quarterly Journal of Speech* 88 (2002): 444–54.

Degler, Carl. *At Odds: Women and the Family in America from the Revolution to the Present*. Oxford: Oxford University Press, 1980.

Dekker, Herman. "Is Abortion Becoming Ethical?" *Medical Life: A Journal of Contemporary and Historical Medicine* 27, no. 11 (1920): 193–201.

Deleuze, Gilles. *Bergsonism*. Translated by Hugh Tomlinson and Barbara Habberjam. New York: Zone Books, 1988.

———. *The Fold: Leibniz and the Baroque*. Translated with a foreword by Tom Conley. Minneapolis: University of Minnesota Press, 1993.

Deleuze, Gilles, and Félix Guattari. *A Thousand Plateaus: Capitalism and Schizophrenia*. Translated with a foreword by Brian Massumi. Minneapolis: University of Minnesota Press, 1987.

Deluca, Kevin Michael. *Image Politics: The New Rhetoric of Environmental Activism*. New York: Guilford Press, 1999.

Derrida, Jacques. *Archive Fever: A Freudian Impression*. Translated by Eric Prenowitz. Chicago: University of Chicago Press, 1995.

———. *Dissemination*. Translated by Barbara Johnson. Chicago: University of Chicago Press, 1981.

———. *Truth in Painting*. Translated by Geoff Bennington and Ian McLeod. Chicago: University of Chicago Press, 1987.

Deutscher, Penelope. "Foucault's *History of Sexuality, Volume I*: Re-reading Its Reproduction." *Theory, Culture, Society* 29 (2012): 119–37.
———. "The Inversion of Exceptionality: Foucault, Agamben, and 'Reproductive Rights.'" *South Atlantic Quarterly* 107 (2008): 55–70.
Devereux, George. "A Typological Study of Abortion in 350 Primitive, Ancient, and Preindustrial Societies." In Rosen, *Therapeutic Abortion*, 97–152.
Dibrell. "Discussion." In *Transactions of the Arkansas Medical Society, 28th Annual Session, Jonesboro, Arkansas, April 30, May 1–2, 1903*, 272–73. Little Rock, Ark.: Thompson Litho. and Printing, 1904.
Dickinson, Robert L. "Discussion." Discussion of Frederick J. Taussig's "Effects of Abortion on the General Health and Reproductive Function of the Individual." In National Committee, *Abortion*, 39–57.
———. Foreword to *Abortion, Spontaneous and Induced: Medical and Social Aspects*, by Frederick J. Taussig, 7–9. St. Louis, Mo.: C. V. Mosby, 1936.
———. Foreword to *Medical History of Contraception*, by Norman E. Himes, xxxi–xxxii. New York: Gamut Press, 1963.
———. "Mailability of Medical Literature on Therapeutic Abortion and Contraception." *New York State Medical Journal* 29, no. 16 (1929): 1019.
———. "Relation of Committee on Maternal Health to the Sanger Birth Control Clinic." Memorandum. March 17, 1924. National Committee on Maternal Health Collection, Countway Library of Medicine, Harvard University, BMS c78, box 1, folder 22.
Dillon, Michael, and Julian Reid. *The Liberal Way of War: Killing to Make Life Live*. New York: Routledge, 2009.
Dixon-Jones, Mary A. "Criminal Abortion: Its Evil and Its Sad Consequences." *Medical Record* 46 (1894): 9–16.
Dolan, Brian, ed. *Malthus, Medicine, and Morality: "Malthusianism" After 1798*. Amsterdam: Editions Rodopi B. V., 2000.
Donnelly, Joseph P. "Are There Medical Indicators for Therapeutic Abortions?" *Journal of the Medical Society of New Jersey* 52, no. 3 (1955): 112–18.
Dorsett, Walter B. "Criminal Abortion in Its Broadest Sense." *Journal of the American Medical Association* 51 (1908): 957–61.
Downie, Regina M. "An Interpretation of Vital Statistics in Relation to Birth Control and Abortion." In *Transactions of the Sixty-Fourth Annual Meeting of the Alumnae Association of the Women's Medical College of Pennsylvania*, 26–31. Philadelphia: Alumnae Association of the Women's Medical College of Pennsylvania, 1939.
duBois, Page. *Torture and Truth: The New Ancient World*. New York: Routledge, 1991.
Dubos, René, and Jean Dubos. *The White Plague: Tuberculosis, Man, and Society*. Foreword by David Mechanic. Introduction by Barbara Gutman Rosenkrantz. New Brunswick: Rutgers University Press, 1987.
Dubow, Sara. *Ourselves Unborn: A History of the Fetus in Modern America*. New York: Oxford University Press, 2011. Kindle edition.
Duden, Barbara. *Disembodying Women: Perspectives on Pregnancy and the Unborn*. Translated by Lee Hoinacki. Cambridge, Mass.: Harvard University Press, 1994.
Dunn, Halbert L. "Frequency of Abortion: Its Effect on Maternal Mortality Rates." In National Committee, *Abortion*, 1–14.
Dyer, Frederick N. *Champion of Women and the Unborn: Horatio Robinson Storer, M.D.* Canton, Mass.: Science History, 1999.
Elias, Norbert. *The Civilizing Process: The History of Manners and State Formation and Civilization*. Translated by Edmund Jephcott. Oxford: Blackwell, 1994.

Eliasberg, W. G. "The Prenatal Psychotic Patient." In Rosen, *Therapeutic Abortion*, 213–18. New York: Julian Press, 1954.

———. "Psychiatry in Prenatal Care and the Problem of Abortion." *Medical Woman's Journal*, January–February 1951, 27–30.

Ely, William B. "The Ethics of Criminal Abortion." *Western Medical Review* 17 (1905): 97–102.

Esposito, Roberto. *Bios: Biopolitics and Philosophy*. Translated with an introduction by Timothy Campbell. Minneapolis: University of Minnesota Press, 2008.

———. *Immunitas: The Protection and Negation of Life*. Translated by Zakiya Hanafi. Cambridge, U.K.: Polity Press, 2011.

Farrell Brodie, Janet. *Contraception and Abortion in Nineteenth-Century America*. Ithaca: Cornell University Press, 1994.

"Fear Makes the Pro-abortionists Say the Most Outrageous Things." *National Right to Life News*, Spring 2012. http://www.nrlc.org/archive/news/2012/201202/Fear.pdf.

Ferguson, Robert Thrift. "Abortion and Abortionists." *Southern Medicine and Surgery* 93 (1931): 889–92.

Fernald, W. J. "A Sociological View of Criminal Abortion." *Illinois Medical Journal* 5, no. 2 (1903): 57–64.

Field, Mark G. "The Re-legalization of Abortion in Soviet Russia." *New England Journal of Medicine* 255, no. 9 (1956): 421–27.

Findley, Palmer. "The Slaughter of Innocents." *American Journal of Obstetrics and Gynecology* 3 (1922): 35–37.

Finn, Lisa. "Risky Subjects: Constructions and Categorizations of Women in Health Care." Ph.D. diss., University of Rochester, 2004.

Fish, E. F. "Criminal Abortion." *Milwaukee Medical Journal* 17 (1909): 106–9.

Fisher, Russell S. "Criminal Abortion." *Journal of Criminal Law and Criminology* 42, no. 2 (1951): 242–49.

Foley, Megan. "Peri Ti? Interrogating Rhetoric's Domain." *Philosophy and Rhetoric* 46 (2013): 241–46.

Foucault, Michel. *Archaeology of Knowledge and The Discourse on Language*. Translated by A. M. Sheridan Smith. New York: Pantheon, 1972.

———. *The Birth of Biopolitics: Lectures at the Collège de France, 1978–1979*. Edited by Michel Senellart. Translated by Graham Burchell. New York: Palgrave-Macmillan, 2008.

———. *The Birth of the Clinic: An Archaeology of Medical Perception*. Translated by A. M. Sheridan Smith. New York: Vintage, 1994.

———. "Governmentality." In *Power*, edited by James D. Faubion, translated by Robert Hurley and others, 201–22. Vol. 3 of *Essential Works of Michel Foucault, 1954–1984*. New York: New Press, 1994.

———. *The Hermeneutics of the Subject: Lectures at the College de France, 1981–1982*. Edited by Frédéric Gros. Translated by Graham Burchell. New York: Palgrave-Macmillan, 2005.

———. *The History of Sexuality*. Vol. 1, *An Introduction*. Translated by Robert Hurley. New York: Vintage, 1978.

———. "Nietzsche, Genealogy, History." In *Language, Counter-memory, Practice: Selected Essays and Interviews by Michel Foucault*, edited by Donald F. Bouchard, translated by Donald F. Bouchard and Sherry Simon, 139–64. Ithaca: Cornell University Press, 1977.

———. "On the Genealogy of Ethics: An Overview of Work in Progress." In Hubert L. Dreyfus and Paul Rabinow, *Michel Foucault: Beyond Structuralism and Hermeneutics*, 2nd ed., 229–52. Chicago: University of Chicago Press, 1983.

————. *The Order of Things: An Archaeology of the Human Sciences.* New York: Vintage, 1994.

————. *Power/Knowledge: Selected Interviews and Other Writings, 1972–1977.* Edited by Colin Gordon. Translated by Colin Gordon, Leo Marshall, John Mepham, and Kate Soper. New York: Pantheon, 1980.

————. *Security, Territory, Population: Lectures at the Collège de France, 1977–1978.* Edited by Michel Senellart, François Ewald, Alessandro Fontana, and Arnold I. Davidson. Translated by Graham Burchell. New York: Palgrave-Macmillan, 2007.

————. *"Society Must Be Defended": Lectures at the Collège de France, 1975–1976.* Edited by Michel Senellart, François Ewald, Alessandro Fontana, and Arnold I. Davidson. Translated by David Macey. New York: Picador, 2003.

————. "What Is Critique?" In *The Politics of Truth,* edited by Sylvère Lotringer, translated by Lysa Hochroth and Catherine Porter, 41–81. With an introduction by John Rajchman. Los Angeles: Semiotext(e), 2007.

Fox, Leon Parrish. "Abortion Deaths in California." *American Journal of Obstetrics and Gynecology* 98, no. 5 (1967): 645–53.

Fox Keller, Evelyn. *Secrets of Life, Secrets of Death: Essays on Language, Gender, and Science.* New York: Routledge, 1992.

Frackman, H. David. "The Present Practice of Contraception and Abortion." *American Medicine* 41, no. 3 [n.s., 30, no. 3] (1935): 162–63.

Franklin, Sarah. "Stem Cells R Us: Emergent Life Forms and the Global Biological." In *Global Assemblages: Technology, Politics, and Ethics as Anthropological Problems,* edited by Aihwa Ong and Stephen J. Collier, 59–78. Malden, Mass.: Blackwell, 2005.

Freudenberg, K. "Frequency of Abortion Deaths." *München Medizin Wochenschr* 79 (1932): 758.

Fried, Marlene Gerber. "Abortion in the United States—Legal but Inaccessible." In *Abortion Wars: A Half-Century of Struggle, 1950–2000,* edited by Rickie Solinger, 208–26. Berkeley: University of California Press, 1998.

Friedman, George Alexander. "Abortion and the Law." *Medical Times* 84, no. 6 (1956): 658–66.

Funkhouser, H. Gray. "Historical Development of the Graphical Representation of Statistical Data." *Osiris* 3 (1937): 269–404.

Galbraith, Anna M. "Are the Dangers of the Menopause Natural or Acquired? A Physiological Study." In *Transactions of the Twenty-Fourth Annual Meeting of the Alumnæ Association of the Woman's Medical College of Pennsylvania,* 39–64. Philadelphia: Alumnæ Association of the Woman's Medical College of Pennsylvania, 1899.

Gallagher, Catherine. *The Body Economic: Life, Death, and Sensation in Political Economy and the Victorian Novel.* Princeton: Princeton University Press, 2006.

Gampell, Ralph J. "Legal Status of Therapeutic Abortion and Sterilization in the United States." *Clinical Obstetrics and Gynecology* 7 (1964): 22–24.

Garber, Marjorie. "Compassion." In *Compassion: The Culture and Politics of an Emotion,* edited by Lauren Berlant, 15–27. New York: Routledge, 2004.

Gathorne-Hardy, Jonathan. *Sex the Measure of All Things: A Life of Alfred C. Kinsey.* Bloomington: Indiana University Press, 1998.

Gebhard, Paul H., Wardell B. Pomeroy, Clyde E. Martin, and Cornelia V. Christenson. *Pregnancy, Birth, and Abortion.* New York: Harper and Bros., 1958.

Ghent, H. C. "Criminal Abortion or Foeticide, and the Prevention of Conception." *Texas Courier-Record of Medicine* 23, no. 5 (1906): 1–16.

————. "Criminal Abortion or Foeticide, and the Prevention of Conception." *Texas Courier-Record of Medicine* 23, no. 6 (1906): 1–10.

Gigerenzer, Gerd, Zeno Swijtink, Theodore Porter, Lorraine Daston, John Beatty, and Lorenz Krüger. *The Empire of Chance: How Probability Changed Science and Everyday Life*. Cambridge, U.K.: Cambridge University Press, 1989.

Gilbert, Scott F., ed. *A Conceptual History of Modern Embryology*. Baltimore: Johns Hopkins University Press, 1991.

Gilman Srebnick, Amy. *The Mysterious Death of Mary Rogers: Sex and Culture in Nineteenth-Century New York*. New York: Oxford University Press, 1995.

Gleason, Rachel. *Talks to My Patients: Hints on Getting Well and Keeping Well*. New York: M. L. Holbrook, 1895.

Gold, Edwin M., Carl L. Erhardt, Harold Jacobziner, and Frieda G. Nelson. "Therapeutic Abortions in New York City: A 20-Year Review." *American Journal of Public Health* 55 (1965): 964–72.

Gold, Rachel Benson, and Elizabeth Nash. "Troubling Trend: More States Hostile to Abortion Rights as Middle Ground Shrinks." *Guttmacher Policy Review* 15, no. 1 (2012). http://www.guttmacher.org/pubs/gpr/15/1/gpr150114.html.

Goldman, Hal. "'A Most Detestable Crime': Character, Consent, and Corroboration in Vermont's Rape Law, 1650–1920." In Smith, *Sex Without Consent*, 178–203.

Goodell, William. "Introductory." In *Clinical Gynæcology: Medical and Surgical for Students and Practitioners*, edited by John M. Keating and Henry C. Coe, 1–25. Philadelphia: J. B. Lippincott, 1895.

Goodno, John A., Irvin M. Cushner, and Paul E. Molumphy. "Management of Infected Abortion: An Analysis of 342 Cases." *American Journal of Obstetrics and Gynecology* 85, no. 1 (1963): 16–23.

Gordon, Linda. *The Moral Property of Women: A History of Birth Control Politics in America*. Urbana: University of Illinois Press, 2007.

———. *Pitied but Not Entitled: Single Mothers and the History of Welfare*. New York: Free Press, 1994.

———. "Teenage Pregnancy and Out-of-Wedlock Birth: Morals, Moralism, Experts." In *Morality and Health*, edited by Allan M. Brandt and Paul Rozin, 251–70. New York: Routledge, 1997.

Gorney, Cynthia. *Articles of Faith: A Frontline History of the Abortion Wars*. New York: Simon and Schuster, 1998.

Goss, Stanley J., William G. Slate, and Richard H. Paul. "Induced Abortion: Clinical and Laboratory Evaluation." *Pacific Medicine and Surgery* 73 (1965): 325–30.

Gould, Stephen Jay. *The Mismeasure of Man*. Rev. and exp. ed. New York: W. W. Norton, 1996.

———. *Ontogeny and Phylogeny*. Cambridge, Mass.: Harvard University Press, 1977.

Govier, Trudy. "Forgiveness and the Unforgivable." *American Philosophical Quarterly* 36 (1999): 59–75.

Graham, Harvey. *Eternal Eve: The History of Gynecology and Obstetrics*. Garden City, N.Y.: Doubleday, 1951.

Grant, John M. "Criminal Abortion." *Interstate Medical Journal* 13 (1906): 513–18.

Greeley, Arthur V. "Abortion: Pathology, Prevention, Treatment." *Journal of the Medical Society of New Jersey* 57, no. 1 (1960): 26–31.

Green, Frank K. "Feticide." *American Medicine* 20 (1914): 590–94.

Greene, Ronald Walter. "Another Materialist Rhetoric." *Critical Studies in Mass Communication* 15 (1998): 21–41.

———. *Malthusian Worlds: U.S. Leadership and the Governing of the Population Crisis*. Boulder: Westview Press, 1999.

———. "Rhetorical Materialism: The Rhetorical Subject and the General Intellect." In Biesecker and Lucaites, *Rhetoric*, 43–65.

———. "Rhetorical Pedagogy as a Postal System: Circulating Subjects Through Michael Warner's 'Publics and Counterpublics.'" *Quarterly Journal of Speech* 88, no. 4 (2002): 434–43.

Greenhill, J. P. *Obstetrics.* 11th ed. Philadelphia: W. B. Saunders, 1955.

Greenley, T. D. "Is the Practice of Producing Abortion Common Among Medical Men?" *Louisville Monthly Journal of Medicine and Surgery* 11, no. 6 (1904): 184–86.

Grossman, Daniel, Kelsey Holt, Melanie Peña, Diana Lara, Maggie Veatch, Denisse Córdova, Marji Gold, Beverly Winikoff, and Kelly Blanchard. "Self-Induction of Abortion Among Women in the United States." *Reproductive Health Matters* 18, no. 36 (2010): 136–46.

Grosz, Elizabeth. *Volatile Bodies: Toward a Corporeal Feminism.* Bloomington: University of Indiana Press, 1994.

Guttmacher, Alan F. "Abortion: Odyssey of an Attitude." *Family Planning Perspectives* 4, no. 4 (1972): 5–7.

———. "The Psychiatric and Socio-psychiatric Indications for Abortion." Panel discussion. May 3, 1956. Alan Guttmacher Papers, Countway Library of Medicine, Harvard University, HMS c155, box 9, folder 27.

———. "The Shrinking Non-psychiatric Indications for Therapeutic Abortion." In Rosen, *Therapeutic Abortion*, 12–21.

———. "Social Problems of Gynecology and Obstetrics." *West Virginia Medical Journal* 39 (1943): 300–306.

———. Testimony Before Subcommittee on Criminal Laws and Procedures of the U.S. Senate Committee on the Judiciary. May 3, 1973. Alan Guttmacher Papers, Countway Library of Medicine, Harvard University, HMS c155, box 10, folder 56.

———. "Therapeutic Abortion: The Doctor's Dilemma." *Journal of the Mt. Sinai Hospital of New York* 21, no. 3 (1954): 111–21.

———. "The United States Medical Profession and Family Planning." In *Family Planning and Population Programs: A Review of World Developments*, edited by Bernard Berelson, Richmond K. Anderson, Oscar Harkavy, John Maier, W. Parker Mauldin, and Sheldon J. Segal, 455–63. Chicago: University of Chicago Press, 1966.

Hacking, Ian. *The Taming of Chance.* New York: Cambridge University Press, 1990.

Halbwachs, Maurice. *On Collective Memory.* Translated and edited by Lewis A. Coser. Chicago: University of Chicago Press, 1992.

Hale, Edwin M. *The Great Crime of the Nineteenth Century. Why Is It Committed? Who Are the Criminals? How Shall They Be Detected? How Shall They Be Punished?* Chicago: C. S. Halsey, 1867.

———. *A Systematic Treatise on Abortion.* Chicago: C. S. Halsey, 1866.

Hall, E. A. "Discussion." *Northwest Medicine* 5 (1907): 311.

Hall, Lesley A. "Malthusian Mutations: The Changing Politics and Moral Meanings of Birth Control in Britain." In Dolan, *Malthus, Medicine, and Morality*, 141–63.

Hall, Robert E. "Abortion: A Non-Catholic View." In *Ethical Issues in Medicine: The Role of the Physician in Today's Society*, edited by E. Fuller Torrey, 75–85. Boston: Little, Brown, 1968.

———. "Abortion in American Hospitals." *American Journal of Public Health* 57, no. 11 (1967): 1933–36.

Hamilton, Virginia. "Some Sociologic and Psychologic Observations on Abortion: A Study of 527 Cases." *American Journal of Obstetrics and Gynecology* 39, no. 6 (1940): 919–28.

Hamlin, Christopher, and Kathleen Gallagher-Kamper. "Malthus and the Doctors: Political Economy, Medicine, and the State in England, Ireland, and Scotland, 1800–1840." In Dolan, *Malthus, Medicine, and Morality*, 115–40.

Hammett, O. H. Letter to the editor. *American Journal of Clinical Medicine*, 1910, 772–73.

Happe, Kelly E. *The Material Gene: Gender, Race, and Heredity After the Human Genome Project*. New York: New York University Press, 2013.

Haraway, Donna Jeanne. *Crystals, Fabrics, and Fields: Metaphors That Shape Embryos*. Berkeley, Calif.: North Atlantic Books, 2004.

———. *Primate Visions: Gender, Race, and Nature in the World of Modern Science*. New York: Routledge, 1989.

———. *Simians, Cyborgs, and Women: The Reinvention of Nature*. New York: Routledge, 1991.

Harter, Carl L., and Joseph D. Beasley. "A Survey Concerning Induced Abortion in New Orleans." *American Journal of Public Health* 57, no. 11 (1967): 1937–47.

Hartmann, Betsy. *Reproductive Rights and Wrongs: The Global Politics of Population Control*. Rev. ed. Boston: South End Press, 1995.

Hasian, Marouf Arif, Jr. *Rhetorical Vectors of Memory in National and International Holocaust Trials*. East Lansing: Michigan State University Press, 2006.

———. *The Rhetoric of Eugenics in Anglo-American Thought*. Athens: University of Georgia Press, 1996.

Hawhee, Deborah, and Christina J. Olson. "Pan-historiography: The Challenge of Writing History Across Time and Space." In *Theorizing Histories of Rhetoric*, edited by Michelle Ballif, 90–105. Carbondale: Southern Illinois University Press, 2013.

Hawkins, G. M. "The Abortion Problem—the Sociologic Side." *American Journal of Clinical Medicine*, 1910, 769–73.

Hecht, Jacqueline. "'Be Fruitful and Multiply' to Family Planning: The Enlightenment Transition." *Eighteenth-Century Studies* 32 (1999): 536–51.

Hefferman, Roy J., and William A. Lynch. "What Is the Status of Therapeutic Abortion in Modern Obstetrics?" *American Journal of Obstetrics and Gynecology* 66 (1953): 335–45.

Heiermann, F. "Ethical and Religious Objections to Criminal Abortion." *Toledo Medical and Surgical Reporter* 31, no. 4 (1905): 233–36.

Hershey, Nathan. "As Society's View Change, Law Changes." *American Journal of Nursing* 67, no. 11 (1967): 2310–12.

Higham, John. *Strangers in the Land: Patterns of Nativism, 1860–1925*. New Brunswick: Rutgers University Press, 1962. Kindle edition.

Hillis, David S. "Experience with One Thousand Cases of Abortion." *Surgery, Gynecology and Obstetrics* 38 (1924): 83–87.

Hodann, Max. "The New Birth Control and Abortion Law in Iceland." *Marriage Hygiene* 3, no. 2 (1936): 180–84.

Hodes, Martha. "Fractions and Fictions in the United States Census of 1890." In Stoler, *Haunted*, 240–70.

Hodge, Hugh L. "Foeticide, or Criminal Abortion: A Lecture Introductory to the Course on Obstetrics and Disease of Women and Children." *American Journal of the Medical Sciences* 59, no. 117 (1870): 223–24.

———. *On Criminal Abortion*. Philadelphia: T. K. and P. G. Collins, 1854.

———. *Principles and Practice of Obstetrics*. Philadelphia: Blanchard and Lea, 1864.

Hodgson, Dennis. "The Ideological Origins of the Population Association of America." *Population and Development Review* 17, no. 1 (1991): 1–34.

Hoitt, E. G. "Criminal Abortion." *Boston Medical and Surgical Journal* 135 (1896): 541–43.

Holmes, John Haynes, Rose Pastor Stokes, Helen Campbell, and Joseph Lorren. "'Why Race-Suicide with Advancing Civilization?' A Symposium." *Arena* 41 (1909): 189–96.

Holmes, Rudolph W. "Discussion." In "Statistical Analysis of One Thousand Abortions," by Jalmar H. Simons. *American Journal of Obstetrics and Gynecology* 37 (1939): 840–49.

Holmes, Rudolph Weiner. "Criminal Abortion: A Brief Consideration of Its Relation to Newspaper Advertising; A Report of a Medico-legal Case." *Illinois Medical Journal* 7 (1905): 29–34.

Holmgren, Margaret. *Forgiveness and Retribution: Responding to Wrongdoing.* New York: Cambridge University Press, 2012.

Hood, Mary G. *For Girls and the Mothers of Girls: A Book for the Home and the School Concerning the Beginnings of Life.* Indianapolis: Bobbs-Merrill, 1914.

Hopwood, Nick. "A History of Normal Plates, Tables, and Stages in Vertebrate Embryology." *International Journal of Developmental Biology* 51 (2007): 1–26.

———. "Producing Development: The Anatomy of Human Embryos and the Norms of Wilhelm His." *Bulletin of the History of Medicine* 74, no. 1 (2000): 29–79.

———. "Visual Standards and Disciplinary Change: Normal Plates, Tables, and Stages in Embryology." *History of Science* 43, pt. 3, no. 141 (2005): 239–303.

Hubbard, S. Dana. "Abortion in New York City." *Monthly Bulletin of the Department of Health of the City of New York* 8, no. 9 (1918): 207–10.

"Hugh L. (Hugh Lenox) Hodge (1796–1873)." University of Pennsylvania Archives and Records Center. http://www.archives.upenn.edu/people/1700s/hodge_hugh_1.html.

Hull, N. E. H., and Peter Charles Hoffer. *Roe v. Wade: The Abortion Rights Controversy in American History.* 2nd ed. Lawrence: University Press of Kansas, 2010.

Hurley, T. W. "The Prevention of Conception—Abortions, Justifiable and Criminal." In *Transactions of the Arkansas Medical Society, 28th Annual Session, Jonesboro, Arkansas, April 30, May 1–2, 1903.* Little Rock, Ark.: Thompson Litho. and Printing, 1904.

Igo, Sarah E. *The Averaged American: Surveys, Citizens, and the Making of a Mass Public.* Cambridge, Mass.: Harvard University Press, 2008.

Imber, Michael. "The First World War, Sex Education, and the American Social Hygiene Association's Campaign Against Venereal Disease." *Journal of Educational Administration and History* 16, no. 1 (1984): 47–56.

Irwin-Zarecka, Iwona. *Frames of Remembrance: The Dynamics of Collective Memory.* New Brunswick, N.J.: Transaction, 1994.

Jacobi, Abraham. "The Best Means of Combating Infant Mortality." *Journal of the American Medical Association* 58, no. 23 (1912): 1735–44.

Jacobi, L. "Infanticide, Abortion, and Prevention of Conception." *Medico-pharmaceutical Critic and Guide* 15, no. 12 (1912): 451–64.

Jacobson, Matthew Frye. *Barbarian Virtues: The United States Encounters Foreign Peoples at Home and Abroad, 1876–1917.* New York: Hill and Wang, 2000.

Janovski, Nikloas A., Louis Wiener, and William B. Ober. "Soap Intoxication Following Criminal Abortion." *New York State Journal of Medicine* 63 (1963): 1461–87.

Jenkins, Richard L. "The Significance of Maternal Rejection of Pregnancy for the Future Development of the Child." In Rosen, *Therapeutic Abortion,* 269–75.

Jensen, Robin E. *Dirty Words: The Rhetoric of Public Sex Education, 1870–1924.* Urbana: University of Illinois Press, 2010.

Jesse, R. W., and Frederick J. Spencer. "Abortion—the Hidden Epidemic." *Virginia Medical Monthly* 95 (1968): 447–56.

Jetter, Walter W., and Francis T. Hunter. "Death from Attempted Abortion with a Potassium Permanganate Douche." *New England Journal of Medicine* 240 (1949): 794–98.

Joffe, Carole. *Doctors of Conscience: The Struggle to Provide Abortion Before and After "Roe v. Wade."* Boston: Beacon Press, 1995.

Johnson, Joseph Taber. "Abortion and Its Effects." *American Journal of Obstetrics* 33 (1896): 86–97.

Jones, James H. *Alfred C. Kinsey: A Public/Private Life.* New York: W. W. Norton, 1997.

Jones, Rachel K., and Jenna Jerman. "Abortion Incidence and Service Availability in the United States, 2011." *Perspectives on Sexual and Reproductive Health* 46, no. 1 (2014). http://www.guttmacher.org/pubs/journals/psrh.46e0414.pdf.

Jones, William H. *On the Management of Labour in Contracted Pelvis.* London: Robert Hardwicke, 1767.

Kaplan, Laura. *The Story of Jane: The Legendary Underground Feminist Abortion Service.* Chicago: University of Chicago Press, 1995.

Keemer, Edward. *Confessions of a Prolife Abortionist.* Detroit: Velco Press, 1980.

Kerényi, Karl. "Mnemosyne—Lesmosyne: On the Spring of 'Memory' and 'Forgetting.'" Translated by Magda Kerényi. *Spring: An Annual of Psychology and Jungian Thought,* 1977, 120–30.

Kevles, Daniel J. *In the Name of Eugenics: Genetics and the Uses of Human Heredity.* New ed. Cambridge, Mass.: Harvard University Press, 1995.

Kisch, E. Heinrich. *The Sexual Life of Woman in Its Physiological and Hygienic Aspect.* New York: Allied, 1966.

Kleegman, Sophia. "Planned Parenthood: The Influence of Public Health and Family Welfare." In Rosen, *Therapeutic Abortion,* 254–65.

Konikow, Antoinette F. *Physician's Manual of Birth Control.* New York: Buchholz, 1931.

Kopp, Marie. *Birth Control in Practice: Analysis of 10,000 Case Histories of the Birth Control Clinical Research Bureau.* New York: Robert M. McBride, 1934.

Korentzwitt, Edith. "The Modern Aspects of Birth Control." Unpublished paper. 1939. Allegheny Special Collection on Women Physicians, Women's Medical College, Allegheny University.

Kosmak, George M. "Introductory Remarks." In National Committee, *Abortion,* 133.

Kross, Anna. "The Abortion Problem Seen in Criminal Courts." In National Committee, *Abortion,* 107–14.

———. "Discussion." Discussion of John Harlan Amen's "Some Obstacles to Effective Legal Control of Criminal Abortions." In National Committee, *Abortion,* 134–47.

Kukla, Rebecca. *Mass Hysteria: Medicine, Culture, and Mothers' Bodies.* Lanham, Md.: Rowman and Littlefield, 2005.

Kummer, Jerome M. "Post-abortion Psychiatric Illness—a Myth." *American Journal of Psychiatry* 119 (1963): 980–83.

———. "Therapeutic Abortion Law Confusion." *Journal of the American Medical Association* 195, no. 2 (1966): 140–44.

Kummer, Jerome M., and Zad Leavy. "Criminal Abortion: A Consideration of Ways to Reduce Incidence." *California Medicine* 95, no. 3 (1961): 170–75.

Kunzel, Regina G. *Fallen Women, Problem Girls: Unmarried Mothers and the Professionalization of Social Work, 1890–1945.* New Haven: Yale University Press, 1993.

Laclau, Ernesto. *On Populist Reason.* London: Verso, 2007.

Ladova, Rosalie M. "Discussion." *Illinois Medical Journal* 7 (1905): 40–44.

Lake, Randall A. "The Metaethical Framework of Anti-abortion Rhetoric." *Signs: Journal of Women in Culture and Society* 11, no. 3 (1986): 478–99.

Lanham, Richard A. *A Handlist of Rhetorical Terms.* 2nd ed. Berkeley: University of California Press, 1991.

Laqueur, Thomas. "Mourning, Pity, and the Work of Narrative in the Making of 'Humanity.'" In *Humanitarianism and Suffering: The Mobilization of Empathy*, edited by Richard Ashby Wilson and Richard D. Brown, 31–57. New York: Cambridge University Press, 2009.

Latour, Bruno. *An Inquiry into Mode of Existence*. Translated by Catherine Porter. Cambridge, Mass.: Harvard University Press, 2013.

———. *The Pasteurization of France*. Translated by Alan Sheridan and John Law. Cambridge, Mass.: Harvard University Press, 1988.

———. *Politics of Nature*. Translated by Catherine Porter. Cambridge, Mass.: Harvard University Press, 2004.

LeBeuf, Louis G. "The Attitude of the Medical Profession Towards Race Suicide and Criminal Abortion." *New Orleans Medical and Surgical Journal* 57 (1904): 3–18.

Le Goff, Jacques. *History and Memory*. Translated by Steven Rendall and Elizabeth Claman. New York: Columbia University Press, 1992.

Lewis, Denslow. "Clinical Lecture on Obstetrics and Gynecology—Sociological Considerations Relative to Criminal Abortion, Infanticide and Illegitimate Pregnancy." *Chicago Clinical Review* 5 (1895): 85–96.

Lidz, Theodore. "Reflections of a Psychiatrist." In Rosen, *Therapeutic Abortion*, 276–83.

Lindquist Dorr, Lisa. "'Another Negro-Did-It Crime': Black-on-White Rape and Protest in Virginia, 1945–1960." In Smith, *Sex Without Consent*, 247–64.

Lockridge, Patricia. "Woman's Home Companion: Paper on Abortion." January 12, 1947. National Committee on Maternal Health Collection, Countway Library of Medicine, Harvard University, BMS c78, box 17, folder 559.

Louis-Fischer, Jean. "Laurent Chabry and the Beginnings of Experimental Embryology in France." In Gilbert, *Conceptual*, 31–41.

Love, Minnie C. T. "Criminal Abortion." *Colorado Medicine* 1 (1903): 55–60.

Lovett, Laura L. *Conceiving the Future: Pronatalism, Reproduction, and the Family in the United States, 1890–1938*. Chapel Hill: University of North Carolina Press, 2007.

Luker, Kristin. *Abortion and the Politics of Motherhood*. Berkeley: University of California Press, 1984.

Lynch, John. "Stem Cells and the Embryo: Biorhetoric and Scientism in Congressional Debate." *Public Understanding of Science* 18 (2009): 309–24.

Lyon, Fred A. "Abortion Laws." *Minnesota Medicine* 50 (1967): 17–22.

Lyons, J. H. "The Moral Qualifications of the Physician." *Northwest Medicine* 5 (1907): 289–96.

Maienschein, Jane. "The Origins of *Entwicklungsmechanik*." In Gilbert, *Conceptual*, 43–61.

Malthus, Thomas R. *An Essay on the Principle of Population*. Edited by Geoffrey Gilbert. Oxford: Oxford University Press, 2004.

Mapes, C. C. "Criminal Abortion or Fœticide." *Medical Age* 14 (1896): 677–85.

Markham, H. C. "Fœticide and Its Prevention." *Journal of the American Medical Association* 11 (1888): 805–6.

Marsh, Steward, and Augusta Webster. "Vaginal Hemorrhage from Potassium Permanganate." *Obstetrics and Gynecology* 3, no. 2 (1954): 169–71.

Mason, Carol. *Killing for Life: The Apocalyptic Narrative of Pro-life Politics*. Ithaca: Cornell University Press, 2002.

Mason Pieklo, Jessica. "For Too Many, Accessing Abortion Is Already an 'Undue Burden.'" *RH Reality Check*, March 11, 2014. http://rhrealitycheck.org/article/2014/03/11/many-accessing-abortion-already-undue-burden/.

Massey, Doreen. *For Space*. London: SAGE, 2005.

Massumi, Brian. "National Enterprise Emergency: Steps Toward an Ecology of Powers." *Theory, Culture, and Society* 26 (2009): 153–85.

May, Elaine Tyler. *America and the Pill: A History of Promise, Peril, and Liberation.* New York: Basic Books, 2010. Kindle edition.

Mayer, Max D., William Harris, and Seymour Wimpfheimer. "Therapeutic Abortion by Means of X-Ray." *American Journal of Obstetrics and Gynecology* 32 (1936): 945–57.

Mbembe, Achille. "Necropolitics." Translated by Libby Meintjes. *Public Culture* 15, no. 1 (2003): 11–40.

McArdle, Thomas E. "The Physical Evils Arising from the Prevention of Conception." *American Journal of Obstetrics* 21 (1888): 935–39.

McCann, Carole R. *Birth Control Politics in the United States, 1916–1945.* Ithaca: Cornell University Press, 1994.

———. "Malthusian Men and Demographic Transitions: A Case Study of Hegemonic Masculinity in Mid-Twentieth-Century Population Theory on Malthus." *Frontiers: A Journal of Women's Studies* 30 (2009): 142–71.

McCann, Frederick J. "Criminal Abortion and Measures Necessary to Reduce the Sale of Abortifacient Drugs." *Medical Press,* February 6, 1929, 111–12.

McClintock, Anne. *Imperial Leather: Race, Gender, and Sexuality in the Colonial Contest.* New York: Routledge, 1995.

McCollom, William. "Criminal Abortion." *Journal of the American Medical Association* 26 (1896): 257–59.

McDonough, James F. "Vaginal Bleeding from Potassium Permanganate as an Abortifacient." *New England Journal of Medicine* 232, no. 7 (1945): 189–90.

McGee, Michael Calvin. "The 'Ideograph': A Link Between Rhetoric and Ideology." *Quarterly Journal of Speech* 66 (1980): 1–16.

———. "A Materialist's Conception of Rhetoric." In Biesecker and Lucaites, *Rhetoric,* 17–42.

McIver, Julius, and J. Collier Rucker. "A Survey of Abortions at Parkland Hospital." *Texas State Journal of Medicine* 37 (1941/42): 221–23.

McNair, Robert H. "Status of the Abortionist in the Modern Social Order." *New York Medical Journal* 107 (1918): 503.

Meckel, Richard A. *Save the Babies: American Public Health Reform and the Prevention of Infant Mortality, 1850–1929.* Baltimore: Johns Hopkins University Press, 1990.

Messer, Ellen, and Kathryn E. May. *Back Rooms: Voices from the Illegal Abortion Era.* Amherst, N.Y.: Prometheus Books, 1994.

Meyer, Arthur William. "The Frequency and Cause of Abortion." *American Journal of Obstetrics and Gynecology* 2 (1921): 138–52.

Millar, William M. "Human Abortion." *Human Biology* 6, no. 2 (1934): 271–307.

Miller, Charles. Draft of review of *Abortion in the United States* from *Medical Economics* and Mary Steichen Calderone's response to the editors. Mary Steichen Calderone Papers, Schlesinger Library, Radcliffe Institute for Advanced Study, Harvard University, call no. 179, box 3, folder 24.

"Model Penal Code Council Draft No. 16." November 23, 1957. American Law Institute Model Penal Code Collection, Biddle Law Library, University of Pennsylvania, box 5, folder 16.

"Model Penal Code Preliminary Draft." November 28, 1958. American Law Institute Model Penal Code Collection, Biddle Law Library, University of Pennsylvania, box 6, folder 16.

"Model Penal Code Proposed Official Draft." July 30, 1962. American Law Institute Model Penal Code Collection, Biddle Law Library, University of Pennsylvania, box 7, folder 17.

"Model Penal Code Tentative Draft No. 9." May 8, 1959. American Law Institute Model Penal Code Collection, Biddle Law Library, University of Pennsylvania, box 7, folder 8.

Mohanram, Radhika. *Black Body: Women, Colonialism, and Space.* Minneapolis: University of Minnesota Press, 1999.

Mohr, James C. *Abortion in America: The Origin and Evolution of National Policy*. Oxford: Oxford University Press, 1978.

Morgan, Lynn M. *Icons of Life: A Cultural History of Human Embryos*. Berkeley: University of California Press, 2009.

Moses, Bessie L. *Contraception as a Therapeutic Measure*. Baltimore: Williams and Wilkins, 1936.

Murdock, Harry M. "Experiences in a Psychiatric Hospital." In Rosen, *Therapeutic Abortion*, 198–206.

Murphy, John B. "Symposium on Criminal Abortion." *Medical News* 86 (1905): 188–92.

Murtha, Tara. "Pennsylvania Woman Arrested for Ordering Abortion-Inducing Pills On-line." *RH Reality Check*. http://rhrealitycheck.org/article/2014/02/20/pennsylvania-woman-arrested-ordering-daughter-abortion-inducing-pills-online/.

Nadesan, Maija Holmer. *Governmentality, Biopower, and Everyday Life*. New York: Routledge, 2008.

NARAL Prochoice America Foundation. "Who Decides? The Status of Women's Reproductive Rights in the United States." 21st ed. NARAL Prochoice America, 2012. http://www.prochoiceamerica.org/assets/download-files/2011-who-decides.pdf.

National Committee on Maternal Health. *The Abortion Problem*. Baltimore: Williams and Wilkins, 1944.

"National Committee on Maternal Health, Inc.: History." Draft manuscript. May 26, 1942. National Committee on Maternal Health Collection, Countway Library of Medicine, Harvard University, BMS c78, box 10, folder 341.

"N.C. Rep. Pittman: Planned Parenthood Is 'Murder for Hire.'" *Independent Tribune*, August 5, 2012. http://www2.independenttribune.com/.

Nealon, Jeffrey T. *Foucault Beyond Foucault: Power and Its Intensification Since 1984*. Stanford: Stanford University Press, 2008.

Nebinger, Andrew. *Criminal Abortion: Its Extent and Prevention*. Philadelphia: Collins, 1870.

Neisser, Ulric. "Remembering as Doing." *Behavioral and Brain Sciences* 19 (1996): 203–4.

Nelken. "Discussion." *New Orleans Medical and Surgical Journal* 57 (1907): 319–20.

Newman, James R. "A Conference on Abortion as a Disease of Societies." *Scientific American*, January 1959, 2–4. Mary Steichen Calderone Papers, Schlesinger Library, Radcliffe Institute for Advanced Study, Harvard University, call no. 179, box 3, folder 24.

Nietzsche, Friedrich. *The Genealogy of Morals*. Translated by Ian Johnston. Arlington, Va.: Richer Resources, 2009. Kindle edition.

———. "On Truth and Lies in an Extra-Moral Sense." In *Friedrich Nietzsche on Rhetoric and Language*, edited and translated by Sander L. Gilman, Carol Blair, and David J. Parent, 246–57. New York: Oxford University Press, 1989.

Nobel, Helen. "Abortion: Its Maternal Mortality and Morbidity." Thesis. 1939. Allegheny Special Collection on Women Physicians, Women's Medical College, Allegheny University.

Nochlin, Linda. *The Body in Pieces: The Fragment as a Metaphor of Modernity*. London: Thames and Hudson, 1994.

Noll, Mark A. *A History of Christianity in the United States and Canada*. Grand Rapids, Mich.: William B. Eerdmans, 1992. Kindle edition.

"Norway." United Nations, Department of Economic and Social Affairs, Population Division. http://www.un.org/esa/population/publications/abortion/doc/norway.doc.

Nowlin, J. B. W. "Criminal Abortion." *Southern Practitioner* 9, no. 5 (1887): 177–82.

O'Callaghan, Peter J. "The Moral and Religious Objections to Inducing Abortion." *Illinois Medical Journal* 7 (1905): 24–29.

O'Donnell, D. A., and W. L. Atlee. "Report on Criminal Abortion." *Transactions of the American Medical Association* 22 (1871): 239–58.

Olick, Jeffrey K. "Collective Memory: Two Cultures." *Sociological Theory* 17 (1999): 333–48.

———. *The Politics of Regret: On Collective Memory and Historical Responsibility*. New York: Routledge, 2007.

Olick, Jeffrey K., and Joyce Robbins. "Social Memory Studies: From 'Collective Memory' to the Historical Sociology of Mnemonic Practices." *Annual Review of Sociology* 24 (1998): 105–40.

Olson, Henry J. "The Problem of Abortion." *American Journal of Obstetrics and Gynecology* 45 (1943): 672–78.

Oppenheimer, Jane M. "Curt Herbst's Contributions to the Concept of Embryonic Induction." In Gilbert, *Conceptual*, 63–89.

Oreman, Jennie G. "The Medical Woman's Temptation and How to Meet It." *Woman's Medical Journal* 11, no. 3 (1901): 87–88.

OSMA Committee on Maternal Health. "Maternal Deaths Involving Criminal Abortion." *Ohio State Medical Journal* 57 (1961): 1024–26.

———. "Maternal Deaths with Septic Shock After Criminal Abortion." *Ohio State Medical Journal* 65 (1969): 601–3.

Overstreet, Edmund W. Foreword to *Clinical Obstetrics and Gynecology* 7 (1964): 11–13.

Packer, Herbert L., and Ralph J. Gampell. "Therapeutic Abortion: A Problem in Law and Medicine." *Stanford Law Review* 11 (1959): 417–55.

Palmer, Rachel Lynn, and Sarah K. Greenberg. *Facts and Frauds in Woman's Hygiene: A Medical Guide Against Misleading Claims and Dangerous Products*. New York: Vanguard Press, 1936.

Parish, W. H. "Criminal Abortion." *Medical and Surgical Reporter* 68 (1893): 644–49.

Parsons, Mary. "The Written Law in Reference to the Unborn Child." *Washington Medical Annals* 9 (1910–11): 153–60.

Paterfamilias. "'Race Suicide' and Common Sense." *North American Review* 176 (1903): 892–900.

Patterson, Andrea. "Germs and Jim Crow: The Impact of Microbiology on Public Health Policies in Progressive Era American South." *Journal of the History of Biology* 42, no. 3 (2009): 529–59.

Pattison, H. A. "Abortion." *Illinois Medical Journal* 11 (1907): 652–58.

Pavey, Charles W. "The Conservative Treatment of Abortion." *Ohio State Medical Journal* 33 (1937): 164–66.

Pearl, Raymond. "Fertility and Contraception in New York and Chicago." *Journal of the American Medical Association* 108 (1937): 1385–90.

Pendleton, E. M. "The Comparative Fecundity of the Black and White Races." *Boston Medical and Surgical Journal* 44, no. 19 (1851): 365–66.

Person, A. G. "Discussions." *Texas Courier-Record of Medicine* 23, no. 6 (1906): 11–13.

Petchesky, Rosalind Pollack. *Abortion and Woman's Choice: The State, Sexuality, and Reproductive Freedom*. Rev. ed. Boston: Northeastern University Press, 1990.

Philbrick, I. C. "Social Causes of Criminal Abortion." *Western Medical Review* 17 (1905): 102–10.

Pink, Louis H. "Motherhood as an Insurance Risk." In National Committee, *Abortion*, 148–54.

Pirkner, E. H. F. "The Problem of Race Suicide: A Problem Rather of National Hygiene and Prophylaxis Than Political Economy." *American Medicine* 15 [complete series] (1909): 372–83.

Plass, E. D. "Personal Report on Questionnaire of Iowa Physicians." In Taussig, *Abortion*, 25, 364, 366, 502.

Ploss-Bartels. "Abortion or Intentional Miscarriage." *American Journal of Urology and Sexology* 8, no. 6 (1917): 256–74.

Pollitt, Katha. "Prochoice Puritans." *Nation*, January 26, 2006. http://www.thenation.com /article/prochoice-puritans.

Poovey, Mary. "The Abortion Question and the Death of Man." In *Feminists Theorize the Political*, edited by Judith Butler and Joan W. Scott, 240–56. New York: Routledge, 1992.

———. *A History of the Modern Fact: Problems of Knowledge in Sciences of Wealth and Society.* Chicago: University of Chicago Press, 1998.

Popenoe, Paul, ed. "The Abortion Problem." *Family Life Education* 5, no. 4 (1945): 1–2.

Porter, Roy. *The Greatest Benefit to Mankind: A Medical History of Humanity.* New York: W. W. Norton, 1997.

———. "The Malthusian Moment." In Dolan, *Malthus, Medicine, and Morality*, 57–72.

Porter, Theodore M. *The Rise in Statistical Thinking, 1820–1900.* Princeton: Princeton University Press, 1986.

"Press Release." Draft. February 29, 1952. American Law Institute Model Penal Code Collection, Biddle Law Library, University of Pennsylvania, box 1, folder 16.

Quintilian. *Institutes of Oratory.* Edited by Lee Honeycutt. Translated by John Shelby Watson. N.p.:n.p. Amazon Digital Services, 2010. Kindle edition.

Rapaport, Judith L. "American Abortion Applicants in Sweden." *Archives of General Psychiatry* 13 (1965): 24–33.

Rapp, Rayna. *Testing Women, Testing the Fetus: The Social Impact of Amniocentesis in America.* New York: Routledge, 1999.

Reagan, Leslie J. *Dangerous Pregnancies: Mothers, Disabilities, and Abortion in Modern America.* Berkeley: University of California Press, 2010.

———. *When Abortion Was a Crime: Women, Medicine, and Law in the United States, 1867–1973.* Berkeley: University of California Press, 1997.

Reagan, Ronald. "Abortion and the Conscience of the Nation." *Human Life Review*, Spring 1983. http://www.humanlifereview.com/index.php/archives/54-special-archives-spring -1983/115.

Reed, Charles B. "Therapeutic and Criminal Abortion." *Illinois Medical Journal* 7 (1905): 26–29.

Revel, Judith. "Identity, Nature, Life: Three Biopolitical Deconstructions." *Theory, Culture, Society* 26 (2009): 45–54.

Rich, Frank. "Stag Party: The GOP's Problem Is That It Has a Serious Problem with Women." *New York Magazine*, March 25, 2013. http://nymag.com/news/frank-rich /gop-women-problem-2012-4/.

Ricoeur, Paul. *Memory, History, Forgetting.* Translated by Kathleen Blamey and David Pellauer. Chicago: University of Chicago Press, 2004.

Riddle, John M. *Contraception and Abortion from the Ancient World to the Renaissance.* Cambridge, Mass.: Harvard University Press, 1992.

Robb, George. "Marriage and Reproduction." In *The Modern History of Sexuality*, edited by H. G. Cocks and Matt Houlbrook, 87–108. Hampshire, U.K.: Palgrave-Macmillan, 2006.

Robinson, Victor. *Pioneers of Birth Control in England and America.* New York: Voluntary Parenthood League, 1919.

Robinson, William J. "Abortion Historically and Ethnologically Considered." *American Journal of Urology and Sexology* 15, nos. 2–3 (1919): 78–86, 109–17.

————. "The Ethics of Abortion." *New York Medical Journal* 100 (1914): 897.

————. *The Law Against Abortion: Its Perniciousness Demonstrated and Its Repeal Demanded.* New York: Eugenics, 1933.

Rock, John. "Abortion." *New Journal of Medicine* 223, no. 25 (1940): 1020–27.

Rogers, Edmund J. A. "The Attitude of the Profession Toward Abortion." *Colorado Medical Journal and Western Medical and Surgical Gazette* 9, no. 4 (1903): 149–51.

Roemer, Ruth. "Abortion Law: The Approaches of Different Nations." *American Journal of Public Health* 57, no. 11 (1967): 1906–22.

Romm, May E. "Psychoanalytic Considerations." In Rosen, *Therapeutic Abortion*, 209–12.

Rongy, A. J. *Abortion: Legal or Illegal?* New York: Vanguard Press, 1933.

————. "Abortion and Birth Control: A Critical Study." *American Medicine* 37 [n.s., 26] (1931): 400–408.

Roosevelt, Theodore. "On Motherhood." March 13, 1905. http://www.nationalcenter.org/TRooseveltMotherhood.html.

Rose, Nikolas. *Governing the Soul: The Shaping of the Private Self.* 2nd ed. London: Free Association, 1999.

————. *Inventing Ourselves: Psychology, Power, and Personhood.* Cambridge, U.K.: Cambridge University Press, 1998.

————. *Politics of Life: Biomedicine, Power, and Subjectivity in the Twenty-First Century.* Princeton: Princeton University Press, 2007.

Rosen, Harold. "The Emotionally Sick Pregnant Patient." In Rosen, *Therapeutic Abortion*, 219–43.

————, ed. *Therapeutic Abortion: Medical, Psychiatric, Legal, Anthropological, and Religious Considerations.* New York: Julian Press, 1954.

Rosenberg, Charles E. "Pathologies of Progress: The Idea of Civilization as Risk." *Bulletin of the History of Medicine* 72 (1998): 714–30.

Ross, Edward A. "Western Civilization and the Birth-Rate." *American Journal of Sociology* 12 (1906–7): 607–32.

Ross, Loretta J. "African-American Women and Abortion: A Neglected History." *Journal of Health Care for the Poor and Underserved* 3 (1992): 274–84.

Rothman, Sheila M. *Living in the Shadow of Death: Tuberculosis and the Social Experience of Illness in American History.* Baltimore: Johns Hopkins University Press, 1995.

Rothstein, William G. *Public Health and the Risk Factor: A History of an Uneven Medical Revolution.* Rochester: University of Rochester Press, 2003.

Rout, Ettie. "Contraception." *American Medicine* 41, no. 3 [n.s., 10, no. 3] (1935): 134–35.

Rubin, I. C., and Josef Novak. *Integrated Gynecology: Principles and Practice.* New York: McGraw-Hill, 1956.

Rubin, Isadore. "Illegal Abortion . . . Disease of Society." *Sexology: Sex Science Illustrated,* January 1959, 348–53.

Russell, Montgomery. "Criminal Abortion." *Northwest Medicine* 5 (1907): 296–304.

Saletan, William, and Katha Pollitt. "Is Abortion Bad?" *Truthout,* February 1, 2006. http://archive.truthout.org/article/w-saletan-and-k-pollitt-is-abortion-bad.

Sanger, Margaret. *Margaret Sanger: An Autobiography.* New York: W. W. Norton, 1939.

————. *Woman and the New Race.* New York: Truth, 1920.

Sangmeister, Henry J. "A Survey of Abortion Deaths in Philadelphia from 1931 to 1940 Inclusive." *American Journal of Obstetrics and Gynecology* 46 (1943): 755–59.

Saur, Prudence B. *Maternity: A Book for Every Wife and Mother.* Rev. ed. Chicago: L. P. Miller, 1888.

Savel, Lewis E. "Adjudication of Therapeutic Abortion and Sterilization." *Clinical Obstetrics and Gynecology* 7 (1964): 14–21.

Saxon, Wolfgang. "Robert E. Hall, 70, Campaigner for Liberalized Abortion Laws." *New York Times*, October 13, 1995. http://www.nytimes.com/1995/10/13/obituaries/robert-e-hall-70-campaigner-for-liberalized-abortion-laws.html.

Scherman, Quinten. "Therapeutic Abortion." *Obstetrics and Gynecology* 11 (1958): 323–35.

Schermer, Irvin. "Abortion and the Law." *Journal-Lancet* 62 (1942): 223–24.

Schiappa, Edward. *Protagoras and Logos: A Study in Greek Philosophy and Rhetoric.* 2nd ed. Columbia: University of South Carolina Press, 2003.

Schindler, Solomon. "'Why Race-Suicide with Advancing Civilization?' A Reply." *Arena* 41 (1909): 301–3.

Schroeder, Theodore. "Physiologic Aspect of Birth Control." *Medico-legal Journal* 39 (1922): 16–21.

Schwartz, Leo S. "The Treatment of Uterine Injuries: With a Report of Seven Cases." *American Journal of Obstetrics and Gynecology* 17 (1929): 66–74.

Schwartz, Richard A. "Psychiatry and the Abortion Laws: An Overview." *Comprehensive Psychiatry* 9, no. 2 (1968): 99–115.

Scott, Charles E. "The Appearance of Public Memory." In *Framing Public Memory*, edited by Kendall R. Phillips, 147–56. Tuscaloosa: University of Alabama Press, 2004.

Scott, James Foster. "Criminal Abortion." *American Journal of Obstetrics* 33 (1896): 72–86.

Scudder, Samuel H. "David Humphreys Storer." *Proceedings of the American Academy of Arts and Sciences* 27 (May 1891): 388–91.

Sheean, J. M. "The Common and Statute Law of Illinois." *Illinois Medical Journal* 7 (1905): 37–39.

Shipps, Hammell P. "Some Aspects of the Abortion Problem." *Journal of the Medical Society of New Jersey* 41, no. 8 (1944): 311–15.

Simmel, Georg. *The Sociology of Georg Simmel.* Translated and edited by Kurt H. Wolff. Glencoe, Ill.: Free Press, 1950.

Simon, Alexander. "Psychiatric Indications for Therapeutic Abortion and Sterilization." *Clinical Obstetrics and Gynecology* 7 (1964): 67–81.

Simondon, Gilbert. *Two Lessons on Animal and Man.* Translated by Drew S. Burk. Minneapolis: Univocal, 2011.

Simons, Jalmar H. "Statistical Analysis of One Thousand Abortions." *American Journal of Obstetrics and Gynecology* 37 (1939): 840–49.

Smith, A. Lapthorn. "Higher Education of Women and Race Suicide." *Popular Science Monthly* 66 (1905): 466–73.

Smith, Merril D., ed. *Sex Without Consent: Rape and Sexual Coercion in America.* New York: New York University Press, 2001.

Smith-Rosenberg, Caroll. *Disorderly Conduct: Visions of Gender in Victorian America.* New York: Oxford University Press, 1985.

Solinger, Rickie. *The Abortionist: A Woman Against the Law.* New York: Free Press, 1994.

———, ed. *Abortion Wars: A Half-Century of Struggle, 1950–2000.* Berkeley: University of California Press, 1998.

———. *Beggars and Choosers: How the Politics of Choice Shapes Adoption, Abortion, and Welfare in the United States.* New York: Hill and Wang, 2001.

———. "'A Complete Disaster': Abortion and the Politics of Hospital Abortion Committees, 1950–1970." *Feminist Studies* 19 (1993): 241–68.

———. Introduction to *Abortion Wars: A Half-Century of Struggle, 1950–2000*, edited by Rickie Solinger, 1–9. Berkeley: University of California Press, 1998.

————. *Pregnancy and Power: A Short History of Reproductive Politics in America*. New York: New York University Press, 2005.

————. *Wake Up Little Susie: Single Pregnancy and Race Before Roe v. Wade*. New York: Routledge, 1994.

Somers, A. B. "Measures for the Prevention of Criminal Abortion." *Western Medical Review* 17 (1905): 110–13.

Sontag, Susan. *Illness as Metaphor and AIDS and Its Metaphors*. New York: Anchor Books, 1990.

Sontheimer, Morton. "Abortion in America Today." *Woman's Home Companion*, October 1955, 44–45, 96.

Spelman, Elizabeth V. *Fruits of Sorrow: Framing Our Attention to Suffering*. Boston: Beacon Press, 1997.

Spengler, Joseph J. "Notes on Abortion, Birth Control, and Medical and Sociological Interpretations of the Decline of the Birth Rate in Nineteenth Century America." *Marriage Hygiene* 2, nos. 1–3 (1935): 43–53, 158–69, 288–300.

Spivak, Gayatri Chakravorty. "Can the Subaltern Speak?" In *Marxism and the Interpretation of Culture*, edited by Cary Nelson and Lawrence Grossberg, 271–316. Urbana: University of Illinois Press, 1988.

————. *A Critique of Postcolonial Reason: Toward a History of the Vanishing Point*. Cambridge, Mass.: Harvard University Press, 1999.

Squier, Raymond. "Discussion." Discussion of George M. Cooper's "The Possibilities of a Statewide Program on Abortion Control." In National Committee, *Abortion*, 170–73.

Stafford, Barbara Maria. *Body Criticism: Imaging the Unseen in Enlightenment Art and Medicine*. Cambridge, Mass.: MIT Press, 1993.

Stengers, Isabelle. *Thinking with Whitehead*. Translated by Michael Chase. Foreword by Bruno Latour. Cambridge, Mass.: Harvard University Press, 2011.

Stern, Alexandra Minna. *Eugenic Nation: Faults and Frontiers of Better Breeding in Modern America*. Berkeley: University of California Press, 2005.

Stevenson, E. H. "Tetanus Following Criminal Abortion." *National Eclectic Medical Journal* 17 (1925/26): 258–61.

Stevenson, Lee B. "Maternal Death and Abortion: Michigan, 1955–1964." *Michigan Medicine* 66 (1967): 287–91.

Stewart, Roger. "An Analysis of 1,772 Abortions and Miscarriages with a Consideration of Treatment and Prevention." *American Journal of Obstetrics and Gynecology* 29 (1935): 872–75.

Stix, Regine K. "A Study of Pregnancy Wastage." *Milbank Memorial Fund Quarterly* 13 (1935): 347–65.

Stix, Regine K., and Dorothy G. Wiehl. "Abortion and Public Health." *American Journal of Public Health* 28 (1938): 621–28.

Stockham, Alice B. *Tokology: A Book for Every Woman*. Chicago: Sanitary, 1885.

Stoler, Ann Laura. *Carnal Knowledge and Imperial Power: Race and the Intimate in Colonial Rule*. Berkeley: University of California Press, 2002.

————, ed. *Haunted by Empire: Geographies of Intimacy in North American History*. Durham: Duke University Press, 2006.

————. *Race and the Education of Desire: Foucault's "History of Sexuality" and the Colonial Order of Things*. Durham: Duke University Press, 1995.

————. "Tense and Tender Ties: The Politics of Comparison in North American History and (Post) Colonial Studies." In Stoler, *Haunted*, 23–67.

Stone, Abraham. "Discussion." Discussion of George M. Cooper's "The Possibilities of a Statewide Program on Abortion Control." In National Committee, *Abortion*, 172.

Stone, Hannah, and Abraham Stone. *A Marriage Manual: A Practical Guide-Book to Sex and Marriage.* New York: Simon and Schuster, 1935.

Stopes, Marie Carmichael. *Wise Parenthood: A Practical Sequel to "Married Love": A Book for Married People.* London: G. P. Putnam's Sons, 1919.

Storer, D. Humphreys. "Two Frequent Causes of Uterine Disease." *Journal of the Gynaecological Society of Boston* 7 (March 1872): 194–203.

Storer, H. R. "Contributions to Obstetric Jurisprudence." *New York Medical Journal* 3, no. 18 (1866): 422–33.

———. *Criminal Abortion: Its Nature, Its Evidence, and Its Law.* Boston: Little, Brown, 1868.

———. *The Criminality and Physical Evils of Forced Abortions.* American Medical Association, 1865.

———. *Is It I?: A Book for Every Man.* Boston: Lee and Shepard, 1868.

———. *On Criminal Abortion in America.* Philadelphia: J. B. Lippincott, 1860.

———. *Why Not?: A Book for Every Woman.* Boston: Lee and Shepard, 1868.

Storer, Horatio R., Thomas W. Blatchford, Hugh L. Hodge, Edward H. Barton, A. Lopez, Charles A. Pope, Wm. Henry Brisbane, and A. J. Semmes. "Report on Criminal Abortion." *Transactions of the American Medical Association* 13 (1859): 75–79.

Stormer, Nathan. *Articulating Life's Memory: U.S. Medical Rhetoric About Abortion in the Nineteenth Century.* Lanham, Md.: Lexington Books, 2003.

———. "Articulation: A Working Paper on Rhetoric and *Taxis*." *Quarterly Journal of Speech* 90 (2004): 257–84.

———. "Recursivity: A Working Paper on Rhetoric and *Mnesis*." *Quarterly Journal of Speech* 99 (2013): 27–50.

———. "*Why Not?*: Memory and Counter-Memory in 19th-Century Abortion Rhetoric." *Women's Studies in Communication* 24, no. 1 (2001): 1–29.

St. Romain, Murphy J., and Frank G. Nix. "Chemical Burns of the Vagina." *Journal of the Louisiana State Medical Society* 107 (1955): 268–72.

Studdiford, William Emery. "The Common Medical Indications for Therapeutic Abortion." *Bulletin of the New York Academy of Medicine* 26, no. 11 (1950): 721–25.

Sturken, Marita. "The Remembering of Forgetting: Recovered Memory and the Question of Experience." *Social Text* 57 (1998): 103–25.

"Summarizing Statement by the Abortion Conference." Draft. November 23, 1955. Mary Steichen Calderone Papers, Schlesinger Library, Radcliffe Institute for Advanced Study, Harvard University, call no. 179, box 2, folder 15.

Suttner, C. N. "A Plea for the Protection of the Unborn." *Northwest Medicine* 5 (1907): 305–10.

Sydenstricker, Edgar. "The Changing Concept of Public Health." *Milbank Memorial Fund Quarterly* 13 (1935): 301–10.

Taussig, Fred J. "Abortion: Cause, Prevention, Treatment." *American Journal of Nursing* 39, no. 8 (1938): 857–63.

———. "Abortion and Its Relation to Fetal and Maternal Mortality." *American Journal of Obstetrics and Gynceology* 33 (1937): 711–14.

———. "Abortion in Relation to Fetal and Maternal Welfare." *American Journal of Obstetrics and Gynecology* 22 (1931): 729–38.

———. "Abortion in Relation to Fetal and Maternal Welfare." In *Fetal, Newborn, and Maternal Morbidity and Mortality: Report of the Subcommittee on Factors and Causes of Fetal, Newborn, and Maternal Morbidity and Mortality*, White House Conference on Child

Health and Protection, chaired by Hugo Ehrenfest, 446–72. New York: D. Appleton-Century, 1933.

———. "The Abortion Problem in Russia." *American Journal of Obstetrics and Gynecology* 22 (1931): 134–39.

———. *Abortion, Spontaneous and Induced: Medical and Social Aspects.* St. Louis, Mo.: C. V. Mosby, 1936.

———. "The Control of Abortion." *New England Journal of Medicine* 216, no. 3 (1937): 109–14.

———. "The Control of Criminal Abortion as Influenced by the Present War." *Interstate Medical Journal* 23 (1916): 772–78.

———. "Discussion." Discussion of P. K. Whelpton's "Frequency of Abortion: Its Effects on the Birth Rates and Future Population of America." In National Committee, *Abortion,* 28–38.

———. "Effects of Abortion on the General Health and Reproductive Function of the Individual." In National Committee, *Abortion,* 39–48.

———. "Frequency of Abortion." *St. Louis Medical Review* 58 (1909): 46–47.

———. *The Prevention and Treatment of Abortion.* St. Louis, Mo.: C. V. Mosby, 1910.

———. "What to Teach the General Practitioner Concerning the Treatment of Abortion and Miscarriage." *Surgery, Gynecology and Obstetrics* 8 (1906): 514.

Taylor, Howard C. "Summary and Recommendation of the Conference." In National Committee, *Abortion,* 174–75.

Thacker, Eugene. "The Shadows of Atheology: Epidemics, Power, and Life After Foucault." *Theory, Culture, Society* 26 (2009): 134–521.

"Therapeutic Abortion." Memorandum. N.d. Mary Steichen Calderone Papers, Schlesinger Library, Radcliffe Institute for Advanced Study, Harvard University, call no. 179, box 2, folder 20.

Thiberge. "Criminal Abortion." *New Orleans Medical and Surgical Journal* 57 (1907): 314–18.

Thomas, T. Gaillard. *Abortion and Its Treatment, from the Stand-Point of Practical Experience: A Special Course of Lectures Delivered at the College of Physicians and Surgeons, New York Session of 1889–'90.* New York: D. Appleton, 1896.

———. *Practical Treatises on the Diseases of Women.* 6th ed. Philadelphia: Lea Brothers, 1891.

Thorndike, Edward L. "The Decrease in the Size of American Families." *Popular Science Monthly* 63 (1903): 64–70.

Tietze, Christopher. "Abortion as a Cause of Death." *American Journal of Public Health* 38 (1948): 1434–41.

———. "Abortion in Europe." *American Journal of Public Health* 57, no. 11 (1967): 1923–32.

———. "Introduction to Abortion Statistics." In *Pregnancy Wastage: Proceedings of a Conference Sponsored by the Committee on Human Reproduction, National Research Council, in Behalf of the National Committee on Maternal Health, Inc.,* edited by Earl T. Engle, 135–45. Springfield, Ill.: Charles C. Thomas, 1953.

———. "Mortality with Contraception and Induced Abortion." *Studies in Family Planning* 1 (1969): 6–8.

———. "Therapeutic Abortion in New York City, 1943–1947." *American Journal of Obstetrics and Gynecology* 60, no. 1 (1950): 146–52.

Tietze, Christopher, and Sarah Lewit. "Abortion." *Scientific American* 220, no. 1 (1969): 21–27.

Tillman, Laura. "Crossing the Line: Women on the US-Mexico Border Seek Alternatives to Embattled Abortion Clinics." *Nation,* August 26, 2010. http://www.thenation.com/article/154166/crossing-line.

Todorov, Tzvetan. *Memory as a Remedy for Evil.* Translated by Gila Walker. London: Seagull Books, 2010.

United States Department of Labor, Children's Bureau. *Maternal Mortality in Fifteen States*, Bureau Publication no. 223. Washington, D.C.: Government Printing Office, 1934.

Vandergriff, William. "Intravaginal Use of Potassium Permanganate as an Abortifacient: The Error in Diagnosis." *Obstetrics and Gynecology* 28, no. 2 (1966): 155–57.

Van De Warker, Ely. "Detection of Criminal Abortion." *Journal of the Gynæcological Society of Boston* 5 (October and December 1871): 229–45, 350–70.

Velpeau, Alfred A. L. M. *An Elementary Treatise on Midwifery; Or, Principles of Tokology and Embryology*. Translated by Charles D. Meigs. Edited by William Harris. Philadelphia: Lindsay and Blakiston, 1845.

Vivian, Bradford. "Jefferson's Other." *Quarterly Journal of Speech* 88 (2002): 284–302.

———. "Neoliberal Epideictic: Rhetorical Form and Commemorative Politics on September 11, 2002." *Quarterly Journal of Speech* 92 (2006): 1–26.

———. *Public Forgetting: The Rhetoric and Politics of Beginning Again*. University Park: Pennsylvania State University Press, 2010.

Walzer, Arthur E. "Logic and Rhetoric in Malthus's *Essay on the Principle of Population*, 1798." *Quarterly Journal of Speech* 73 (1987): 1–17.

Wanamaker, F. D. "The Lay Use of Potassium Permanganate as an Abortifacient." *American Journal of Obstetrics and Gynecology* 69, no. 2 (1955): 259–64.

Warner, John Harley. *The Therapeutic Perspective: Medical Practice, Knowledge, and Identity in America, 1820–1885*. Cambridge, Mass.: Harvard University Press, 1986.

Warner, Michael. "The Mass Public and the Mass Subject." In *Habermas and the Public Sphere*, edited by Craig Calhoun, 377–401. Cambridge, Mass.: MIT Press, 1992.

———. *Publics and Counterpublics*. New York: Zone Books, 2002.

Waters, Chris. "Sexology." In *The Modern History of Sexuality*, edited by H. G. Cocks and Matt Houlbrook, 41–63. Hampshire, U.K.: Palgrave Macmillan, 2006.

Watkins, Raymond E. "A Five-Year Study of Abortion." *American Journal of Obstetrics and Gynecology* 26 (1933): 161–72.

Weiss, E. A. "Some Moral and Ethical Aspects of Feticide." *American Journal of Obstetrics and the Diseases of Women and Children* 67 (1913): 72–81.

Welsh, Margaret. "The Problem of Abortion." Thesis. 1937. Allegheny Special Collection on Women Physicians, Women's Medical College, Allegheny University.

Wetherill, H. G. "Remedies." *Colorado Medical Journal and Western Medical and Surgical Gazette* 9, no. 4 (1903): 151–52.

Whelpton, P. K. "Discussion." Discussion of P. K. Whelpton's "Frequency of Abortion: Its Effects on the Birth Rates and Future Population of America." In National Committee, *Abortion*, 28–38.

———. "Frequency of Abortion: Its Effects on the Birth Rates and Future Population of America." In National Committee, *Abortion*, 15–27.

Whitehead, Alfred North. *Process and Reality*. Corrected ed. Edited by David Ray Griffin and Donald W. Sherburne. New York: Free Press, 1978.

Wife of a Christian Physician. "Why Not? A Book for Every Woman: A Woman's View." *Boston Medical and Surgical Journal* 75, no. 14 (1867): 273–76.

Wiklund, Susan. *This Common Secret: My Journey as an Abortion Doctor*. New York: PublicAffairs, 2007.

Wile, Ira S. "Birth Control: Creation vs. Propagation." *American Medicine* 41, no. 3 [n.s., 30, no. 3] (1935): 141–47.

Willson, J. Robert, Clayton T. Beecham, Isador Forman, and Elsie Reid Carrington. *Obstetrics and Gynecology*. St. Louis, Mo.: C. V. Mosby, 1958.

Winslow, C.-E. A. "Efficiency in the Public-Health Campaign." *North American Review* 197, no. 691 (1913): 761–73.

Winter, John T. "Criminal Abortion." *American Journal of Obstetrics* 38 (1898): 85–92.

Witherspoon, J. Thornwell. "An Analysis of 200 Cases of Septic Abortion Treated Conservatively." *American Journal of Obstetrics and Gynecology* 26 (1933): 367–74.

Wolfe, Cary. *Before the Law: Humans and Other Animals in a Biopolitical Frame.* Chicago: University of Chicago Press, 2013. Kindle edition.

World Health Organization. "History of the Development of the ICD." http://www.who .int/classifications/icd/en/HistoryOfICD.pdf.

Wynne, Frank B. "Abortion." *Medico-legal Journal* 39 (1922): 21–23.

Yarros, Rachelle S. "From Obstetrics to Social Hygiene." *Medical Woman's Journal* 33, no. 11 (1926): 305–9.

———. *Modern Woman and Sex: A Feminist Physician Speaks.* New York: Vanguard Press, 1933.

Young, Brian. "Malthus Among the Theologians." In Dolan, *Malthus, Medicine, and Morality,* 93–113.

Zakin, David, William H. Godsick, and Benjamin Segal. "Foreign Bodies Lost in the Pelvis During Attempted Abortion with Special Reference to Urethral Catheters." *American Journal of Obstetrics and Gynecology* 70, no. 2 (1955): 233–51.

Zeisler, Sigmund. "The Legal and Moral Aspects of Abortion." *Surgery, Gynecology and Obstetrics* 10 (1910): 538–41.

Zelizer, Barbie. "Reading the Past Against the Grain: The Shape of Memory Studies." *Critical Studies in Mass Communication* 12 (1995): 214–39.

Zerubavel, Eviatar. *Time Maps: Collective Memory and the Social Shape of the Past.* Chicago: University of Chicago Press, 2003.

Index

Typeset by
BOOKCOMP

Printed and bound by
SHERIDAN BOOKS

Composed in
ADOBE JENSON PRO, BERLING NOVA SANS PRO

Printed on
NATURES NATURAL

Bound in
ARRESTOX LINEN